"With its diverse perspectives and actionable insights, *Contemporary Issues in Human Services: Special Topics for Clinical Practice, Public Health, and Social Justice* serves as a dynamic guide for fostering critical thinking, advocacy, and leadership. It equips readers to analyze and predict trends, address systemic issues, and become effective agents of change. A must-read for those dedicated to advancing equity and innovation in human services, this book offers both inspiration and practical tools for creating meaningful impact."

**Monique Howard**, *EdD, MPH, Senior Director of Women's Health Initiatives, Center for Global Women's Health*

"For instructors aiming to educate and graduate the next generation of Human Service professionals, *Contemporary Issues in Human Services: Special Topics for Clinical Practice, Public Health, and Social Justice* is the essential book. This compilation of readings will provide valuable insights and practical tools for Human Service professionals. Here, Dr. James Wadley brings together writings from a diverse pool of experts to shed light on topics like interprofessional collaboration (a future-focused trend in healthcare), best practices for supporting marginalized populations (a key factor in promoting equality), and human development-based approaches to serving individuals at various life stages (a best practice for targeted, tailored care)."

**Jeannette M. Wade**, *PhD, Associate Professor and Program Director of Human Health Sciences, University of North Carolina at Greensboro*

"This book is a must have for human service and public health practitioners. It offers transformative strategies for a variety of human service settings that equips professionals with the tools needed for complex situations. I can't wait to share this book with my students and my colleagues. Awesome, indeed!"

**Kamilah Woodson**, *PhD, Professor of Human Development and Psychoeducational Studies, Howard University*

# Contemporary Issues in Human Services

This text informs human services students and practitioners on complex contemporary issues in the human services, public health, and clinical social work fields, allowing them to be more agile and better-prepared agents and leaders of change.

Dr. James C. Wadley brings together a collection of critical perspectives from the top human service practitioners, administrators, advocates, and leaders in the field. Chapters consider contemporary issues such as social justice, sexuality, ability and disability, policy formation, pedagogy, mental health, sociopolitical perspectives, constructions of race and gender, and social positioning and identities. This text helps readers in human services, public health, and social work fields expand their understanding about service access and coordination, resource delivery, and the potential implications for a variety of populations and settings. Each chapter offers an opportunity to engage professionals, students, clients, and constituents in meaningful dialogue about sensitive issues that impact a range of communities and individuals. This book also offers a wealth of strategies, insights, interventions, and suggestions for students and practitioners to consider while working with a myriad of populations.

This book is an invaluable resource for human service professionals, social workers, policymakers, mental health practitioners, and community behavioral health professionals, as well as undergraduate and graduate students.

**James C. Wadley, PhD,** is a professor in the Human Services Department at Lincoln University. He is the Editor-in-Chief of the *Journal of Black Sexuality and Relationships* and founder and principal of the Association of Black Sexologists and Clinicians.

# Contemporary Issues in Human Services

## Special Topics for Clinical Practice, Public Health, and Social Justice

**Edited by James C. Wadley**

Foreword by Candace Robertson-James

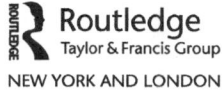

Routledge
Taylor & Francis Group

NEW YORK AND LONDON

Designed cover image: cienpies © Getty Images

First published 2026
by Routledge
605 Third Avenue, New York, NY 10158

and by Routledge
4 Park Square, Milton Park, Abingdon, Oxon, OX14 4RN

*Routledge is an imprint of the Taylor & Francis Group, an informa business*

ISBN: 978-1-032-87171-4 (hbk)
ISBN: 978-1-032-86514-0 (pbk)
ISBN: 978-1-003-53125-8 (ebk)

DOI: 10.4324/9781003531258

Typeset in Sabon
by codeMantra

## Dedication

This book is dedicated to my family, friends, and colleagues who supported me with this project and throughout my professional career.

# Contents

*Acknowledgments*                                                    *xiii*
*List of Contributors*                                                *xiv*
*Foreword*                                                           *xxiv*

Introduction                                                            1
JAMES C. WADLEY

SECTION I
Leading Conversations about Clinical Practice in Human Services          3

1  Therapists' Grief: Creativity as Part of an Essential Ethical Practice   5
   REBECCA ARNOLD

2  Trauma-Informed Human Service Practices                              15
   DEIRDRE O'SULLIVAN, JENNIFER L. HANNA,
   AND SHYRUN KARANDIKAR

3  Sense of Belonging in Interprofessional Collaboration               25
   LUANNE SHAW AND SCOTT SHAW

4  Partner Abuse in Domestic and Dating Relationships: How Trauma
   Impacts the Brain, the Family, and Functioning                      38
   CORINNE D. WARRENER

5  The Power of Play: Exploring the Efficacy of Play Therapy in Child Abuse Cases   52
   MICHELLE M. PLISKE

6  Digital Community Explorations: How Can Incel Community Insights
   Inform Generalist Human Services Practice in the Digital Era?        65
   CAYETANA CALDERON-SMITH

7  Connected Recovery™: Therapeutic Navigation of Problematic and
Out-of-Control Sexual Behavior                                        78
LANEY KNOWLTON

SECTION II
Leading Conversations about Public Health and Human Services          91

8  The Intersection of Public Health and Human Services               93
NEIL E. DUCHAC, JILL S. MINOR, AND JONAH N. DUCHAC

9  One Health and Human Services: A Course in Land-Based Care Work    105
MELINA McCONATHA AND NIKKI DIGREGORIO

10  Navigating Parental Challenges in Child Welfare: Strategies for Enhancing
Family Resilience                                                    118
DEVIN SENON-GARCIA WADLEY

11  Nothing without Us! Working in Community with Disabled Persons     127
MIA OCEAN, MEAGAN CORRADO, MELISSA HIRSCHI,
AND LASHIRAH WARREN GLENN

12  Supporting Graduate Students' Mental Health: Addressing Challenges for
Underrepresented Communities                                          140
ADRIAN RODRIGUEZ

13  Shifting the Narrative in Healthcare: From "Limited English Proficiency"
to "Limited Linguistic and Cultural Competence"                      151
NEDA MOINOLMOLKI

14  Reframing Adolescent Development through the Lens of Cascading
Collective Trauma                                                    158
DAYA PATTON

15  Treating Adults Living with Perinatally Acquired HIV              171
ANGELA M. WILBON

16  Human Services and Sexuality Consultation: The Need to Move beyond
Clinical Discomfort in Talking about Sex                             188
ANASTASIA GORDEN

17  The Impact of Loss, Death, and Bereavement across the Lifespan    197
MICHELLE M. PLISKE

SECTION III
Leading Conversations: Cultural Considerations and Social Justice    211

18  Edge Dancers: Mixed Heritage Identity Negotiation of Multiracial/Ethnic
    Students in Higher Education—Are They Welcome in Human Services
    Departments?    213
    MIKEL HOGAN

19  Health Equity: Addressing a Social Justice Imperative for Black,
    Indigenous, and People of Color (BIPOC) through a Population Health
    Framework    225
    DARRIN E. WRIGHT

20  Death Customs: Cross-Cultural Issues of Grief and Bereavement    236
    ROLANDA L. WARD, ISIAH MARSHALL JR.,
    PEDRO M. HERNANDEZ, AND PATRICE R. JENKINS

21  A "Real-World" Social Work Analysis of Child and Family Welfare:
    Implications for Culturally Competent Interventions to Address
    21st-Century Issues    251
    IRMA J. GIBSON

22  Being Still … Reflections about Professionalism, Friendship, and
    Internalized White Supremacy in Human Services    272
    JASALYNNE NORTHCROSS

23  Access to Artificial Intelligence (AI) Art: Healing Trauma and
    Transforming Children and Youth in Marginalized Communities—Leading
    Human Service Conversations: Cultural Considerations and Social Justice    275
    TREVA GRAY JONES

24  Creating a Beloved Community: A Radical Approach to Unlearning Racism    286
    TRACY ROBINSON WHITAKER

25  Multiculturalism in Human Services: Challenges and Solutions    294
    BEVERLY EDWARDS

SECTION IV
Leading Conversations about Human Services and Education    301

26  Creative Means to Address Mental Health in the African American
    Community: Arts, Advocacy, and Awareness    303
    DENISE F. BROWN

27  Addressing Empathy Deficits in College-Age Students Utilizing Social
Work Pedagogy amid Social Shifts                                          315
SANDRA R. WILLIAMSON-ASHE

28  The New Homeschool Movement: What Human Services Professionals
Need to Know                                                             325
EMILEE PRINS AND SCOTT SHAW

SECTION V
Leading Conversations about Human Services Trends                        339

29  Human Service Transformations and Emergent Trends                    341
JAMES C. WADLEY

*Index*                                                                  355

# Acknowledgments

I would like to take this opportunity to acknowledge and thank my colleagues at Lincoln University who believed in me several years ago to become a faculty member in the Human Services Department and who supported me every step of the way. The role gave me a chance to learn about the academy, develop a myriad of human service courses, and teach students about the challenges and changes in the field. Last year, I was awarded a faculty development grant that allowed for the idea of this book to come to fruition. I am honored to have received the award and am happy that this book may serve as a cornerstone for our department. The book creates scores of possibilities for us to continue to grow as a program and empower constituents across the region. I hope this book can do the same for other human service programs around the world.

Finally, I would like to thank my Lincoln University students (Tiffinie Carter, Jason China, Alice Holmes, Sierra Jones, Kristina Lane, Elisha Richardson, Sadiyah, Marsha Brown, Indiya Frazier, Alecia Miller, and Heather Myers) for their stories, patience, and support. I received their stories and experiences as "gifts" and I am certain that they will emerge as leaders within our field.

# Contributors

## Editor

**Dr. James C. Wadley** is a tenured Professor in the Counseling and Human Services Department at Lincoln University. As a scholar-practitioner, he is a licensed professional counselor and maintains a private practice in the States of Pennsylvania and New Jersey. He is the Director of the Sex Therapy Program at Council for Relationships and serves as a mental health consultant to the Philadelphia 76ers.

He is the founding editor of the scholarly, interdisciplinary journal, the *Journal of Black Sexuality and Relationships*. Dr. Wadley's vision and efforts have created a scholarly medium that is now available at over 1,300 institutions globally. In addition, as founder and principal of the Association of Black Sexologists and Clinicians, he has hosted/chaired relational and sexual health conferences in Cape Town, Prague, Havana, San Pedro, St. George's (Grenada), Montreal, Montego Bay, Philadelphia, Chicago, Ft. Lauderdale, and St. Thomas (US Virgin Islands). His professional background in human sexuality education, educational leadership, and program development has enabled him to galvanize scholars and practitioners in the field of sexology around the world.

His research and publication interests include sexual decision-making among young adults, masculinity development, conceptions of fatherhood by non-custodial fathers, and HIV/AIDS prevention. He has written undergraduate and graduate courses and authored 22 courses for the Master of Science in Counseling program for Lincoln University (PA). In addition, he recently co-authored 13 doctoral-level courses for the Theological Seminary of Puerto Rico. In 2015, Dr. Wadley earned his NBCC-International Mental Health Facilitator certification after spending time with Rwandan therapists, discussing the impact of genocide and trauma in the early 1990s. In 2016, he helped develop curricula and conducted a sexuality education course at the University of Muhimbili in Tanzania for the nursing and midwifery program. Later that year, he developed and taught an applied research methods course at the Cape Peninsula University of Technology in Cape Town, South Africa. In 2017, Dr. Wadley's work and advocacy domestically and abroad enabled him to complete his first documentary, "Raw to Reel: Race, Drugs, and Sex in Trenton, New Jersey," which captures some of the challenges that emerge in addiction and recovery. In 2018, Dr. Wadley co-edited *The Art of Sex Therapy Supervision* (Routledge), a book devoted to the clinical experiences of supervisors and supervisees in the field of sex therapy. The book won AASECT's 2019 Book of the Year Award. In 2020, his book *The Handbook of Sexuality Leadership: Inspiring Community Engagement, Social Empowerment, and Transformational Influence* (Routledge) carves a new path for sexuality educators, counselors, and therapists in that it serves as an invitation for re-conceptualizing the consultative and leadership roles that sexuality professionals engage in. In 2021, he co-edited a book, *An Intersectional Approach to Sex Therapy: Centering the Lives of Indigenous, Racialized, and People of Color*, which draws attention to the experiences of BIPOC sex therapists and educators. In 2024, Dr. Wadley's book *The Professional's Guide to Sexuality Consultation: An Exploration of Entrepreneurship, Strategic Planning, and Business Influence* continues a needed discussion about navigating best business practices in the field of sexuality. Finally, in 2024, Dr. Wadley was awarded the SASH Patrick J. Carnes Lifetime Achievement Award.

Dr. Wadley received his Doctorate of Philosophy degree in Education from the University of Pennsylvania with a concentration in Educational Leadership and Human Sexuality Education. He earned a Master of Science in Education degree in School Psychology from the University of Kentucky after completing his BA in Psychology from Hampton University. He holds a clinical postgraduate certificate from Thomas Jefferson University/Council for Relationships in Philadelphia. In 2020, Dr. Wadley also earned a Performance Leadership Certificate from Cornell University and his MBA from Keystone College. As a result, he has helped leaders engage in courageous and transformative dialogue about corporate social responsibility and strategic change. Finally, he is an AASECT Certified Sex Therapist Supervisor as well as a SASH Certified Sexuality and Wellness Therapist Supervisor. These credentials and a wealth of domestic and international clinical experiences have catapulted him to be one of the nation's best marriage, family, and sexuality clinicians.

## Contributors

**Rebecca Arnold, PhD,** is a registered, board-certified (ATR-BC), and licensed art therapist (CLAT). She received her PhD in Expressive Therapies through Lesley University, where her dissertation focus was an exploration of the influences of grief and loss on creativity and visual art making in professional artists. She is a published author and was the founding director of the graduate art therapy program at Cedar Crest College in Allentown, Pennsylvania. She is currently an Associate Professor and the Clinical Coordinator for the Master of Arts in Art Therapy and Counseling program at Albertus Magnus College in New Haven, Connecticut.

**Denise F. Brown, DHS,** is a Philly native and an alumna of the second oldest HBCU, Cheyney University. Denise Brown obtained her bachelor's in Social Relations, a Master's in Criminology from the Indiana University of Pennsylvania, and a doctorate in Human Services with a Specialization in Clinical Social Work from Walden University. Denise spent a decade in social work/mental health therapy and 12 years teaching at the university level. Now, as a tenured Professor at Lincoln University, Denise's major research goals are in the study of artistic advocacy, mental health, inclusivity, and diversity.

**Cayetana Calderon-Smith** is a license-eligible professional counselor (MSEd, MPhilEd, The University of Pennsylvania) and a classically trained designer and design researcher (BFA, The School of the Art Institute of Chicago). She fuses participant-observer and digital ethnographic methods with applied clinical practice to explore mental health sequelae driven by problematic internet use. Her focus on at-risk and/or outlier digital communities scales to offer generalist clinical and systemic insight for practitioners. Cayetana presents at local and national conferences, most recently at GPACA (Philadelphia) and AICAD (Los Angeles). She is an Early Career board member of ACBS, Philadelphia.

**Meagan Corrado, DSW, LCSW**, is an Assistant Professor in the Graduate Social Work Department at West Chester University. Meagan specializes in clinical work with urban youth of color who have experienced trauma. She uses storytelling, art, music, poetry, and play therapy in her practice. Meagan's own experiences with trauma inspired her to develop the Storiez trauma narrative intervention. Storiez supports youth in creatively reflecting on their past experiences and developing a future vision. Meagan has also designed training curriculum and provided trauma-informed consultation for a wide range of systems and organizations.

**Nikki DiGregorio, PhD**, is an Assistant Professor in the Family Studies and Community Development Department at Towson University. She has over ten years of experience building partnerships with local organizations and community members in rural southeast Georgia and the greater Baltimore area of Maryland to improve accessibility and availability of human services for historically underserved groups. Her primary scholarship examines the interplay between human development, policy, gender and sexual diversity, and the environment. In her research and practice, she believes collaborative engagement can be transformative for individuals and communities, and she works to leverage knowledge, understanding, and empirical research to inform meaningful change.

**Jonah N. Duchac, MDiv**, is a full-time student pursuing his PhD in Organizational Leadership at Regent University. He has published several works on servant leadership, as well as his thesis *But None Comes Further: An Examination and Hypothetical Implementation of a Kierkegaardian View of Faith*. In his free time, Jonah enjoys spending time with friends and family.

**Neil E. Duchac, DrPH, EdD, PhD**, is an Associate Professor and Executive Director of the Academy for Inclusive Learning and Social Growth, an Inclusive Post-Secondary Education Program at Kennesaw State University. For the past 30 years, he has worked in the human services field in various settings. Professionally, he is a licensed professional counselor and certified school counselor. Additionally, he is a national certified counselor, approved clinical supervisor, and human services board-certified professional.

**Dr. Beverly Edwards** is currently the MSW Program Director and Associate Professor in the School of Social Work at Fayetteville State University. She teaches in the Master's in Social Work degree program. She has practiced in the profession of social work at the micro-, mezzo-, and macrolevels with children and families and policy implementation and development for over three decades. Her research interests include social emotional learning, social work ethics and rural practice, health disparities, spirituality, and issues impacting people of color. Additionally, Dr. Edwards has authored several publications in her area of research interests.

**Irma J. Gibson, PhD, MSW**, is an Associate Professor of Social Work at Florida Agricultural and Mechanical University (FAMU). She teaches across the BSW program curriculum and joined the FAMUly in Fall 2019 after teaching seven years at Albany State University and six years at Savannah State University, respectively, and 21 years of clinical and administrative practice with the federal government, nationally and internationally. She is a study abroad program coordinator who facilitates summer courses annually and crosses global borders to culturally connect the U.S. and the Trinidad and Tobago child and family welfare systems. Research interests include child and family welfare, poverty, homelessness, intimate partner violence, PTSD, veterans' affairs, and international social work.

**Lashirah Warren Glenn, MSW, LSW, CTRS,** is a licensed social worker and certified recreational therapist. She specializes in working with older adults and the aging population. Previously, Lashirah has worked with older adults in long-term care and adult day settings, helping them reengage with recreation and leisure activities as their abilities change. Lashirah also assisted older adults in exploring new interests and hobbies to maintain or increase their quality of life. Additionally, Lashirah has experience working with adults with intellectual and developmental disabilities.

**Dr. Anastasia Gorden** is currently a teaching faculty member as well as the Director of New Student Support for Antioch University's Masters of Arts in Clinical Psychology Program. Dr. Gorden's focus includes teaching and providing faculty support in helping new students prepare and adjust to the start of their program. Dr. Anastasia Gorden comes to us as a dedicated mental health advocate with a history of commitment to promoting diversity, equity, and inclusion for BIPOC and LGBTQ+ communities both personally and professionally.

Dr. Gorden earned her doctorate in Couples and Family Therapy from Alliant International University, her Master's in Clinical Psychology from the Chicago School of Professional Psychology, and her BA in African American and African Studies from the University of California, Davis.

Dr. Gorden provides an experiential learning environment to create hands-on experience through role plays and class demonstrations, exploring vignettes and case samples, while also facilitating a collaborative learning environment that embodies group assignments and class discussion topics.

Her research has focused on exploring racial-sexual stereotypes and the impact it has on sexual expression, with the following publications below:

- Gorden, A. M., Seshadri, G., Glebova, T., & Nylund, D. K. (2024). Sensate focus: Addressing potential preconceived notions of black sexuality. *Sexual and Relationship Therapy*, 1–25. https://doi.org/10.1080/14681994.2024.2366506
- Gorden, A. (2021). Sensate focus: Addressing potential preconceived notions of black sexuality (Publication No. 28720764) [Doctoral dissertation, Alliant International University]. ProQuest Dissertations Publishing.
- Gorden, A. M., & Seshadri, G. (2018) Institute for family and sexuality studies. In J. Lebow, A. Chambers, & D. Breunlin (Eds.). *Encyclopedia of Couple and Family Therapy*. Springer, Cham. https://doi.org/10.1007/978-3-319-15877-8_634-1

**Jennifer L. Hanna, PhD,** is an Assistant Teaching Professor in the Department of Educational Psychology, Counseling, and Special Education at Penn State University and a national-certified counselor. She has years of experience working in various bachelors-level human services positions, and her teaching focuses largely on undergraduate education with clinical support to graduate students.

**Dr. Pedro M. Hernandez** is an Associate Professor at the Jackson State University School of Social Work.

**Melissa Hirschi, PhD, LCSW,** is an Associate Professor of Social Work and the Director of the Bachelor of Social Work program at Utah Valley University. Melissa's passions have led to work that focuses on individuals living with mental illness, substance use, and peer support services, individuals living with HIV, and persons with disabilities across the lifespan. Melissa has partnered with advocacy and support organizations and secured funding for financial justice to compensate peer support specialists for their role in our community.

**Mikel Hogan, PhD,** an applied anthropologist, is a Professor and was a 17-year chair of the Human Services Department at CSU Fullerton. Her fields of research and practice are applied anthropology in health; education; pedagogy; mixed heritage identity; the intersection of race, ethnicity, class, and gender relations; and four cultural-dialogic skills presented in the fourth edition of her book *Four Skills of Cultural Diversity Competence* (2013). Her other publications appear in *Applied Anthropology, Health*, and *Human Services* journals. Dr. Hogan has membership in the American Anthropological Association, Society for Applied Anthropology (a Fellow), the Society for Medical Anthropology, the Council on Anthropology and Education, and the National Organization for Human Services Education.

**Dr. Patrice R. Jenkins** is an Associate Professor and Interim Associate Dean at the Jackson State University School of Social Work. Rev. Kimberly Gladden is the pastor of ZionQuest Fellowship and a Louisville Institute Pastoral Study Projects grantee, which funded this study.

**Dr. Treva Gray Jones, LCSW,** is a caring, professional, and hardworking clinician who finds meaning in seeking to improve the lives of children, youth, adults, families, and seniors in Metro Atlanta, GA, and surrounding areas. With more than 22 years of working directly in the community, Treva has experience as a manager of behavioral health in an inpatient unit and crisis stabilization unit for two years and mental health supervisor and forensic experience as a victim/witness advocate where she worked for close to eight years in a specialized unit for victims of trauma in DeKalb County government, specializing in families, communities, and victims of violence. She is certified in Cognitive Behavior Intervention for Substance Abuse by the Cincinnati Corrections Institute. She was also certified as a victim witness assistance program coordinator by the Criminal Justice Coordinating Council in 2006 and has worked with children, adolescents, and adults. She obtained her doctorate in Trauma-Informed Social Work at Barry University in Miami Shores, Florida, and at Clark Atlanta University's Whitney M. Young, Jr. School of Social Work, where she obtained her Master's in Health/Mental Health. She earned her undergraduate degree at Southern University at New Orleans, where she studied generally in the area of Business and Substance Abuse Counseling.

**Shyrun Karandikar, BA,** is currently a Master's student in the Counselor Education program at Penn State University. She is focused on working with minority, disabled, and underserved populations to provide culturally competent and equitable mental health support, aiming to address disparities, promote wellness within these communities, and integrate counseling practices into healthcare settings to ensure comprehensive and accessible mental health services.

**Dr. Laney Knowlton** is a licensed marriage and family therapist supervisor (LMFT-S), author, and public speaker. She has worked in the field of mental health since 2009, specializing in problematic sexual behaviors (PSB) and betrayal trauma. Laney has a PhD in Clinical Sexology. She is a CSAT-S (certified sex addiction therapist supervisor), a CCPS (certified clinical partner specialist), a CPTT-S (certified partner trauma therapist supervisor), an AASECT certified sex therapist, an CCRS (certified connected recovery specialist), and a CCBRT (certified couple betrayal recovery therapist). She is trained in multiple trauma treatment models. Her expertise includes counseling for individuals, couples, and groups, along with directing recovery programs and training other clinicians. She has presented at professional conferences ranging from local to international levels, including SASH, ACA, AAMFT, the IITAP Symposium, and TAMFT. She is on the faculty of the International Institute of Trauma & Addiction Professionals (IITAP). She developed the Connected Recovery™ model of therapy, which connects the treatment of PSB, Betrayal Trauma, Relational Counseling through an Emotionally Focused Therapy lens, and Sex Therapy. She has published multiple books, including *Facing Hope*, which helps individuals and relationships create emotional safety through truth after betrayal. She owns Connected Recovery Training (a training program that offers various levels of certification and training in her model and in trauma awareness and treatment) and Knowlton Counseling, and co-owns NorthStar Relational Consultants in the Dallas/Fort Worth area of TX, where she lives with her husband and six children.

**Dr. Isiah Marshall** Jr. is a Professor and Dean of the Ethelyn R. Strong School of Social Work at Norfolk State University.

**Melina McConatha, PhD,** is a queer ecologist, rewilder, and educator at Lincoln University—the first degree granting historically Black university. She lives in a yurt with her multi-species family on land once cared for by the Lenni-Lenape. Melina's current scholarship explores care, reparations, and collective liberation in open spaces.

**Jill S. Minor, EdD, LSC,** is an Assistant Professor in Counselor Education at Marshall University. She is trained as both a clinical mental health counselor and a school counselor. Over the past 20 years, Dr. Minor has worked across mental health disciplines, actively advocating for mental wellness and the counseling profession at local, state, and national levels.

**Dr. Neda Moinolmolki** is an Assistant Professor of Psychology at Albertus Magnus College. She received her PhD in Human Development and Family Studies and has been teaching in the field for over ten years. She is committed to applied, strength-based, participatory action research centered on underserved and marginalized populations. Dr. Moinolmolki's dedication to research is evident in her active publication record and the various honors she has received, including the Distinguished Contribution to the Science of Psychology Award from the Connecticut Psychological Association and the Early Career Research Award from the Southeastern Psychological Association.

**Jasalynne Northcross, LCSW,** is based in Washington, DC. She is a sex and relationship therapist and doctoral student at the Howard University School of Social Work. She is passionate about helping individuals and couples release fear and shame and experience healthy and fulfilling sexual experiences. Ms. Northcross wants to engage rising social workers who are interested in helping Black people transform their intimate relationships. She is currently pursuing the American Association of Sexuality Educators, Counselors, and Therapists (AASECT) sex therapy certification.

**Deirdre O'Sullivan, PhD,** is an Associate Professor in the Department of Educational Psychology, Counseling, and Special Education at Penn State University. Her current research focuses on trauma, substance use, and disability. She teaches undergraduate and graduate classes as well as supervises doctoral students in the researcher-practitioner model.

**Mia Ocean, PhD, LCSW, LMFT,** is an Associate Professor in the School of Social Work at Wichita State University, adjunct faculty at the University of Maryland Global Campus, and a staff writer for The Squeaky Wheel, a disability-focused satire publication. Previously, Mia taught human services, addictions studies, sociology, and psychology at open-door minority-serving colleges and served as an Americans with Disabilities Act coordinator at a public university. Mia lives with multiple dynamic disabilities, and her anti-oppressive, participatory scholarship centers community-generated policy and practical solutions.

**Daya Patton, PhD,** is a professor of Counselor Education at The State University of New York at Oneonta. Dr. Patton holds a Doctor of Philosophy in Human Services from Walden University, a Master of Education in Counseling from American Public University, a Master of Arts in Liberal Studies from East Tennessee State University, and a Bachelor of Arts in Political Science from Hampton University. Dr. Patton is a Licensed Clinical Mental Health Counselor, Licensed Clinical Addiction Specialist, Certified Clinical Supervisor, Licensed Professional School Counselor, and a Human Services Board Board-Certified Practitioner. Dr. Patton has over 15 years of experience working with youth in educational settings. Her research and teaching interests include addiction counseling, adolescent development, trauma-informed counseling, race and social justice, and youth delinquency.

**Dr. Michelle M. Pliske** is an Assistant Professor of Social Work at Pacific University in Forest Grove, OR. Dr. Pliske's research uses qualitative design to explore the effects of adversity, social determinants of health, and relational-cultural theory in application to education, supervision, and direct clinical care. She is a licensed clinical social worker and registered play therapy supervisor. Dr. Pliske is the clinical director for outpatient mental health services at the Firefly Institute and currently serves on the board of directors for the National Association of Social Work in Washington, DC. Dr. Pliske provides clinical supervision across disciplines and specializes in pediatric mental health care.

**Emilee Prins, MA, MSW,** is an Assistant Professor of Human Services at Grace Christian University, Grand Rapids, MI, USA. She is actively involved in social work practice and community engagement, including working in clinical practice in mental health and substance abuse.

**Candace Robertson-James, DrPH,** is an Associate Professor, Director of the Bachelor's and Master's of Public Health Programs, and Chair of the Department of Urban Public Health and Nutrition at LaSalle University. She has taught numerous public health courses, including introduction to public health, research methods, race, ethnicity and public health, social and behavioral health, and global health. She led and evaluated community participatory research initiatives involving multiple sectors (health, community, school, faith, etc.), promoting health in diverse and underserved communities for over 15 years. Dr. Robertson-James has also participated in research, exploring the role of experiences of racism and discrimination in health risks as well as the role of faith institutions in sexual and relationship violence risk reduction and prevention interventions. She served as the program evaluator for programs integrating HIV risk reduction into domestic violence services, as well as health education and promotion initiatives targeting various groups of women, including women with a history of incarceration. She authored a children's book in 2019, titled *Reflections of Me*, to promote a positive self-concept in girls of color based on her research with Black women and is the founder of the Ruach Lab, a faith-inspired space that aims to engage, empower, and equip individuals and families to promote wellness.

**Dr. Adrian Rodriguez** is an Associate Professor of Human Services at California State University, Fullerton. He specializes in counseling theories and techniques; self-awareness through group dialogue; case analysis and intervention techniques; co-occurring disorders; and serving Veterans and their families. His current research with his student research team focuses on the impact of stress on the graduate school aspirations of undergraduate college students. He also investigates how adverse childhood experiences, attachment styles, and PTSD influence college students' relationship dynamics and conflict management styles with their professors as well as their internship and professional supervisors.

**Luanne Shaw, DNP, RN, CEN,** is Assistant Professor of Nursing in the Kirkhof College of Nursing at Grand Valley State University. Luanne has spoken nationally and internationally on topics of healthcare leadership, interprofessional collaboration, and social determinants of health.

**Scott Shaw, PhD, EdD, DMin, LPC, LMSW,** is Dean and Professor in the School of Business Innovation and Public Service at Grace Christian University, Grand Rapids, MI, USA. Scott is a licensed professional counselor (LPC) and licensed master social worker (LMSW—Clinical & Macro) and has worked in the human services field for over 30 years. Scott has spoken internationally on topics of leadership, interprofessional collaboration, public policy, and social determinants of health. He has worked in mental health, addictions, family preservation, and trauma.

**Devin Senon-Garcia Wadley, MSW,** is a CUA case management specialist at Bethanna Children's Services in Philadelphia. He completed his Master of Social Work degree at LaSalle University. Professionally, Devin is dedicated to supporting children and families in Philadelphia's child welfare system. In this role, Devin applies a wealth of knowledge and skills to advocate for and assist those in need. His knowledge, expertise, and compassion continue to make a difference for traditionally marginalized and underrepresented communities.

**Dr. Rolanda L. Ward** is a Professor of Social Work and Director of the Ostapenko Center for Race, Equity, & Mission at Niagara University.

**Corinne D. Warrener, PhD,** is an Associate Professor of Social Work at Clark Atlanta University. She earned her Master's and PhD in Social Work from Rutgers, the State University of New Jersey. Her area of expertise is intimate partner violence, including domestic violence, dating violence, sexual assault, and trauma. Dr. Warrener has several years of practice experience, including working in child protection and foster care, schools, and domestic violence services. She has experience doing individual and group therapy, community outreach and education, and prevention work, mainly in the area of dating violence and domestic violence.

Her research is focused on topics such as perpetration of violence, financial abuse, and economic disadvantages of divorced/separated women. She recently worked on a project around veteran suicide and oxytocin with the Laboratory for Darwinian Neuroscience at Emory University, funded by the American Foundation for Suicide Prevention. She is currently working on an NIJ-funded project to examine campus climate and sexual assault at HBCUs.

**Dr. Tracy Robinson Whitaker** is an Associate Professor and the Associate Dean for academic and student advancement at the Howard University School of Social Work. Dr. Whitaker's research interests are diversity and inclusion within the profession and the workplace. In 2021, she served as the co-chair of the Council on Social Work Education's Task Force to Advance Anti-Racism and is certified in Diversity, Equity, and Inclusion in the Workplace by the University of South Florida. Dr. Whitaker serves as a board member for the Community Partnership for the Prevention of Homelessness in Washington, DC. She is an alumna of Howard University.

**Angela M. Wilbon, DSW,** a licensed clinical social worker, earned her BSW and MSW from the University of Iowa, and a doctorate from Howard University School of Social Work. With over two decades of experience, her expertise spans diverse demographics. She spent 17 years at Children's National Hospital, offering mental health services to acute and chronically ill patients while supporting their families. Ms. Wilbon serves as a psychotherapist in a private group practice. Lastly, Angela provides workshops and training across the District of Columbia metropolitan area, imparting knowledge to childcare facilities, social services agencies, and various non-profits.

**Dr. Sandra R. Williamson-Ashe** is a tenured Associate Professor in the Ethelyn R. Strong School of Social Work at Norfolk State University and serves in the Office of the Provost as the academic affairs recruitment coordinator. She completed her Master of Social Work degree at Norfolk State University and her doctorate in higher education administration and leadership from the George Washington University. She has served in several senior-level university administrative positions, including assistant to the director of the Virginia Beach higher education center, associate vice president for student affairs at Norfolk State University, and vice president for enrollment management and student affairs at Virginia Union University. As a proponent of leadership, she has published several peer-reviewed book chapters on leadership and articles that improve collegiate pedagogy, group work, ethics, student success, and redefining the Black woman.

Dr. Williamson-Ashe has served as a Commonwealth of Virginia gubernatorial appointment to the Council on Aging, a Virginia Beach Mayoral appointment to the e-government commission, Social-Emotional Learning Advisory Council, Chesapeake Public Schools, Association of Black Social Workers, and appointed to the Chesapeake Citizens Juvenile Advisory Council.

She is a graduate of the ACE Virginia Network of Women Senior Leadership Seminar series, an Honorary Member of the Golden Key International Honour Society, a Senior Faculty Fellow of the Robert S. Nusbaum Honors College, and has completed certifications for DARE to LEAD, CSWE site visitation, and ACUE Effective College Instruction.

**Darrin E. Wright, PhD, LMSW,** is an Associate Professor and Associate Dean in Social Work at Fayetteville State University in Fayetteville, NC. He formerly held the position of Director of Practicum Education at Clark Atlanta University, Whitney M. Young Jr. School of Social Work. Dr. Wright has been in academia for nearly two decades. Dr. Wright has worked in various leadership and service capacities in the corporate world, academia, non-profit human services, and the U.S. Air Force Reserves. He has occupied several leadership positions at the national and international levels of social work education.

Dr. Wright earned a BA in Forensic Psychology from John Jay College of Criminal Justice in Manhattan, NY; a Master's in Social Work from Columbia University's School of

Social Work in Manhattan, NY; and a PhD in Social Work Policy, Planning, and Administration from Clark Atlanta University, Atlanta, GA, with a minor in Public Health Administration from Morehouse School of Medicine, Atlanta, GA. He is a licensed social worker with several certifications in addictions and trauma-informed care and a true colors personal success coach/consultant.

His areas of practice expertise, research interests, and publications are focused on integrated behavioral health practice, community-based partnerships and interventions, international social work (primarily in the English-speaking Caribbean), workforce development opportunities in behavioral health, leadership in social work, and African-centered approaches to social work education and practice. He has presented his areas of expertise and research interests at numerous national and international conferences.

# Foreword

## Contemporary Issues in Human Services

*Candace Robertson-James, DrPH, MPH*

One does not have to explore too many headlines to quickly become overwhelmed. From wondering how artificial intelligence influences the workforce, everyday life, healthcare, or therapy to wildfires, war, affordable housing crises, book bans, space docking experiments, and more, our society changes quickly, and while we make great advances that will forever change our world as we know it, we also face continued and new crises and challenges. Educators and practitioners alike are tasked with learning, relearning, and unlearning concepts and practices necessary to truly understand how to promote health and wellness in diverse communities. It's imperative that we understand how these emerging and future trends allow opportunities to further operationalize concepts of equity and justice as we continue to work to create the conditions that promote health and wellness for all people.

Our world is more diverse than ever, and human services and public health organizations and practitioners alike have increasingly come to appreciate that diversity in all its various forms. But many gaps remain in our ability to meet the needs of diverse groups. Historical inequities, prejudices, discrimination, biases, and norms have often shaped perspectives that have informed institutions meant to serve the entire population, often causing them to prioritize and value some experiences while criticizing and demonizing others. Some groups continue to struggle to be known, seen, valued, and appreciated, even as societal and mainstream cultural pressures to mute certain voices and render others invisible remain. This text critically engages professionals across the country to discuss emergent lessons in how human service and public health agencies can go beyond merely supporting people of differing abilities, education, employment, identities, income and wealth statuses, orientation, race/ethnicities, immigration statuses, and adversity to create systems that promote empowerment.

This discourse assesses how organizations can aptly serve as both mirrors and windows. Mirrors allow us to aptly consider the communities we serve, including their aspirations, desires, challenges, and needs. They allow us to critically reflect on the situations and circumstances we observe while we consider our role in promoting equity and justice. They call us to assess our role in recognizing both the achievements and successes gained, as well as existing barriers and failures. Mirrors force us to stop and reflect on ourselves, our institutions, our practices, our beliefs, our limitations, and our opportunities as we move forward. They cause us to consider new areas of learning and unlearning and embolden us with the courage to explore how we can make a difference. Concurrently, we can evaluate how we utilize practices that are limiting and inequitable. Thus, leadership is a necessity for change and growth. Human service and public health practitioners need to be able to challenge inequities that continue to marginalize disadvantaged populations and uphold white supremacy and colonialism. These mirrors give us an opportunity to reflect not only on policies and practices that need to be modified but also on areas of understanding that need to adjust. They cause us to question, consider, critique, and evaluate our systems, and they inspire us to put aside band aid approaches and reach instead for new tools. These mirrors represent critical junctures for us all. As a human service or public health practitioner, what might you see in your mirror?

Windows, however, allow us to see the communities we serve more clearly. We have an opportunity to share in their experiences and possibly go beyond understanding and discussing determinants of health to engaging in meaningful interventions and practices that promote healthy decision making. A deeper understanding and constructive conversations may include attention to the assets and challenges faced by communities. Windows may allow us to articulate the role of policy violence, cultural racism, and historical and collective trauma in present-day experiences and challenges. They compel us to acknowledge how effective human services and public health organizations can dismantle the impact of structural inequalities and rely on the power of collaboration and partnership to address emergent aspirations and concerns as we work together to redesign systems. These windows prevent us from judging too quickly. They cause us to further investigate root causes across the lifespan and implement evidence-based strategies. The chapters included within this text provide continued insight into the lived experiences of various groups through reflective case examples and research. These windows invite us to center voices from diverse groups as they allow marginalized communities to narrate their own stories. They call us to commit to knowing our communities through the lens of their assets as well as their challenges. They inspire us to contest the deficit-laden language inherent in many of our systems and frameworks and, instead, celebrate the resilience, strength, and hopes of the groups we serve. They compel us to consider not only existing situations but also the needs and desires that emerge from our changing landscape.

We are not oblivious to the importance of this moment in history. Approximately one in five adults, representing over 59 million people, lives with a mental illness. Moreover, at least half of individuals over 12 have used an illicit drug at least once, and drug overdose is a leading cause of death in people under 45. The National Center for PTSD reports that approximately 60% of men and 50% of women will encounter at least one traumatic event during their lifetime. Suicide is recognized as a leading cause of death, and more than half of Americans are grieving the loss of a loved one from many causes. We are in a climate crisis that is having dire consequences for many communities, and while the poverty rate is 11% for the nation, great racial/ethnic disparities exist, leading to rates that are doubled for Black and Latinx populations. Moreover, as poverty rates persist, income among affluent individuals continues to rise, and wage inequities continue to exist. Racial gaps in wealth continue to be observed and are sizeable. An increasing number of people are experiencing homelessness and housing insecurity, and over 47 million people experience food insecurity. We are in the midst of a loneliness epidemic that is associated with a number of health, social, and behavioral risks. This compendium gives us an opportunity to reflect upon social challenges, interventions used, and resources needed to offer compassion and support to our constituents and clients.

At this pivotal moment, characterized by a mix of significant challenges and notable advancements, we must pause to consider the unique opportunities before us. This text serves as a guide for that exploration. Use it as both a mirror and a window. Let this guide act as a beacon in an effort to lead human service and public health professionals and educators into the future.

# Introduction

*James C. Wadley*

The field of human services continues to evolve, and professionals have to be skilled, intuitive, and accessible to their constituents. When I returned from sabbatical and was invited to teach a Special Topics in Human Services course for my department, I knew that my students would need to be exposed to a variety of emergent issues in our field in order for them to become knowledgeable and capable of meeting the needs of their clients and agencies. The course was developed after discussions with several professionals in the field and reviews of some of the current and historical literature related to human service policy, delivery, and administration. Moreover, it was important to develop a course that centers the experiences of traditionally marginalized groups (e.g., BIPOC, disabled, LGBTQ, lower socioeconomic status) in an effort to expand my students' understanding of systemic issues that may impact the mental and relational health of the populations that they might represent or serve.

By the end of the course, some of the feedback that I received from my students was that they would have wanted additional time and space to discuss a variety of topics in greater detail. While the course offered small and large group discussions, activities, and service learning projects, students shared that they needed additional time to reflect, process, and work toward integrating new material into their personal and professional experiences. Also, students suggested several additional topics (e.g., health, spirituality, sexuality, aging) that were not included within the course. I reminded them that we only had a semester to cover as many areas as we could and that we could not cover everything. Students also indicated in their evaluations that the course offered them an opportunity to engage in discussions that ultimately gave them an idea about how they might set up their own mental health private practice; develop management strategies for a drug/alcohol treatment facility; create innovative behavioral and mental health policy; advocate for the disadvantaged; and conceptualize new approaches for leadership and community engagement. The Special Topics course was an opportunity for students to expand their understanding of human services, resource delivery, and interventions for a variety of populations and settings. Most of my students in the class already had a job within the field of human services, and they were able to apply course learnings to their current roles and positions. The course gave students an opportunity to enhance their critical thinking skills and insight so that they could develop the capacity to "see around the corner" by analyzing and predicting trends within and outside of the field. Using class storytelling as a means of information gathering and processing, students were able to continue their journey toward becoming agents of change. They reflected on their personal and professional experiences, considered the history and evolution of human service delivery and their knowledge of service provision, and projected what needs would emerge for their constituents.

DOI: 10.4324/9781003531258-1

With that in mind, a call for proposals and manuscripts was sent out nationwide to human service professionals and educators to help shed light on current and future trends in the field. There was a tremendous response and enthusiasm for the preparation of a compendium that could address an array of topics. The invite was for practitioners and advocates to write about their research, clinical experience, advocacy, and activism so that college students and professionals could learn more about how to effectively reach a variety of populations.

Given the diverse array of submitted manuscripts, the book is organized into five sections: Leading Conversations about Clinical Practice in Human Services; Leading Conversations about Public Health and Human Services; Leading Conversations about Human Services and Education; Leading Conversations about Cultural Considerations and Social Justice; and Leading Conversations about Human Services Trends.

The first section, Leading Conversations about Clinical Practice in Human Services, centers the mental and relational health experiences of practitioners and their constituents. The second installment for this book, Leading Conversations about Public Health and Human Services, focuses on macro- and micro-level entities that seek to provide support, accommodation, and advocacy for disenfranchised populations and communities. The third section, Leading Human Service Conversations: Cultural Considerations and Social Justice, contains chapters that take into account the necessity of employing nuanced considerations and interventions for individuals and families to meet their needs. The fourth portion of this book, Leading Conversations about Human Services and Education, invites us to reflect on pedagogy, research, and gender. The final chapter of this book comprises the Leading Conversations about Human Service Trends and gives readers an opportunity to reflect on emergent needs of the field and traits needed for effective delivery.

I feel proud and honored to be a part of this human service community and initiative, as the book contains over two dozen chapters. I am grateful to the contributors who shared their thoughts and experiences and worked with us in an effort to conceptualize and talk about the fluidity of change in the field. This book serves as a generational medium for human service practitioners to discuss contemporary topics in the field for years to come.

# Section I

# Leading Conversations about Clinical Practice in Human Services

# 1 Therapists' Grief

## Creativity as Part of an Essential Ethical Practice

*Rebecca Arnold*

## Introduction

Individuals, families, and whole cultures experience both personal and collective loss. One way this can occur is through the death of a significant individual, creating a changed relationship between the deceased and those left behind (Bonanno et al., 2008; Kessler, 2019; Rando, 1995). Over a lifetime, losing a loved one is inevitable (Drescher, 2013), whether the death was anticipated or unexpected because of war, suicide, natural disaster, or other tragedy. However, at any age, there seems to be no loss as significant as that which is experienced from the loss of who we knew ourselves to be. Attempts to understand this "dissonance" or inconsistency within the self (Fortino et al., 2021, p. 99) and "how our life story has changed" (O'Connor, 2022, p. 136) can lead one to question if they are still the same person after the loss experience.

Bereavement authors have not only suggested the importance of a whole body approach to understanding grief (Gudmundsdottir, 2009) but also described how the brain grieves and manages (or does not) the loss of closeness with the deceased (O'Connor, 2022). Coping with loss can depend largely on our ability to deal with such a ubiquitous change, which often focuses on the lost relationship, how we understand it, and how we knew ourselves within it (Arnold, 2023; Davis, 2008). Complications of grief can develop into feeling disconnected from and confused about the world in which the bereaved continues to live without their loved one.

This chapter focuses on the use of creativity for self-care in bereavement, specifically directed at professionals working in human service fields. A brief review of the literature will examine the ethical underpinnings of self-care in mental health and medical practices and provide a foundation for creativity as a natural grief response. Art making, in particular, will be presented as a specific application and "ethical imperative" (Barnett et al., 2007) for ongoing professional self-care. A personal account of my own bereavement experience and subsequent grief response is included to increase the collective conversations about therapists' grief. Overall, this writing intends to re-engage those in the helping professions with creative aspects they may already embrace, ones that may be lying dormant, or as a way of inviting new opportunities for self-exploration. Reflective questions at the end of this chapter invite bereaved professionals to examine their current creative capacities and offer recommendations for incorporating new artistic processes in their already-established self-care routines.

## Ethical Underpinnings

At the forefront of any therapeutic encounter is a collaborative approach that aligns the therapist and client in a relationship with one another (Baier et al., 2020). The work is not

DOI: 10.4324/9781003531258-3

only about honoring the experiences of the client through attentiveness and compassion but also for the therapist to engage in the often-harder work of self-inquiry. Grieving therapists who overlook personal experiences of loss may develop ineffective countertransference responses in their client relationships, thereby experiencing increased self-criticism and feelings of guilt. Coenen (2018) suggested that previous patterns of coping with adversity might not be effective when experiencing overwhelming grief. In addition, research on grief and art making is increasing, perhaps in large part due to the recent multigenerational experience of the COVID-19 pandemic (Anaxagorou, 2023; Davis, 2021; Legari, 2022). Therefore, it becomes important for therapists to consider new ways to express their personal emotional landscape to continue an ethical practice.

Unique to therapeutic work is the persistent possibility of self-disclosure and the impossibility of leaving oneself out of the therapeutic relationship. Bressi and Vaden (2017) considered self-care to be "rooted in a relational frame" and called for a reconsideration of ways those in the helping professions can thrive while working with those who are suffering (p. 37). However, it is often difficult for those working in human service fields to recognize when they are disclosing personal material that crosses ethical boundaries (Johnsen & Ding, 2021). More importantly, research has suggested that there is likely to be a significant impact on the therapeutic relationship when the one providing care is themselves experiencing grief symptoms (Broadbent, 2013; Hayes et al., 2007; Kouriatis & Brown, 2013–2014; Pearce et al., 2021; Swinden, 2023; Tsai et al., 2010). Felberbaum (2010) poignantly wrote about how grief impacted professional responsibilities after the death of a parent. This author described tearfulness and exhaustion when interacting with patients, which negatively affected the therapeutic care that was being provided.

Most professionals, such as those who work in psychology, nursing, social work, counseling, and the creative arts therapies, are often educated in self-care practices while completing their graduate or doctoral-level education (Bamonti et al., 2014; Detrick, 2021; Padilla, 2024; Self et al., 2018). In many ways, self-care is promoted as a vital part of professional ethics (Barnett et al., 2007; Coaston, 2017; Linton & Koonmen, 2020; Mirick, 2022; Newell & Nelson-Gardell, 2014; Wise et al., 2012), yet most suggestions for self-care practices embed art making or creative action into categories such as "activities" or "hobbies." A more specific application of visual art making will be introduced in this text as beneficial to an ethical practice.

## Creativity as a Natural Grief Response

The arts have been identified as powerful restorative tools in healthcare (Corriero et al., 2024; Forgeard, 2019; Frantz, 2016; Gabora & Kaufman, 2010). In fact, image making can offer more expansive ways to identify and understand our emotions more often than what verbal language can represent (Gillies et al., 2005), especially in times of grief (e.g. Archambault, 2021; Arnold, 2019; Iliya & Harris, 2016; Iype, 2010; Lev, 2022; Metzl & Shamai, 2021). However, Kossak (2015) acknowledged an awareness that people more often value product over process (pp. 20–21). Yet, creativity for self-care and the particular use of visual art can assist an individual in uncovering personal symbols, increasing personal awareness through explorations of metaphor, and inviting curative benefits through the simple act of non-verbal expression of thoughts and emotions.

Exploring the world and our place in it through creative action is an "essential attribute" shared by all humanity (Halprin, 1997, p. 49). More recently, Baker (2023) expanded on this notion writing that people "are wired for story, symbols, art, and imagery ... that resonate with us on a deep emotional and psychological level, and that can inspire us to take action, even in the face of obstacles" (para 2). These two authors provide an opportunity to examine the benefits of art making during bereavement. For instance, therapists who respond to loss by engaging in their innate creativity may find new understandings of the grief experience. Likewise, professional art therapists have found profound benefit from using the visual arts "as an informal practice" for personal exploration, specifically for supporting "health equilibrium" (Fish, 2012, pp. 138–139). Moon (2016) identified three distinct ways in which the uses of art making can be helpful in professional art therapy practice, including establishing empathy in regard to the therapeutic relationship, providing an outlet for tense emotional content, and acting as a catalyst for discussion in supervision (p. 48). Therefore, creative action not only invites insight and promotes "meaning making" (Beaumont, 2013) after the loss experience, but applications of art making can also help maintain a sense of attachment (Kosminsky & Jordan, 2016; O'Connor, 2022) and continuing and transformational bonds (Jonsson & Walter, 2017; Mathijssen, 2017; Scholtes & Browne, 2014) with the deceased through both product and process.

Although grief symptoms are unique to the individual, mourners often seek ways to convey their experiences to others (Metzl & Shamai, 2021; O'Connor, 2022; Sanstrom, 2012). For instance, applications of grief rituals have become more prevalent in the research literature (Sas & Coman, 2016; Wojtkowiak et al., 2021). More specifically, being able to share created artwork or using art products as a catalyst for discussion has been noteworthy in the bereavement literature on the uses of creativity in grief (Andrus, 2022; Arnold, 2023; Metzl & Shamai, 2021). Several collective expressions of grief by way of installation pieces and collaborative projects that stand as memorials to the dead are also identified in the literature (Castle & Phillips, 2003; Kirkpatrick, 2017; Klorer, 2014; Margry & Sánchez-Carretero, 2011; van Lil, 2012; Wagoner & Brescó de Luna, 2022), providing the bereaved with various ways of expressing and sharing grief. Percy (2014) suggested trying new ways of coping (such as engaging in creative practices) so that one could grapple with the "attachment dilemma" (p. 151). Transformation may occur for the bereaved as newly acquired behaviors develop that invite positive emotional, cognitive, and physiological changes (O'Connor, 2022, p. 136) through both individual expression and collective witnessing.

## Visual Art Making as a Form of Self-Care

Prior to my mother's death in August 2015, I was full of art, imagery, and imagination. My mom championed my creative efforts throughout my life by providing art supplies in my youth and supporting my artistic pursuits in higher education. Initially, my interest in becoming an art therapist stemmed from a desire to make art with others, which itself grew from a deep faith in creativity and the visual arts. Yet, after my mother's death, I experienced my emotions as strangers that, ultimately, caused me to abandon my creative voice. This loss of activity further affected my work as a professional and as an educator. I felt like a fraud as I continued to run my art therapy groups or taught my graduate art therapy students about the varied benefits of making art. During the early stages of being a bereaved therapist, I was able to connect to others to talk about my grief but was detached from my familiar creative processes and could not use art materials as effortlessly as I once had.

I had not allowed myself to grieve for my mother and found that abandoning the profound, natural way of coping I had experienced in the past with art making was worsening my bereavement symptoms. For one full year, I did not make art, which limited the way

I was able to release my sadness or the fears and uncertainties of living that I began experiencing. Instead, I was attempting to avoid feeling this loss by not engaging with my creative capacities, and this caused my emotions to pour over into my work and family obligations. It all seemed reasonable at the time, since I still had both personal and professional responsibilities that needed my full attention. Specifically, my children were still growing and needed parenting, I was continuing to work in clinical practice and needed to be emotionally available to my clients, and I was still the director of a graduate art therapy program and responsible for student achievement. Along with all that, I had entered a doctoral program, which only increased my unconscious self-neglect. However, as my coursework deepened, I focused my writing assignments on topics such as *grief and loss*, *the grieving clinician*, and *creativity* after profound loss. During one of my explorations into the literature, words from Levine's (2004) text challenged me to move into my own emptiness so that the work of grieving could occur, for it would be "upon this canvas of nothing" that my character could be rebuilt (p. 194).

### When Grief Strikes

My mother was 64 when she died after suspected lung cancer had spread to her brain. Two years prior to that, she had been complaining of discomfort under her shoulder blade, which was later found to be a malignant mass that had encapsulated one of her ribs. Because the mass could not be removed, she began radiation treatments just after the New Year in 2014. I was my mother's only child and readily took responsibility for getting her to and from all of her appointments. My familiarity with the medical field also automatically turned her attention to me during procedural conversations whenever she was asked about her current condition, her medical history, or potential future treatment options. The cancer took over quickly, and radiation gave way to weekly chemotherapy appointments.

A year before my mom's diagnosis, my husband had started a new career that required long hours, and I had just been hired to develop and direct a new graduate art therapy program at a college local to where we were living. My mom moved closer to us so she could help with childcare, but once chemotherapy began, her energy level and developing confusion did not allow her to continue in this role. At the time she began to decline, we moved her into our house, and a few months before her death, she was admitted to hospice. We lived too far from my maternal family or my in-laws for anyone else to help ease childcare needs, but several close friends were available when balancing those responsibilities became more and more difficult. Hospice care also offered additional support for her medical needs and declining physical abilities but on a preplanned schedule.

Relationally, my experiences with my mother affected me in two distinct ways. The first was during her illness. As her physical health rapidly declined, and unbeknownst to her medical team, the cancer had begun attacking her brain, causing her moods and behaviors to change significantly. She became more agitated and stopped using her assistive devices for walking, which caused her to fall frequently. Subsequently, she became less aware of her decline, which made her even more dependent on physical care to move from her bed or chair or off the floor. She struggled to go to the bathroom on her own and required physical assistance for that, as well as medication administering, which changed my sense of self. The relationship had changed without much warning, and I found I was reacting to my mom in much the same ways I did with my own children—I was parenting her.

The second way my relational self was affected was after my mother died. The artist and creator I knew myself to be went dormant, and this once staple in my life seemed non-existent. I became a shadowed silhouette in a pond's reflection, and art became a painful experience that reminded me of the loss of my only parent. In my responsibilities to others, I ignored any need to release these feelings for fear I would be an unavailable parent to my children. I also struggled not to become a gooey, unprofessional mess to my art therapy clients or incoherent to the graduate students I taught. Instead, the emotions slipped out of me in conflicting ways. I was short-tempered with my family but longed to spend as much time with them as possible. I was less insightful and creative with my art therapy clients but reacted more sympathetically to the issues that brought them into treatment. Moreover, although I was able to still extend compassion toward my students, I found I also had a desire for them to be more certain and secure in their coursework and internship experiences, needing me less.

## Creative Processes Explored

Eventually, I moved into a purposeful creative process that met my self-care needs and re-established art making as a meaningful practice in my life. The following will provide an overview of three specific art-making processes, including photography, altered book making, and installation art, with brief explorations of each material as a healing component for my grief.

### Photography

I have always loved photography, focusing on this and painting while I was in art school. During my doctoral education, it felt easy to use this medium to create images that defined my grief through metaphor, and also this style of working provided a creative process that required me to just take pictures (Jiménez-Alonso & De Luna, 2021, p. 94). Using my iPhone, I began snapping shots as I walked to and from my classes. One day, I found solace staring at an empty park bench on the sidewalk before finally taking a picture of it. This image became the impetus for my research flyer and my continuing work as a bereaved practitioner and budding researcher. I continued taking images and video footage of benches in various spaces and environmental conditions, and an important relationship grew between images of *the empty bench* and my grief. This relationship was quickly realized as a notable personal symbol of bereavement for me.

### Altered Books

Unlike photography, this process did not come as easily to me. I disliked what I thought of as "ruining a beautiful book" but found a tattered un-shelved one free in the entryway of the library that caught my eye, titled *Is There No Place on Earth for Me?* by Susan Sheehan. The book achieved a similar effect, as a blank canvas would have if I had chosen to paint. I did not need to purchase special art media or spend hours in a store searching for the perfect supplies. Instead, I chose creative materials that were easy to find and use, including decorative bags and condolence cards I had received in the first weeks of my bereavement. I found simple tools around my home, such as markers, pencils, and pens that were stored in my kitchen drawers and the bedrooms of my children. Magazines from the recycle bin and my daughter's watercolor set provided additional avenues of making simple expressions. I used the pages to create blackout poetry (Ramser, 2020); I sewed into them with thread and scrap wire; I went for walks in nature to collect leaves, feathers, and stones to glue into them; and I spent time rummaging through my mom's old papers and belongings to incorporate her writings and other items that connected us in life.

Although altered books had previously held little interest for me, this commonly used practice in art therapy seemed a relevant way for me to memorialize my mother (Klorer, 2014). The inclusion of visual and poetic dialogue in the making of it not only provided me a safe way to share my grief story with others but also elicited an artistic, narrative sculpture (Klorer, 2014) as well as invited a "rebuilding process" for creative work and my re-emerging identity (Jacobson-Levy & Miller, 2022, p. 195).

### Installation Work

After the first year of my doctoral training, I presented my yearlong altered book project along with my cohort's gallery exhibit. I chose to display my work as an installation (Andrus, 2022) in the university's art gallery. To my delight, I found a one-person bench on campus that was made in the same way and with the same wood materials as the two-seaters and longer benches I had previously photographed. Using it as the basis for my installation piece, I gathered branches and other items from nature and pulled those into the gallery space to create an overall environment. The altered book rested on one of the bench arms as an invitation to gallery visitors to sit, rest, and connect through a common humanity.

### Summary

This chapter reviewed the ethical underpinnings regarding self-disclosure of therapist grief and the potential harm it invites to the therapeutic relationship. Self-care, as a countermeasure, was re-examined as an important part of an ethical practice. Creativity was suggested to be part of human hardwiring and a way to offer practical approaches to restore a sense of self, find meaning, and re-imagine the relationship with the deceased. Lastly, readers were invited to consider the visual arts as a possible creative process that could assist in self-care when dealing with any level of bereavement.

Engaging in creative avenues for self-care may not only increase wellness but may also help expand personal meaning and offer transformative experiences. Through my own example, it was suggested that the use of photography, altered book making, and installation art could be helpful creative explorations of grief symptoms for others. Critical to an ethical therapeutic practice is the ability of the human service professional to examine the self, with the assumption that there is no shortage of techniques to do so. Understanding how grief is experienced and how it might interfere with effective treatment not only is healthy for therapeutic interactions but can also increase the ability to have positive interactions with those outside of clinical practice. My hope is that this text inspires students, new professionals, and established human service practitioners to find their own creative element. It is my belief that engagement with the visual arts or other creative action may provide the grieving therapist with constructive ways to process emotions linked to bereavement, in turn, leading to improved competence in the therapeutic care of others.

### Questions for Reflection

1  What creative activities have been successful in promoting your own self-care? Are there any new ones you would like to try?
2  Are you able to identify any creative materials that are readily available to you in your home, work, or school environment?

3 Create a list of professional values you will not compromise in your work with clients. Then create another one identifying the values you will not compromise in your personal relationships. Where do the lists overlap, and where are they different?
4 What do you believe about your personal strengths, and how might you reflect them in a creative way? (i.e., could you create a collage using magazine images, create an abstract drawing or painting to represent your strengths in color and shape, or maybe take a walk in nature to collect photographs or items to create a small installation in your home or office?)
5 How might you work with your inner critic in a more creative way? Is there also a "compassionate observer" (Neff, n.d.) who needs to have a voice?

## References

Anaxagorou, V. (2023). Building resilience: The (new?) politics of grief and mourning at the time of the pandemic in contemporary art practices. *The International Journal of Social, Political and Community Agendas in the Arts, 18*(1), 39–61. https://doi.org/10.18848/2326-9960/CGP/v18i01/39-61

Andrus, M. (2022). Private to public: Exhibition in art therapy. In C. Brown, & H. Omand (Eds.), *Contemporary practice in studio art therapy* (pp. 194–203). Routledge. https://doi.org/10.4324/9781003095606

Archambault, M. J. (2021). *Continuing bonds through art making: A heuristic exploration of the loss of an attachment figure* [Graduate Projects (Non-thesis)] (Unpublished). Concordia University Montreal. https://spectrum.library.concordia.ca/id/eprint/988747/

Arnold, R. (2019). Navigating loss through creativity: Influences of bereavement on creativity and professional practice in art therapy. *Art Therapy: Journal of the American Art Therapy Association, 37*(1), 1–10. https://doi.org/10.1080/07421656.2019.1657718

Arnold, R. (2023). Grieving artists: Influences of loss and bereavement on visual art making. *The Arts in Psychotherapy, 82*, 1–11. 102001. https://doi.org/10.1016/j.aip.2023.102001

Baier, A. L., Kline, A. C., & Feeny, N. C. (2020). Therapeutic alliance as a mediator of change: A systematic review and evaluation of research. *Clinical Psychology Review, 82*, 101921. https://doi.org/10.1016/j.cpr.2020.101921

Baker, L. (2023, March 16). *Art & symbol as catalysts for personal growth*. Medium. https://bakerlance.medium.com/art-symbol-as-catalysts-for-personal-growth-7315d3a0370c

Bamonti, P. M., Keelan, C. M., Larson, N., Mentrikoski, J. M., Randall, C. L., Sly, S. K., Travers, R. M., & McNeil, D. W. (2014). Promoting ethical behavior by cultivating a culture of self-care during graduate training: A call to action. *Training and Education in Professional Psychology, 8*(4), 253–260. https://doi.org/10.1037/tep0000056

Barnett, J. E., Baker, E. K., Elman, N. S., & Schoener, G. R. (2007). In pursuit of wellness: The self-care imperative. *Professional Psychology: Research and Practice, 38*(6), 603–612. https://psycnet.apa.org/doi/10.1037/0735-7028.38.6.603

Beaumont, S. L., (2013). Art therapy for complicated grief: A focus on meaning-making approaches. *Canadian Art Therapy Association Journal, 26*(2), 1–7. https://psycnet.apa.org/doi/10.1080/08322473.2013.11415582

Bonanno, G. A., Boerner, K., & Wortman, C. B. (2008). Trajectories of grieving. In M. S. Stroebe, R. O. Hansson, H. Schut, & W. Stroebe (Eds.), *Handbook of bereavement research and practice: Advances in theory and intervention* [electronic resource] (pp. 287–307). American Psychological Association. https://doi.org/10.1037/14498-014

Bressi, S. K., & Vaden, E. R. (2017). Reconsidering self care. *Clinical Social Work Journal, 45*(1), 33–38. https://doi.org/10.1007/s10615-016-0575-4

Broadbent, J. R. (2013). 'The bereaved therapist speaks'. An interpretative phenomenological analysis of humanistic therapists' experiences of a significant personal bereavement and its impact upon their therapeutic practice: An exploratory study. *Counselling and Psychotherapy Research, 13*(4), 263–271. https://doi.org/10.1080/14733145.2013.768285

Castle, J., & Phillips, W. (2003). Grief rituals: Aspects that facilitate adjustment to bereavement. *Journal of Loss and Trauma, 8*, 41–71. https://doi.org/10.1080/15325020305876

Coaston, S. C. (2017). Self-care through self-compassion: A balm for burnout. *The Professional Counselor, 7*(3), 285–297. https://doi.org/10.15241/scc.7.3.285

Coenen, C. (2018). *Shattered by grief: Picking up the pieces to become whole again*. Jessica Kingsley.

Corriero, A., Giglio, M., Soloperto, R., Varrassi, G., & Puntillo, F. (2024). Harnessing the healing power of creativity: Exploring the role of art in healthcare through art, dance, and music therapy. *Advancements in Health Research, 1*(1), 42–46. https://doi.org/10.4081/ahr.2024.17

Davis, C. G. (2008). Redefining goals and redefining self: A closer look at posttraumatic growth following loss. In M. S. Stroebe, R. O. Hansson, H. Schut, & W. Stroebe (Eds.), *Handbook of bereavement research and practice: Advances in theory and intervention* (pp. 309–325). American Psychological Association. https://dx.doi.org/10.1037/14498-015

Davis, S. (2021). Perezhivanie, art, and creative traversal: A method of marking and moving through COVID and grief. *Qualitative Inquiry, 27*(7), 767–770. https://doi.org/10.1177/1077800420960158

Detrick, S. M. (2021). *Self-care ethics knowledge and self-care practices: Clinical and counseling psychology doctoral students in early and late phases of training* (Doctoral dissertation). Retrieved from ProQuest Dissertations & Theses. (Order No. 28720973, Fielding Graduate University).

Drescher, K. D. (2013). Grief, loss, and war. In B. A. Moore, & J. E. Barnett (Eds.), *Military psychologists' desk reference* (pp. 251–255). Oxford University Press.

Felberbaum, S. (2010). Memory, mourning and meaning in a psychotherapist's life. *Clinical Social Work Journal, 38*, 269–274.

Fish, B. (2012). Response art: The art of the art therapist. *Art Therapy: Journal of the American Art Therapy Association, 29*(3), 138–143.

Forgeard, M. (2019). Creativity and healing. In J. C. Kaufman, & R. J. Sternberg (Eds.), *The Cambridge handbook of creativity* (2nd ed., pp. 319–332). Cambridge University Press. https://doi.org/10.1017/9781316979839

Fortino, N., Dommert, P., Santiago, N., & Smith, J. (2021). Positive psychological transformation: A mixed methods investigation Into catalysts and processes of meaningful change. *International Journal of Transpersonal Studies, 40*(1), 96–122. https://doi.org/10.24972/ijts.2021.40.1.96

Frantz, G. (2016). Creativity and healing. *Psychological Perspectives, 59*(2), 242–251. https://dx.doi.org/10.1080/00332925.2016.1170567

Gabora, L., & Kaufman, S. B. (2010). Evolutionary approaches to creativity. In J. C. Kaufman, & R. J. Sternberg (Eds.), *The Cambridge handbook of creativity* (pp. 279–300). Cambridge University Press.

Gillies, V., Harden, A., Johnson, K., Reavey, P., Strange, V., & Willig, C. (2005). Painting pictures of embodied experience: The use of nonverbal data production for the study of embodiment. *Qualitative research in psychology, 2*(3), 199–212. https://doi.org/10.1191/1478088705qp038oa

Gudmundsdottir, M. (2009). Embodied grief: Bereaved parents' narratives of their suffering body. *Omega—Journal of Death and Dying, 59*(3), 253–269. https://doi.org/10.2190/OM.59.3.e

Halprin, A. (1997). The process is the purpose. In F. Barron, A. Montuori, & A. Barron (Eds.), *Creators on creating: Awakening and cultivating the imaginative mind* (pp. 44–49). Penguin.

Hayes, J. A., Yeh, Y. J., & Eisenberg, A. (2007). Good grief and not-so-good grief: Countertransference in bereavement therapy. *Journal of Clinical Psychology, 63*(4), 345–355. https://doi.org/10.1002/jclp.20353

Iliya, Y. A., & Harris, B. T. (2016). Singing an imaginal dialogue: A qualitative examination of a Bereavement intervention with creative arts therapists. *Nordic Journal of Music Therapy, 25*(3), 248–272. https://doi.org/10.1080/08098131.2015.1044259

Iype, N. (2010). The experience of grief: An art therapist's exploration. *Canadian Art Therapy Association Journal, 23*(2), 18–35. https://doi.org/10.1080/08322473.2010.11432335

Jacobson-Levy, M., & Miller, G. M. (2022). Creative destruction and transformation in art and therapy: Reframing, reforming, reclaiming. *Art Therapy: Journal of the American Art Therapy Association, 39*(4), 194–202. https://doi.org/10.1080/07421656.2022.2090306

Jiménez-Alonso, B., & De Luna, I. B. (2021). Narratives of loss: Exploring grief through photography. *Qualitative Studies, 6*(1), 91–115. https://doi.org/10.7146/qs.v6i1.124433

Johnsen, C., & Ding, H. T. (2021). Therapist self-disclosure: Let's tackle the elephant in the room. *Clinical Child Psychology and Psychiatry, 26*(2), 443–450. https://doi.org/10.1177/135910452 1994178

Jonsson, A., & Walter, T. (2017). Continuing bonds and place. *Death Studies, 41*(7), 406–415. https://doi.org/10.1080/07481187.2017.1286412

Kessler, D. (2019). *Finding meaning: The sixth stage of grief*. Scribner.

Kirkpatrick, D. (2017). *Grief and loss; living with the presence of absence. A practice based study of personal grief narratives and participatory projects* (Doctoral dissertation). Retrieved from University of the West of England. https://eprints.uwe.ac.uk/29973

Klorer, P. G. (2014). My story, your story, our stories: A community art-based research project. *Art Therapy: Journal of the American Art Therapy Association, 31*(4), 146–154. https://doi.org/10.1080/07421656.2015.963486

Kosminsky, P. S., & Jordan, J. R. (2016). *Attachment-informed grief therapy: The clinician's guide to foundations and applications*. Routledge. https://doi.org/10.4324/9780203798393

Kossak, M. (2015). *Attunement in expressive arts therapy: Toward an understanding of embodied empathy*. Charles C. Thomas Publishing Ltd.

Kouriatis, K., & Brown, D. (2013–2014). Therapists' experience of loss: An interpretative phenomenological analysis. *Omega, 68*(2), 89–109. https://dx.doi.org/10.2190/OM.68.2.a

Legari, S. (2022). Without words: The art and therapy of grief and loss in pandemic times. In M. G. Marini, & J. McFarland (Eds.), *Health humanities for quality of care in times of COVID -19: New paradigms in healthcare* (pp. 47–60). Springer. https://doi.org/10.1007/978-3-030-93359-3_5

Lev, M. (2022). Artmaking resilience: Reflections on art-based research of bereavement and grief. *Creative Arts in Education and Therapy, 8*(1), pp. 126–138. https://caet.inspirees.com/caetojsjournals/index.php/caet/article/view/379

Levine, E. (2004). The practice of expressive arts therapy: Training, therapy and supervision. In S. K. Levine, P. Knill, & E. Levine (Eds.), *Principles and practice of expressive arts therapy: Toward a therapeutic aesthetics* (pp. 171–255), Jessica Kingsley publishers.

Linton, M., & Koonmen, J. (2020). Self-care as an ethical obligation for nurses. *Nursing Ethics, 27*(8), 1694–1702. https://doi.org/10.1177/0969733020940371

Margry, P. J., & Sánchez-Carretero, C. (Eds.). (2011). *Grassroots memorials: The politics of memorializing traumatic death*. Berghahn Books, Inc.

Mathijssen, B. (2017). Transforming bonds: Ritualising post-mortem relationships in the Netherlands. *Mortality, 23*(3), 215–230. https://doi.org/10.1080/13576275.2017.1364228

Metzl, E., & Shamai, M. G. (2021). I carry your heart: A dialogue about coping, art, and therapy after a profound loss. *The Arts in Psychotherapy, 74*, 1–8. https://doi.org/10.1016/j.aip.2021.101801

Mirick, R. G. (2022). Teaching note—Self-care in social work education: An experiential learning exercise. *Journal of Social Work Education, 59*(4), 1281–1286. https://doi.org/10.1080/10437797.2022.2119051

Moon, B. L. (2016). *Art-based group therapy: Theory and practice* (2nd ed.). Charles C Thomas.

Neff, K. (n.d.). *The criticizer, the criticized, and the compassionate observer* [Pamphlet]. Side-by-Side Nutrition. https://tinyurl.com/8vvt2pj2

Newell, J. M., & Nelson-Gardell, D. (2014). A competency-based approach to teaching professional self-care: An ethical consideration for social work educators. *Journal of Social Work Education, 50*(3), 427–439. https://doi.org/10.1080/10437797.2014.917928

O'Connor, M. (2022). *The grieving brain: The surprising science of how we learn from love and loss*. Harper One.

Padilla, J. A. (2024). *Mindfulness and self-compassion: Attuning skills in self-awareness to promote self-care for art therapy practitioners a mixed-methods study using a mandala art directive and acceptance commitment therapy (ACT)* (Master's thesis #18). Dominican University of California. https://scholar.dominican.edu/art-therapy-masters-theses/18/

Pearce, C., Honey, J. R., Lovick, R., Creamer, N. Z., Henry, C., Langford, A., Stobert, M., & Barclay, S. (2021). 'A silent epidemic of grief': A survey of bereavement care provision in the UK and Ireland during the COVID-19 pandemic. *BMJ Open, 11*, 1–10. https://dx.doi.org/10.1136/bmjopen-2020-046872

Percy, P. E. (2014). *Mourning and transformation: A phenomenological study of living through the journey of grief* (Doctoral dissertation). Retrieved from ProQuest Dissertations and Theses. (Order No. 10014516, Pacifica Graduate Institute).

Ramser, E. (2020). *This ocean of texts: The history of blackout poetry* (Doctoral dissertation). https://hdl.handle.net/11274/12438

Rando, T. A. (1995). Grief and mourning: Accommodating to loss. In H. Wass, & R. Neimeyer (Eds.), *Dying: Facing the facts* (pp. 211–241). Taylor & Francis.

Sanstrom, B. (2012). A visual dialogue: What are the inter relational dynamics of grief? *The International Journal of the Humanities, 9*(4), 287–298. https://doi.org/10.18848/1447-9508/cgp/v09i04/43157

Sas, C., & Coman, A. (2016). Designing personal grief rituals: An analysis of symbolic objects and actions. *Death Studies, 40*(9), 558–569. https://doi.org/10.1080/07481187.2016.1188868

Scholtes, D., & Browne, M. (2014). Internalized and externalized continuing bonds in bereaved parents: Their relationship with grief intensity and personal growth. *Death Studies, 39*(2), 75–83. https://doi.org/10.1080/07481187.2014.890680

Self, M. M., Wise, E. H., Beauvais, J., & Molinari, V. (2018). Ethics in training and training in ethics: Special considerations for postdoctoral fellowships in health service psychology. *Training and Education in Professional Psychology, 12*(2), 105–112. https://doi.org/10.1037/tep0000178

Swinden, C. (2023). Working after loss: How bereavement counsellors experience returning to therapeutic work after the death of their parent. *Illness, Crisis & Loss, 31*(2), 364–384. https://doi.org/10.1177/10541373211067670

Tsai, M., Plummer, M. D., Kanter, J. W., Newring, R. W., & Kohlenberg, R. J. (2010). Therapist grief and Functional Analytic Psychotherapy: Strategic self-disclosure of personal loss. *Journal of Contemporary Psychotherapy, 40*, 1–10. https://psycnet.apa.org/doi/10.1007/s10879-009-9116-6

van Lil, K. (2012). Creative qualities of mourning: Artists responding to loss today. *The International Journal of the Arts in Society, 6*(6), 141–155. https://doi.org/10.18848/1833-1866/CGP/v06i06/36112

Wagoner, B., & Brescó de Luna, I. B. D. (2022). Collective grief: Mourning rituals, politics and memorial sites. In A. Køster, & E. Holte Kofod (Eds.), *Cultural, existential, and phenomenological dimensions of bereavement* (pp. 197–213). Routledge. https://doi.org/10.4324/9781003099420-17

Wise, E. H., Hersh, M. A., & Gibson, C. M. (2012). Ethics, self-care and well-being for psychologists: Reenvisioning the stress-distress continuum. *Professional Psychology: Research and Practice, 43*(5), 487–494. https://doi.org/10.1037/a0029446

Wojtkowiak, J., Lind, J., & Smid, G. E. (2021). Ritual in therapy for prolonged grief: A Scoping review of ritual elements in evidence-informed grief interventions. *Frontiers in Psychiatry, 11*, 1–13. https://doi.org/10.3389/fpsyt.2020.623835

# 2 Trauma-Informed Human Service Practices

*Deirdre O'Sullivan, Jennifer L. Hanna,*
*and Shyrun Karandikar*

## A Trauma-Informed Approach

A trauma-informed human service provider is one who delivers services from a trauma-informed perspective, which means they are aware and understand the impacts of contextual features, ecological perspectives, and types of traumas on individuals and work to avoid re-traumatizing them during their work together.

Although trauma-informed providers may know about the many negative ways that trauma impacts people, they also maintain a strength-based approach and know that people can and do recover from trauma with the appropriate support and services. Trauma-informed providers do not necessarily treat the trauma or provide clinical interventions. Training (and possibly certification) is needed for providers to enhance their knowledge and skillset for addressing sensitive issues reported by clients. This chapter focuses on trauma-informed practices that entry-level helping professionals are qualified to provide by building on their existing skills and education. Trauma-informed providers do not have to be trauma survivors themselves to be effective, just as mental health providers and cancer providers can be effective clinicians even if they do not have direct experience with these illnesses.

Rather than asking "What is wrong with you?" as a way of understanding how trauma is impacting a person, a trauma-informed provider asks, "What happened to you?" or "What have you lived through?" to explain the struggles and choices in a person's life. In addition to having this perspective, providers must also be sensitive to the cultural, historical, and personal factors that are relevant for those they serve as well as for themselves. A culturally sensitive, historically knowledgeable, and self-aware trauma-informed provider (1) realizes the widespread impact of trauma and the many sources of trauma; (2) understands the signs and symptoms of trauma in individuals, families, and communities and the potential for systems serving people as sources of trauma; (3) understands the multiple paths toward recovery; (4) responds by integrating knowledge about trauma into the policies, procedures, and practices and actively avoids re-traumatizing; and (5) seeks out self-awareness of their lived trauma and works to heal from these traumatic experiences so they can be an effective service provider.

## Overview of Trauma and Adversity

Traumatic or adverse events can take many forms, can be acute or chronic, and can occur across the lifespan. Trauma is generally thought of as a response to an event or series of events that was perceived to be harmful or life-threatening. While exposure to an event is inherent in trauma, the experience of potentially traumatic events depends on many

DOI: 10.4324/9781003531258-4

individual factors, such as the person's perception of the event, ability to cope, available support, and sensitivity to stress (Shonkoff & Garner, 2012; Shonkoff et al., 2021). Oftentimes, a traumatic experience leaves a lasting impact, affecting functioning across domains, and influences the person's worldview (Harris & Fallot, 2001).

Trauma can occur at any time across the lifespan, and it may result from a one-time event or repeated exposure. A one-time event—such as an auto accident, rape or assault, or natural disaster—may be referred to as acute trauma. Trauma that occurs through repeated exposure—such as living in an abusive family, a combat zone, or a racist society—is called chronic trauma. Complex trauma is prolonged exposure to maltreatment or multiple types of maltreatment or adversity.

Chronic or complex trauma, particularly during sensitive developmental periods, disrupts the body's stress response. Our nervous system is activated in times of high stress to keep us safe, sometimes referred to as the fight-or-flight response. When a child experiences trauma or adversity that results in repeated or prolonged activation of the nervous system, particularly without the presence of a protective adult, they experience toxic stress. The stress response system gets stuck in the "on" position, causing changes to the brain and body in ways that have long-term negative impacts on health (Shonkoff & Garner, 2012).

### Child Maltreatment

Child maltreatment encompasses abuse—broadly, an act of harm targeting a child and committed by a caretaker—and neglect, which is omission of adequate and appropriate care for a child. The Child Abuse Prevention and Treatment Act (PL 93-247), a federal law that provides funding and requires states to maintain systems to protect children from maltreatment, offers the following broad definition of child abuse and neglect, which acts as the basis for each state to independently define maltreatment:

> The term "child abuse and neglect" means, at a minimum, any recent act or failure to act on the part of a parent or caretaker, which results in death, serious physical or emotional harm, sexual abuse or exploitation (including sexual abuse as determined under section 111), or an act or failure to act which presents an imminent risk of serious harm.
>
> (Section 3.2)

Most states define physical abuse, sexual abuse, emotional abuse, and neglect as reportable maltreatment. Maltreatment may occur through commission, an act of doing something, or through omission, neglecting or not doing something to protect or meet a child's needs. In general, states' definitions capture the following (CWIG, 2022):

- Physical abuse includes intentional or unintentional physical injury or harm to the child, including harsh discipline and other physical acts that harm the body.
- Sexual abuse includes sexual acts and touching as well as exploitation of the child.
- Emotional abuse, sometimes referred to as psychological abuse, includes acts that endanger the child's emotional or mental stability, such as humiliation, harsh criticism, and manipulation. Withholding of care, love, and affection constitutes emotional neglect.
- Neglect is failure to provide for the child's needs to the degree that health, well-being, or safety is impaired.

While these definitions provide a useful frame for thinking about events that may be traumatic, events or circumstances that may not meet the legal definition of maltreatment also have the potential to be traumatic. See Figure 2.1 for maltreatment and adversity categories.

## Populations Most at Risk for Trauma Exposure

Some people are more likely to experience traumatic events due to their personal and environmental risk factors. Trauma-informed providers know who experiences higher risk for trauma exposure so that further trauma can be prevented, and so they can connect the individual to services and supports to begin the healing process. The following is an inexhaustive list of populations at higher risk for a range of different traumas:

- Children and adults with disabilities
- Girls and women
- LGBTQ+ and gender non-conforming children and adults
- Minority race children and adults
- People struggling with substance use disorder
- People formerly incarcerated
- People living at or below the poverty level
- Refugees

## Stress Response

When a person is exposed to a stressor, their stress response system is activated. This unconscious physiological process serves a protective function, priming the brain and body to respond to the threat. The stress response activates hormones and various body processes that enable adaptive reactions, such as fight-flight-freeze-fawn (see Figure 2.2). Under normal circumstances, the processes and hormones that make up this response return to normal when they are no longer needed, that is, when stressors are resolved or are within a manageable range.

The pattern of response in children has implications for development and is conceptualized in three categories: positive, tolerable, and toxic (Shonkoff et al., 2012). In a positive stress response, the child's stress process is activated briefly and to a moderate degree before returning to baseline. The support of a caring adult through a stressful event is protective,

**CHILDHOOD MALTREATMENT SUBTYPES:**

PHYSICAL ABUSE, PHYSICAL NEGLECT, PSYCHOLOGICAL ABUSE, PSYCHOLOGICAL NEGLECT, SEXUAL ABUSE

**CHILDHOOD ADVERSITY SUBTYPES:**

DIVORCED/SEPARATED PARENTS, PARENT WITH MENTAL ILLNESS, PARENT WITH SUBSTANCE USE DISORDER, PARENT INCARCERATED, WITNESSING DOMESTIC VIOLENCE

*Figure 2.1* Maltreatment and adversity subtypes.

# TRAUMA RESPONSES

## FIGHT
Sympathetic Nervous System

- Irritability
- Anger
- Aggression
- Moving toward

## FLIGHT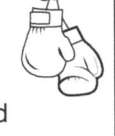
Sympathetic Nervous System

- Anxiety and Fear
- Panic
- Avoiding
- Chronic worry
- Perfectionism

## FREEZE
Dorsal Vagal

- Immobilization or Feeling Stuck
- Collapse
- Spacing out or Dissociation
- Depression
- Shame

## FAWN*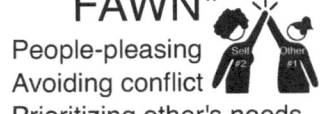

- People-pleasing
- Avoiding conflict
- Prioritizing other's needs over personal needs
- Difficulty setting boundaries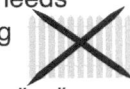
- Difficulty saying "no"

*Figure 2.2* Description of four types of trauma responses.

and children can make sense of and learn from these types of experiences, growing in their abilities to navigate stress. These responses are often elicited by common stressors, like taking a test or facing frustration. Events that are less common and more stressful or threatening, for example, a car accident or the death of a parent, stimulate a bigger stress response (see Figure 2.3). Through relationships with caring adults who support the child to cope and regain a sense of control, the physiological stress response can often be tempered, conceptualized as a tolerable stress response. When a child faces a major stressor or series of stressors without at least one supportive relationship, strong and/or prolonged activation of the stress response results in toxic stress (Shonkoff and Garner, 2012; Shonkoff et al., 2021). The stress response system does not regulate as expected, remaining activated over time and resulting in ongoing exposure to stress hormones, changes in the nervous system, and an immune response. These processes impact brain development during sensitive periods and cause "wear and tear" on the body. Brain chemistry and structure, as well as immune, metabolic, and cardiac functioning, are impaired because of toxic stress (Shonkoff & Garner, 2012).

The impacts of toxic stress work directly and indirectly in the brain and body. For example, exposure to high amounts of stress hormones in utero or in early childhood has a direct impact on the formation of the amygdala, hippocampus, and prefrontal cortex, altering aspects such as size and activity level (Shonkoff & Garner, 2012; Shonkoff et al., 2021). These structural impacts then translate to functional impacts in that these areas of the brain

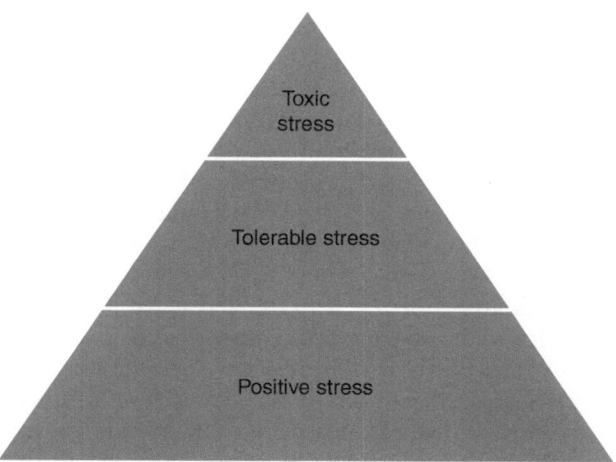

*Figure 2.3* Pyramid of stress ranging from positive to toxic.

are associated with mood, control and regulation, and memory. Indirect impacts of toxic stress work through changing the processes within the brain. For example, an amygdala that has been flooded with stress hormones during development is primed for stress, anxiety, and fear and will initiate or sustain the stress response even when danger is not immediately present.

### Lasting Impacts of Trauma

The relationship between maltreatment or adversity and health outcomes was explored through the landmark Adverse Childhood Experiences (ACES) study (Felitti et al., 1998). The people in this study—over 9,500 respondents who had private health insurance coverage through Kaiser Permanente and had a recent routine care visit—reported through a mailed survey about experiences of maltreatment (physical, sexual, and psychological abuse) and household dysfunction (witnessed violence against their mother/stepmother and/or living with someone who had been incarcerated, had a mental health condition or attempted suicide, or abused substances) that occurred before age 18. Their reports were then examined in the context of their health history. The study found that the more adverse exposures someone had, particularly if they reported four or more exposures, the more likely they were to exhibit health risk factors (e.g., smoking, suicide attempts, substance use, or obesity) and to report certain health conditions (e.g., heart disease and cancer). This is called a dose-response relationship; in this case, dose refers to the number of adverse experiences reported, and response refers to negative health indicators. Subsequent research has supported the seminal findings from this study (Dye, 2018; Noteboom et al., 2021).

Research links adverse and traumatic experiences to mental health outcomes across the lifespan, too (Copeland et al., 2018; Gilbert et al., 2009). Adversity and maltreatment have been shown to correlate with increased mental health symptoms in children (Cross et al., 2017; Kim & Cicchetti, 2010; Turner et al., 2006), adolescents (Lansford et al., 2002; Pierce et al., 2023; Turner et al., 2006), and adults (Banyard et al., 2001; Dye, 2018). Evidence suggests that behavior problems in children and adolescents may be strongly linked to the timing of maltreatment and have a cumulative impact (Dye, 2018; Gilbert et al., 2009). Kids who have experienced maltreatment and exhibit lower levels of emotion regulation also experience more peer rejection (Copeland et al., 2018; Kim & Cicchetti, 2010).

Evidence also points to academic and cognitive impacts following experiences of maltreatment and adversity. An international meta-analysis found relationships between maltreatment and several academic outcomes, including lower grades and graduation rates, more special education involvement, and poorer attendance (Dye, 2018; Gilbert et al., 2009). School-aged children who were involved with the child protection system based on suspected maltreatment were about two times as likely to score lower than the national average on standardized measures of IQ, reading, and math (Crozier & Barth, 2005). In addition to the potential for reduced educational performance and attainment, exposure to adverse and traumatic experiences may hold broader socioeconomic status (SES) implications (Dye, 2018). SES-related factors such as type of occupation, persistence in working (Gilbert et al., 2009), employment status, income, and healthcare coverage have been found to be related to maltreatment and adverse experiences (Zielinski, 2009). People who have experienced maltreatment are more likely to be unemployed, to live in poverty, and to access healthcare through government supports, such as Medicaid (Zielinski, 2009).

## Resilience and Recovery

Resilience refers to the skill of responding to stressful, adverse, or traumatic events. Resiliency includes intrinsic predispositions such as the interplay among genetics, developing brain circuitry, psychological status, and immune responsiveness and external factors in the person's home, school or work, and community (National Scientific Council on the Developing Child NSCDC, 2015; Pierce et al., 2023).

## Strategies to Enhance Resiliency

Resiliency is dynamic and can be developed and enhanced at any age. Research in behavioral and social science suggests that resiliency can be built by facilitating supportive adult-child relationships, providing the opportunity to increase self-efficacy and perceived control, strengthening adaptive skills and self-regulatory capacities, and mobilizing sources of faith, hope, and cultural traditions (NSCDC, 2015).

Children are more likely to develop resiliency when facing significant adversity and/or disadvantages with the support of a trusted, significant adult. The interaction of supportive relationships can provide them with crucial emotional and psychological resources necessary to navigate challenges. The perception of self-efficacy empowers individuals to be self-assured in their perspectives and capacity to manage stressors, navigate complexities, and foster perseverance. Strengthening adaptive skills increases problem-solving and flexibility to adapt personal strategies and responses to changing circumstances and recognize their need for assistance. Self-regulation is the capacity to manage thoughts and emotions and promote self-awareness, well-being, and goal attainment behaviors.

The positive mobilization and integration of sources of faith, hope, and cultural traditions provide individuals with a sense of meaning, purpose, and belonging, which can significantly bolster their ability to navigate adversity. Faith offers a framework for understanding challenges within a broader spiritual context, promoting a sense of trust and reliance on higher powers or guiding principles. Hope instills optimism and perseverance, encouraging individuals to envision better outcomes and persist despite setbacks. Cultural traditions offer a sense of identity and continuity, providing rituals, values, and community support that reinforce resilience through shared beliefs and practices. Integration of each of these strategies should be adapted for the individual to account for their cultural identity, values, beliefs, self-concept, and personal ecological context.

## Reporting Considerations

Ethical guidelines and trauma-informed principles should be considered in conjunction with laws regarding reporting suspected child maltreatment. Professionals who have frequent contact with children are often designated as mandated reporters, meaning that they are legally required to report suspected child maltreatment under penalty of law. In many states, school and childcare personnel, medical professionals, mental health and social service professionals, and law enforcement professionals are groups commonly designated as mandated reporters (CWIG, 2023). Mandated reporters must be familiar with the standard for reporting in their state. Suspicion or reasonable cause to suspect that maltreatment has occurred is the standard for reporting in some states, whereas others require mandated reporters to report when they know of or observe a situation that is likely to lead to endangerment or harm of a child (CWIG, 2023). It is the human service provider's responsibility to know their status as a mandated reporter and to know the procedures for making a report.

Mandated reporters report relevant information when maltreatment is suspected, but they are not responsible for confirming or proving maltreatment. Trained child protection services (CPS) workers evaluate reports and make determinations to screen in (i.e., open a case) when the information meets criteria or to screen out when it does not. Differentiated reporting procedures are recommended in most states so that families that demonstrate less severe forms of neglect or abuse are directed to supportive services so that the needs of the family are met. Examples might include harsh but not abusive parenting; neglect due to poverty; insensitive or impaired parenting due to drug or alcohol use; or domestic violence in the home. The goal in these cases is to provide appropriate support to the families with the intention of keeping these families engaged in services designed to enhance family interactions. Parents or caregivers who demonstrate severe forms of abuse, including physically aggressive forms of punishment, sexual abuse, and severe neglect, are investigated forensically to determine if maltreatment is substantiated and if a crime has been committed. If maltreatment is found to be present, a range of actions may occur, including the removal of the child(ren) from the home to ensure their safety.

Mandated reporting decisions can be complex for many reasons. As noted above, the standard for reporting is not universal, and, further, definitions of maltreatment can be somewhat ambiguous. While some parenting behaviors are almost universally viewed as unacceptable, there are many situations that are less clear in the context of the standard for reporting, given that professionals often have a limited picture. Cases where suspected maltreatment is less overt (e.g., emotional abuse) pose more difficulty for mandated reporters (McTavish et al., 2017).

Mandated reporters are worried about the impact of a report and the potential for negative outcomes related to CPS involvement (McTavish et al., 2017). Children of color, particularly Black and American Indian/Alaska Native children, may be more likely to experience these negative impacts as they are referred at rates disproportionate to their representation in the general population and are also disproportionately represented at later points in the CPS continuum of care (USDHHS, 2020). Culturally sensitive, self-aware, trauma-informed human service providers can balance personal factors, cultural factors, and legal factors in making appropriate reporting decisions and in their work within the system(s) that could be contributing to trauma for some people (e.g., correctional facilities, healthcare facilities, substance use treatment centers).

### Communication Strategies

As for the basic principles of trauma-informed human service care, actively avoiding re-traumatization is essential. To do this, providers must be aware of their language and how language impacts trauma survivors. Based on dialectical behavioral theory (DBT, Linnemann et al., 2022), validating a person's experiences and their reactions to a stimulus is an important form of communication in all work with trauma survivors. Validations are simple but potent and likely skills that many human service providers already know how to do.

There are six levels of validation. *Level 1* is simply active listening and expressing interest and investment by using eye contact, leaning in, nodding, and other uses of body language to express interest in what they are telling you. *Level 2* includes restating what someone has shared, for instance, "I want to make sure I understand ... are you saying you felt ..." *Level 3* validations include articulation of the person's non-verbal body language. For instance, "From your expression and your posture, I can tell you feel defeated" or "scared," "surprised," or whatever emotion you sense they are experiencing but not verbalizing. *Level 4* validations require knowing the person and having some rapport with them as you layer in historical information to help contextualize what they are sharing. For instance, "Based on your past, I can understand why you reacted that way." *Level 5* validations normalize the reaction. For example, "Anyone who experienced what you just shared with me would have done the same thing." And, finally, a *Level 6* validation is sometimes referred to as "radical genuineness" since it can be conveyed only if the human service provider has the same lived experience. For instance, "I understand completely—I've done that same thing myself." This is often effective when service providers in the addiction treatment realm are in recovery themselves from addiction and work as service providers. This level of validation may not be possible, but level 5 validations are just as potent. When a provider listens, believes, and normalizes events that people hold as shameful, they validate their clients' feelings and communicate to them that their response makes sense in the context of their trauma and lives.

It is also important to avoid using invalidating statements that are often well-intentioned but can be re-traumatizing. Invalidating statements include saying things such as "try not to think about it," "don't over-react," "that happened to me too and I'm fine, so you'll be fine too," and "I can't help you if you continue to avoid talking about the hard stuff." There are many ways our words can invalidate another's experience. When in doubt, ask the person if your words hurt or landed wrong. This question communicates your investment in the relationship and your willingness to work to repair it. Repairing a relationship and admitting that you used your words recklessly can be a form of validation in its own way if done with sincerity and humility.

### Conclusion

This chapter summarized the role of a trauma-informed human service provider. Types of traumas and adversities and their impact on the body and brain were explained. The stress response system and how to reduce stress were discussed. Populations at highest risk for trauma exposure were outlined. Strategies for strengthening resiliency were included, as were specific communication strategies.

## Reflective Questions for Consideration

1  Explain how childhood trauma and adversity impact the developing body and mind.
2  What does it mean to be "trauma-informed"? How might your own agency/institution benefit from trauma-informed training?
3  Outline some strategies to enhance resiliency.
4  Describe some communication strategies to implement with trauma survivors. Consider those who have been abused, abandoned, or neglected. How might communication strategies directed toward adolescents be different/similar for adults? Finally, explain the role that identity (e.g., gender, race, sexual orientation, and ability) might play in communication strategies.
5  Explain the ethical responsibilities for mandated reporters. What might be some potential blindspots for reporters?

## References

Banyard, V. L., Williams, L. M., & Siegel, J. A. (2001). The long-term mental health consequences of child sexual abuse: An exploratory study of the impact of multiple traumas in a sample of women. *Journal of Traumatic Stress, 14*(4), 697–715. https://doi.org/10.1023/A:1013085904337

Child Welfare Information Gateway, U.S. Department of Health and Human Services, Children's Bureau (2022). *Definitions of child abuse and neglect.* https://www.childwelfare.gov/topics/systemwide/laws-policies/statutes/define/

Child Welfare Information Gateway, U.S. Department of Health and Human Services, Children's Bureau. (2023). *Mandatory reporters of child abuse and neglect.* https://www.childwelfare.gov/topics/systemwide/laws-policies/statutes/manda/

Copeland, W. E., Shanahan, L., Hinesley, J., Chan, R. F., Aberg, K. A., Fairbank, J. A., ... & Costello, E. J. (2018). Association of childhood trauma exposure with adult psychiatric disorders and functional outcomes. *JAMA Network Open, 1*(7), e184493–e184493.

Cross, D., Fani, N., Powers, A., & Bradley, B. (2017). Neurobiological development in the context of childhood trauma. *Clinical Psychology: Science and Practice, 24*(2), 111.

Crozier, J. C., & Barth, R. P. (2005). Cognitive and academic functioning in maltreated children. *Children & Schools, 27*(4), 197–206. https://doi.org/10.1093/cs/27.4.197

Dye, H. (2018). The impact and long-term effects of childhood trauma. *Journal of Human Behavior in the Social Environment, 28*(3), 381–392.

Felitti, V. J., Anda, R. F., Nordenberg, D., Williamson, D. F., Spitz, A. M., Edwards, V., Koss, M. P., & Marks, J. S. (1998). Relationship of childhood abuse and household dysfunction to many of the leading causes of death in adults. The Adverse Childhood Experiences (ACE) Study. *American Journal of Preventive Medicine, 14*(4), 245–258. https://doi.org/10.1016/s0749-3797(98)00017-8

Gilbert, R., Widom, C. S., Browne, K., Fergusson, D., Webb, E., & Janson, S. (2009). Burden and consequences of child maltreatment in high-income countries. *Lancet (London, England), 373*(9657), 68–81. https://doi.org/10.1016/S0140-6736(08)61706-7

Harris, M., & Fallot, R. D. (2001). Envisioning a trauma-informed service system: A vital paradigm shift. *New Directions for Mental Health Services, 89*, 3–22. https://doi.org/10.1002/yd.23320018903

Kim, J., & Cicchetti, D. (2010). Longitudinal pathways linking child maltreatment, emotion regulation, peer relations, and psychopathology. *Journal of Child Psychology and Psychiatry, and Allied Disciplines, 51*(6), 706–716. https://doi.org/10.1111/j.1469-7610.2009.02202.x

Lansford, J. E., Dodge, K. A., Pettit, G. S., Bates, J. E., Crozier, J., & Kaplow, J. (2002). A 12-year prospective study of the long-term effects of early child physical maltreatment on psychological, behavioral, and academic problems in adolescence. *Archives of Pediatrics & Adolescent Medicine, 156*(8), 824–830. https://doi.org/10.1001/archpedi.156.8.824

Linnemann, P., Berger, K., & Teismann, H. (2022). Associations between outcome resilience and sociodemographic factors, childhood trauma, personality dimensions and self-rated health in middle-aged adults. *International Journal of Behavioral Medicine, 29*(6), 796–806. https://doi.org/10.1007/s12529-022-10061-1

McTavish, J. R., Kimber, M., Devries, K., Colombini, M., MacGregor, J. C. D., Wathen, C. N., Agarwal, A., & MacMillan, H. L. (2017). Mandated reporters' experiences with reporting child maltreatment: A meta-synthesis of qualitative studies. *BMJ open, 7*(10), e013942. https://doi.org/10.1136/bmjopen-2016-013942

National Scientific Council on the Developing Child. (2015). Supportive Relationships and Active Skill-Building Strengthen the Foundations of Resilience: Working Paper 13.

Noteboom, A., Ten Have, M., de Graaf, R., Beekman, A. T., Penninx, B. W., & Lamers, F. (2021). The long-lasting impact of childhood trauma on adult chronic physical disorders. *Journal of Psychiatric Research, 136*, 87–94.

Pierce, H., Jones, M. S., Shoaf, H., & Heim, M. (2023). Early adverse childhood experiences and positive functioning during adolescence. *Journal of Youth and Adolescence, 52*(4), 913–930. https://doi.org/10.1007/s10964-022-01729-8

Shonkoff, J. P., Garner, A. S., Committee on Psychosocial Aspects of Child and Family Health, Committee on Early Childhood, Adoption, and Dependent Care, & Section on Developmental and Behavioral Pediatrics. (2012). The lifelong effects of early childhood adversity and toxic stress. *Pediatrics, 129*(1), e232–e246. https://doi.org/10.1542/peds.2011-2663

Shonkoff, J. P., Slopen, N., & Williams, D. R. (2021). Early childhood adversity, toxic stress, and the impacts of racism on the foundations of health. *Annual Review of Public Health, 42*, 115–134. https://doi.org/10.1146/annurev-publhealth-090419-101940

The Child Abuse Prevention and Treatment Act, 42 U.S.C. § 5101 *et seq.*; 42 U.S.C. § 5116 *et seq.* (1974).

Turner, J. A., Mancl, L., & Aaron, L. A. (2006). Short- and long-term efficacy of brief cognitive-behavioral therapy for patients with chronic temporomandibular disorder pain: a randomized, controlled trial. *Pain, 121*(3), 181–194. https://doi.org/10.1016/j.pain.2005.11.017

U.S. Department of Health & Human Services, Administration for Children and Families, Administration on Children, Youth and Families, Children's Bureau. (2020). *Child maltreatment 2018.* https://www.acf.hhs.gov/cb/research-data-technology/statistics-research/child-maltreatment

Zielinski, D. S. (2009). Child maltreatment and adult socioeconomic well- being. *Child Abuse & Neglect, 33*(10), 666–678. https://doi.org/10.1016/j.chiabu.2009.09.001

# 3 Sense of Belonging in Interprofessional Collaboration

*Luanne Shaw and Scott Shaw*

The purpose of this chapter is to provide a structured approach to exploring the intersection of sense of belonging and interprofessional collaboration within human services, catering to a diverse audience of social service, public health, medical, and nursing professionals.

Sense of belonging has become a "hot topic" in many circles, from minority groups to educational settings and business teams, this concept is gaining support and recognition as an essential element of better environments and performance outcomes. Cornell University, a respected institution of higher education, embraces sense of belonging and describes belonging in terms of feeling secure and supported, accepted, included, and involving an identity as a member of a specific group (Cornell University, 2024, para. 1). Allen et al. (2021) emphasize the "subjective feeling of deep connection" with other persons and the "fundamental human need" for this feeling, which impacts numerous outcomes across determinants of health and behaviors (p. 1). Finally, Strayhorn and Johnson (2023) are leading the conversation and movement around the recruitment and retention of students of color in predominantly white institutions, citing a sense of belonging as a pivotal factor in student success. He stresses the perception of connectedness, "the experience of mattering or feeling cared about," in defining a sense of belonging and its importance in attracting and maintaining a more diverse student body or, in this case, a more diverse and committed team (Strayhorn & Johnson, 2023, para 5 & 6).

Why should we, as human service professionals, care about a sense of belonging? Human service professionals spend a sizable portion of their work in direct contact with individuals and groups of people who are internal and external to their organization. These connections and relationships may be transactional in nature, though they often involve a necessity to engage and collaborate on a deeper level for the achievement of desired outcomes. One's perception of their role and very being, how they sense being accepted or rejected, whether they feel valued and respected, and whether they feel the need to contribute and commit to others all contribute to a sense of belonging and will affect the outcomes of interactions (Academy of Executive Coaching Ltd., 2024; Davis et al., 2022).

Interprofessional collaboration is more than just talking to professionals in other disciplines. Collaboration or collaborative practice occurs when two or more professionals work together, putting individual preferences and needs aside and managing power differentials to achieve improved outcomes for the organization or person(s) being served (Keehn, 2024). Collaborators share a mutual purpose, demonstrate trust and respect for each other's skills and unique knowledge, communicate effectively, and can adapt leadership based on priorities and needs (Keehn, 2024). The Interprofessional Education Collaborative ([IPEC], 2023) is a federally recognized non-profit representing over 20 health profession associations, including public health and social work. IPEC has developed a

DOI: 10.4324/9781003531258-5

competency framework for interprofessional collaboration with four supporting domains: Values and Ethics, Roles and Responsibilities, Communication, and Teams and Teamwork (IPEC, 2023). Each domain includes a defining competency statement and is supported by subcompetencies for each domain, which aim to prepare individuals to "engage in lifelong learning and collaboration to improve person/client care and population health outcomes" (IPEC, 2023, p. 14). The significance of being prepared for collaboration should be evident in the work of human services professionals.

As human service professionals, we cannot work in silos to achieve the desired and necessary outcomes for our patients/clients/communities we serve. The ability to collaborate effectively within our teams and among other disciplines puts the "customer" at the center of care, taking the focus off professional biases, power differentials, and personal agendas. There is a consensus in the literature, among organizations, in current practice that there are benefits to interprofessional collaboration including achieving more in high-performing collaborative teams than individually, serving more "customers" with better quality, addressing complex social issues more comprehensively, and promoting individual and organizational growth (Green & Johnson, 2015; Keehn, 2024; Ohio University, 2024).

The reader can expect to learn more about theoretical frameworks for sense of belonging and interprofessional collaboration with further conceptual exploration. Models for interprofessional collaboration, including their strengths and weaknesses in fostering a sense of belonging with illustrations of successful models, are included. Barriers and facilitators to interprofessional collaboration and sense of belonging are addressed at the individual, organizational, and system levels. Ethical considerations for interprofessional collaboration and ensuring equity and justice in fostering a sense of belonging are considered. Lastly, emerging trends and a call to action in human service professions conclude this chapter.

## Theoretical Framework

### *Social Identity Theory and Sense of Belonging*

Maslow (1962) identified five essential physiological, psychological, and emotional needs that framed his hierarchy of needs. These foundational physiological needs formed the base of his model, including food and shelter, followed by safety (physical and emotional), love and belonging, esteem needs, and eventually self-actualization if the preceding needs were met. This is often visualized as a triangle, with the most essential needs representing the foundation or base and the emotional higher-level (emotional, psychological) needs representing the peak once lower-level needs have been accomplished (Maslow, 1943). Assuming that one's physiological needs have been met (i.e., food, shelter), the role of belonging and feeling connected becomes a critical need in Maslow's model and has significant implications for human services professionals who often tend to the needs of one's clients or patients while also remaining aware of one's own physical and physiological reactions from one's work environment.

Social identity theory was developed by Tajfel and Turner (1979) to highlight the role of group interactions in individual identity formation. Important concepts within social identity theory are group membership within in-groups and how people define out-groups or those with whom they do not share membership and why. Such cognitive processes as prejudice, bias, and discrimination are components of emotional reactions in response to feeling included in an in-group and/or excluded or separated from an out-group. In-groups to which an individual identifies themself can be a significant sense of pride and identity (i.e., employer, team, sports). Social identity theory proposes that being part of an in-group can also foster a sense of belonging, greater purpose, and heightened self-worth and help crystallize identity. This is also evident in response to one's chosen profession, which includes how one identifies oneself professionally following rigorous education, training, licensure processes, and profession-specific codes of ethics that define one's daily practice (i.e., nursing, psychology, social work). One rarely says they have a job in nursing or social work but rather describes their very identity as being a nurse or social worker. One's professional identity creates significant professional cohesion with one's work.

Building upon these theories, a sense of belonging has been developed as its own theoretical construct and persists as a significant factor in understanding the highly contextual response someone has to their environment (Painter, 2013). The sense of belonging has focused on factors that help clarify how connection, how one seeks to have attachments or perceived security and predictability in relationships, is essential to optimal development and success in various professional, educational, and personal settings (Baumeister & Leary, 1995). The sense of belonging has been referred to as an individual's sense of "feeling or sensation of connectedness, and the experience of mattering or feeling cared about, accepted, respected, valued by, and important" (Strayhorn, 2019, p. 4).

### Conceptualization of Interprofessional Collaboration

As an essential component of healthcare and numerous other industries, the education of professionals in these fields to work in teams and collaborate effectively has been incorporated into their programs of study and workplace training to various degrees. The World Health Organization's (WHO) position is based on robust evidence leading up to 2010, demonstrating that interprofessional education facilitates more effective collaborative practice. Therefore, the WHO established a model conceptualization of this relationship. In the model, as present and future health workforces enter their degree or certification programs, they are not equipped to address local health needs and effect change among the fragmented health systems. Integration of interprofessional education during their training provides them with the competencies necessary to become collaborative practice-ready and optimized to strengthen the health systems they work for and improve health outcomes of the populations served (WHO, 2010, p. 18).

The IPEC competency framework (2023) builds upon the WHO model in addition to continuing evidence and expertise from multiple professions and global organizations (Figure 3.1). The competency domains represent critical elements shown to produce the most effective collaboration. Many academic degree programs integrate this framework in their curriculum, while practice settings may offer training derived from the IPEC competencies. Each competency domain is defined as follows (IPEC, 2023, p. 15):

- Values and ethics are demonstrated by working within groups to maintain shared values, ethical conduct, and mutual respect.
- Roles and responsibilities are demonstrated by using one's unique role and expertise to inform individual and population health outcomes.
- Communication is practiced with responsiveness, responsibility, respect, and compassion among team members.
- Teams and teamwork require the application of the scientific values and principles of teamwork and adapting one's role in a variety of team settings.

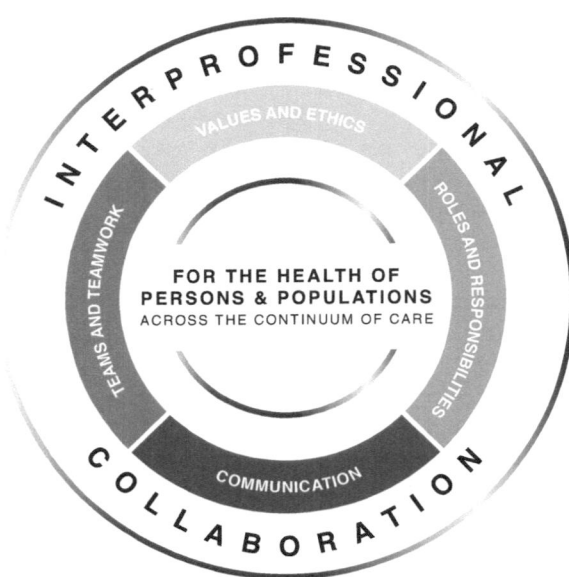

*Figure 3.1* IPEC Core Competencies for Interprofessional Collaborative Practice: Version 3 (2023, p. 15).

### Integration of Sense of Belonging within Interprofessional Collaboration Frameworks

With a sense of belonging emerging as a unique factor in successful individual and team outcomes in the literature, frameworks must adapt or be newly created. The existing IPEC (2023) model does not include the specific concept of sense of belonging but emphasizes values associated with effective teamwork and communication, such as mutual respect, just culture, and well-being. As organizations and systems continue to incorporate policies and practices which recognize and promote diversity, equity, inclusion, and, most recently, belonging (DEIB), two frameworks have been identified in current literature and media, distinguishing a sense of belonging/belonging as an essential element of the conceptual framework for interprofessional collaboration.

Inclusion and belonging, often used interchangeably, have distinct meanings and applicability in the context of interprofessional collaboration. According to the Academy to Innovate Human Resources (AIHR), the key difference between these concepts involves *action* on the part of the employer or team leadership to promote transparent, equitable policies and ensure all members are sought out and listened to in the case of inclusion (Verlinden, 2024). Belonging is then the *feeling* members have of being valued, seen, heard, and respected as part of the team (Verlinden, 2024). This differentiation and definition of belonging aligns with the defining characteristics of sense of belonging in the literature. The model proposed by the AIHR (Figure 3.2) places belonging at the center of organizational or team culture, supported and encased in the concepts of diversity, equity, and inclusion, which are encircled by actions which promote the achievement of belonging.

A second framework offers additional benefit in overcoming barriers to team training alone or separately from DEIB work in achieving a sense of belonging and better outcomes for teams. Davis et al. (2022) propose a framework integrating emotional management with team and/or diversity training to optimize belonging and uniting members through

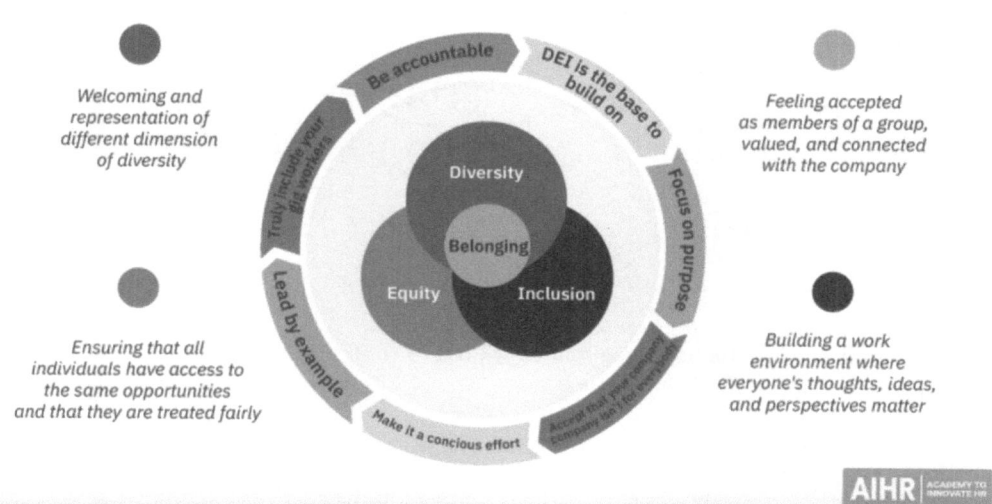

*Figure 3.2* Diversity, equity, inclusion, and belonging framework from the Academy to Innovate Human Resources (Verlinden, 2024, https://www.aihr.com/wp-content/uploads/diversity-equity-inclusion-belonging-1.png).

their differences. In reviewing the state of the science, including 339 empirical articles, Davis et al. (2022) conclude that "opposing motives of the traditionally separate team and diversity trainings with limited focus on shared goals" restrict their effectiveness (p. 112). When emotion and self-regulation strategies are incorporated with training and interventions, the affective component of active learning is optimized and may produce transference beyond the training (Davis et al., 2022). Figure 3.3 represents contextual influences (at system, organizational, and individual levels) on the training and development of skills, which impact the level of belonging achieved and ultimately team and individual performance. The contextual influences are strongly supported by Wei et al. (2022) in their meta-review of collaborative practice based on thematic analysis of 36 studies published between 2010 and 2020. The mediating factor on belonging and outcomes of training, most apparent in the literature reviewed, was the intentional focus on emotional management within training. The frameworks presented inform and instruct human services professionals and agencies on improving the preparation and development of more effective teams and collaboration for improved outcomes.

## Evaluation of Current Models

### Strengths and Weaknesses

Regardless of the model or framework, there are strengths and weaknesses to be considered. One crucial factor is cultural fitness. A famous quote in the business and change

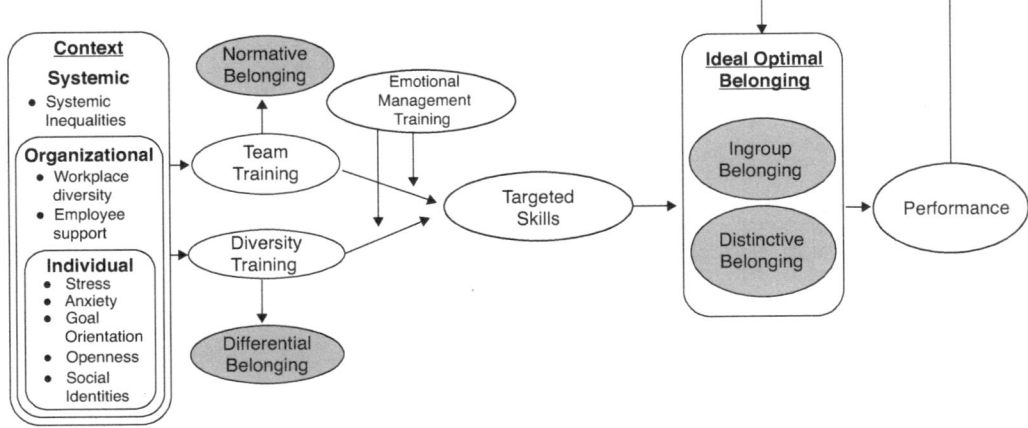

*Figure 3.3* Conceptual team belonging framework (Davis et al., 2022, p. 107).

management worlds, often attributed to Peter Drucker, a leading management theorist and author of his day, though the origin is debated, states "culture eats strategy for breakfast" (Foust, 2024, para. 2). Though the origin of the quote is questionable, the principle is exhaustingly true. Without support from all key stakeholders, buy-in from all affected, and the right context, such as perceived need or urgency to do something differently, a change, philosophy, or value cannot be fully embraced and sustained in a team or organization.

The AIHR (Verlinden, 2024; Figure 3.2) model beautifully represents the ideals of feeling valued and supported within an organization. All efforts surrounding the DEIB principles are focused on creating and maintaining belonging at the core of the organization's being. However, implementing and sustaining this model or culture within a team may be more difficult. If those who lead, manage, finance, and operate within the organization or team do not hold to the values and assumptions of the model, the framework will fail (Wei et al., 2022). There must be mutual purpose and intentional effort on the part of everyone in the organization or on the team toward upholding and enacting the strategies of the framework to successfully produce a sense of belonging among members and greater outcomes. Additionally, some weaknesses of this model could be the length of time needed to fully implement and operationalize it and/or the amount of effort and resources needed to foster and sustain values, especially if a team is frequently changing members.

The conceptual team belonging framework (Davis et al., 2022) brings awareness of contextual factors from the individual to the systemic level, which may impact the degree of trust, respect, and implicit biases of team members. The greatest strength of the model is the intentional management of emotions often triggered during DEIB or team trainings and inclusion of strategies for ongoing emotional management by team members when consensus is not easily achieved or belonging is not sensed by members. There are, however, some clear weaknesses. Training takes time and can involve significant cost if bringing in experts or commercial programs to train members in team values and skills or DEIB. Emotional management can be mentally stressful as well, and there is no guarantee members will all adhere to ground rules or sustain the behaviors and gains made during training. Ongoing support from outside the team may be needed.

## Barriers to Interprofessional Collaboration and Sense of Belonging

### *Individual Barriers*

Barriers to collaboration and one's sense of belonging are as diverse as the world's population. Some common barriers identified in the Conceptual Team Belonging Framework (Davis et al., 2022) include psychological factors, such as one's perceived stress level or anxiety. Everyone will have their own situations in life or at work, which contribute to perceived stress and anxiety. One's firsthand experiences with poor collaboration or feeling excluded or unvalued in a team in the past may also contribute to feelings of stress and anxiety and pose barriers (Wei et al., 2022). Even how one manages, or fails to manage, their own stress or anxiety can impact their ability and desire to effectively contribute to the team or how they perceive their level of belonging to the team. Psychological health and individual preferences for working alone or fear of and discomfort working with others can be significant barriers preventing some individuals from being able to effectively collaborate within teams or be motivated to belong.

Goal orientation may also pose barriers to effective team collaboration and sense of belonging (Davis et al., 2022). When one's personal agenda is at odds with others in the team or with the intended outcomes of the team, collaboration becomes compromised. Fear of losing or diminishing one's disciplinary boundaries or role identity, personally or professionally, could impact their alignment with goals and ability to collaborate with other professional disciplines (Wei et al., 2022). One's individual awareness of their personal and professional values provides valuable insight into their ability to build and sustain effective collaborative relationships. Failure to address, recognize, and consider how these values might conflict with or need to be managed among teams is a form of implicit bias and can lead to conflict. Implicit biases can manifest as language or actions perceived as disrespectful by other team members and create a lack of trust. Poor skills in dialogue, in addition to individual barriers such as implicit biases, can escalate conflict further and sabotage effective collaboration and sense of belonging among team members (Davis et al., 2022; Wei et al., 2022).

### *Organizational and System-Level Barriers*

At the organizational level, barriers stem from the culture, steeped in historical influences, policies, mission and vision, and experiences of past and present team successes or failures. If the organization or agency's team members represent a lack of diversity, hold philosophically different values and purposes, or do not provide strong support for employee inclusion and diversity, team collaboration and sense of belonging will be more challenging (Davis et al., 2022; Wei et al., 2022). Power differentials, whether real or perceived, and a lack of resources further contribute to ineffective collaboration and feelings of isolation or exclusion.

Organizational barriers are strongly influenced by the systems in which they operate, including local, state, and national policies and regulations. Systemic disparities result from a lack of promotion of DEIB and collaboration in laws and regulatory mechanisms, posing significant barriers at all levels. Where funds are directed, invested, or withheld, there is a lack of commitment to effective collaboration and promoting a sense of belonging across systems.

## Facilitation of Interprofessional Collaboration and Sense of Belonging

### *Individual-Level Facilitators*

Personal accountability is essential to embracing and contributing to effective collaboration, recognizing one's own sense of belonging, and helping others to feel they belong to the team. Individuals must recognize their own role and responsibilities and how their personal values, goals, and ability to build trust and show respect to others impact the team. Each discipline brings its own unique body of knowledge and skills to the table. Each representative of their discipline is responsible for their own level of expertise, maintaining competence and relevance in their field and completing their work to the best of their ability within expected timeframes. One must bring professional maturity, humility, and personal insight to the team. Personal accountability includes proficient skills in teamwork, such as knowing when and how to ask for help, how to communicate effectively both verbally and non-verbally in a respectful and culturally sensitive manner, and some strategies to address one's own emotional response to conflict or express concerns when goals and actions do not align with other team members, the organization(s), or the expected work and outcomes of the team (IPEC, 2023; Wei et al., 2022).

### *Organizational/System-Level Facilitators*

### *Training and Education*

Many organizations provide orientation to their new team members, spending varying numbers of hours in training and educating them on organizational structure, processes, and information or skills specific to one's role and expected outcomes, which support the overall mission. Often, training on DEIB, implicit biases, and, sometimes, team building is included. As previously identified, emotional management throughout these trainings and during educational delivery, regardless of how it is administered, is often neglected or lacking. In some cases, despite the amount or quality of training, the culture or "reality" of the organization or team experience is not representative of the values and intention upheld in that training. Recognizing the emotional energy necessary to participate in education and training, especially in team training, is crucial to best facilitate collaboration and a sense of belonging. According to Davis et al. (2022), feeling connected to both the content of training and other team members is needed for more successful results. Anticipating discomfort, potentially negative emotions, or defensiveness from individuals during diversity or implicit bias training can help facilitate better management of facilitator and group responses. When the affective domain of learning, including emotions, is well-managed throughout training and education, team members have a better chance of successful interprofessional collaboration and developing a sense of belonging (Davis et al., 2022; Green & Johnson, 2015).

### *Structural Facilitators*

The organizational flowchart or chain of command/power gradient within an organization, whether a large system or team, sets the foundation and culture for strong or weak collaboration and sense of belonging (Wei et al., 2022). Policies which promote and support a diverse workforce or team, procedures which are inclusive of all voices, and role-modeling by leaders within organizations or teams also contribute to more successful collaboration and a sense of belonging (Davis et al., 2022; Green & Johnson, 2015; Wei et al., 2022). Additional structural facilitators include physical environments that are flexible and encourage open communication and collaboration, mission and vision aligned with the values of DEIB and collaboration, and mechanisms for voicing concerns and sharing opinions which make members feel heard, respected, and valued. Consider open forums, intentional time to connect on professional and personal levels, dedicated agenda items to gain feedback and manage emotional responses during meetings, and even some spot-checking or routine measurement of the "climate" of collaboration or belonging using formal tools/surveys or informal methods, which can be strategies for facilitating collaboration and belonging.

## Exemplars

The COVID-19 pandemic, though not a specific company or team, provides a strong example of negative and positive outcomes of collaboration and the loss of or restoration of a sense of belonging. As individuals faced prolonged periods of physical isolation from their teams, it was necessary to pivot quickly to allow for effective collaboration and innovative strategies to maintain and foster a sense of belonging among them. The literature suggests that "co-location" or the use of a shared space for interaction among members is foundational for building trusting relationships and a sense of belonging (Wei et al., 2022). Technology like telehealth emerged on the provider/service end to stay connected with patients/clients. Platforms such as Zoom or Microsoft Teams became essential, in addition to increased use of media and forms of communication, such as video calling, for co-location to occur, continuing efforts to collaborate and ensure members of teams felt connected and a sense of belonging (Allen et al., 2021).

The Black Lives Matter (BLM) movement exemplifies collaboration and creation of opportunities for belonging "by building social capital that strengthens connections, allows activists to share their messages, and illuminates the inequities existing within and across cultures" (Allen et al., 2021, p. 9). The movement emerged with a strong mutual sense of purpose among Black Americans and people of other racial and ethnic backgrounds who recognized inequities and exclusions that are implicit and explicit in society. The BLM movement embodies strategies Allen et al. (2021) refer to as "bridging and bonding." As a broad array of BLM members were bridged together with a high degree of social reciprocity, they bonded in shared attitudes and interests.

Other organizations and companies provide examples of strategies and practices which are effectively working to promote inclusion. Microsoft initiated an Autism Hiring Program to promote a more diverse team (Ganesh, 2024). Microsoft altered its interview process to ensure inclusive practices more fitting to persons with autism (Microsoft Alumni Network, 2024). Check out Google's https://about.google/belonging/ site, which promotes the company's commitment to belonging, and, according to Ganesh (2024), it offers allyship training to team members, providing a more proactive approach to supporting and advocating for members from traditionally underrepresented groups. Finally, Johnson & Johnson promotes DEIB principles in their strategies, vision, and mission, even establishing a global diversity and inclusion council (Ganesh, 2024; Johnson & Johnson, 2024). These examples provide some hope for larger-scale efforts to promote collaboration and a sense of belonging for teams of all sizes and scope, yet ethical principles and practices must guide these efforts.

## Ethical Considerations

Ethical principles, including justice and beneficence, are directly reflective of effective interprofessional collaboration and a sense of belonging. Justice emulates principles of DEIB by ensuring all team members, regardless of role or discipline and personal characteristics or beliefs, are valued and respected. The concept of equity in team dynamics can be realized in removing barriers, such as ensuring times and methods of meeting are accessible and feasible for all members and ensuring a culture of safety where members do not fear punitive action or are not immobilized by power differentials. Justice is affirmed through efforts to foster and address individual and organizational/system-level facilitators while intentionally identifying, mitigating, and eliminating barriers. In some cases, when the culture and structure of an organization or team do not and will not support the principles and practices of DEIB, upholding justice among team members, it may be necessary for individuals to decide for themselves whether to remain or leave the organization or team. Affecting change is no easy task, especially without support from key stakeholders, including those with power and influence over structural and cultural change.

Beneficence is applied and upheld when all team members feel heard, seen, respected, and valued. Philosophically, teams must decide whether this includes the patient/client/customer as a member of the team and to what degree (Pakkanen et al., 2022). In healthcare, especially the discipline of nursing, person-centered care is a domain of nursing practice and is essential to competency-based education (American Association of Colleges of Nursing [AACN], 2024). Practices such as interdisciplinary rounding and bedside handover in hospitals are intended to benefit the various disciplines and patients through transparent information sharing and planning of care. When the goals and actions of the team benefit all members, each member is more likely to feel a sense of belonging and, therefore, be more motivated and committed to contributing their best. When each member is dedicated to the goals of the team and contributing their best, the results of more effective collaboration are much greater than those any individual member might accomplish on their own, and team synergy is created (Davis et al., 2022) As teams continue to evolve practices around more effective collaboration and building a sense of belonging among members, emerging trends and next steps must be considered.

## Emerging Trends and Call to Action

Some emerging trends to watch and consider implementing include refocused or re-envisioned training and methods of interprofessional education and collaboration and effective strategies to foster a sense of belonging. Kupershmidt et al. (2024) describe an interprofessional education summit involving multiple academic and practice sites, with multiple hubs participating simultaneously to promote education and collaboration within and across health professions. The summit provided phases for participants to react to topics, consider actionable strategies, and harvest further collaboration through discussion and exploration within each profession, across professions, and in large groups. Innovative educational efforts and models, such as the summit model supported by the Association of Schools Advancing Health Professions, can help bridge existing gaps from education to practice and across various industry teams.

Effective collaboration and a sense of belonging require intentional effort and commitment by design. Wei et al. (2022) confirm that system-level effort is needed to evaluate facilitators and barriers at each level and focus attention on policies and organizational culture to have a positive impact on a collaborative environment where team members feel they belong (p. 747). Systems must recruit, retain, and support leaders and members with elevated levels of competency in interprofessional collaboration and facilitation of a sense of belonging. This may require re-training and ongoing education and development for leaders and members.

Calling all human services professionals to action is the first step in furthering efforts to promote stronger interprofessional team collaboration and a sense of belonging. Operationalizing this work may be more challenging. The current literature and media dedicated to collaborative practices and building a sense of belonging have some key strategies to offer.

- Recognize and celebrate contributions and achievements of all members; a simple thank you, whether publicly or in a personal note, can go a long way.
- Recognize biases, whether intentional or inadvertent/implicit, in hiring or inviting practices to teams, and take action to address and change these practices to be more inclusive and equitable.
- Include emotional management in training and ongoing collaboration, taking time to recognize tensions and positive and negative emotional responses.
- Build community and bonding among team members through activities which include intentional connection and are accessible for all members, considering the time, place, attire, child/family friendly or care provisions for those with these considerations, etc.
- Promote a positive work environment, including fostering a healthy work-life balance, inviting physical workspaces, ongoing professional development and opportunities, health and wellness programs or spaces, etc.
- Ensure conflict is addressed promptly and equitably; policies and procedures for inappropriate, discriminatory behaviors should be developed and/or reviewed.
- Build transparency in communication from leadership, from employees or team members, and during collaboration. Note not every decision or task may require collaboration; knowing when collaboration is needed or not is important to determine.
- Assess and evaluate workplace or team collaboration and sense of belonging periodically; it has been said, "What gets measured, gets done" (original source debated). If teams are unaware of members' feelings of belonging or culture of collaboration, it is difficult to make or determine what improvements should be made.

(Davis et al., 2022; Green & Johnson, 2015; He, 2024;
Wei et al., 2022)

Further research and quality improvement work is needed to continue the dissemination and uptake of best practices around interprofessional education, teamwork, and collaboration, as well as fostering a sense of belonging. Studies specific to human services and those which include the patient/client perspective will further the state of science and evidence-based practice. In conclusion, even small actions can improve collaboration and a sense of belonging among interprofessional team members. Consider the following reflective questions in your own teams and practices.

### Questions for Reflection

1 When you think about the teams you participate in or will need to interact with, what is the culture toward collaboration and the sense of belonging you perceive?
2 Do the teams you participate in include the client (or patient, customer)? If so, how does the team ensure the client feels included and has a sense of belonging to the team? If not, what are the barriers or rationale?
3 Do you see diversity and inclusion represented in your organization, teams, and structure? If so, how is this reflected in the teamwork you participate in? If not, is there a process to express concerns safely or suggest a policy change?

4  What might be some individual, team, organizational, or system-level barriers and facilitators you are experiencing?
5  What are three practices or structural processes that might further improve interprofessional collaboration and sense of belonging in your teams?

## References

Academy of Executive Coaching Ltd. (2024). *Why the sense of belonging is crucial to teamwork.* https://www.aoec.com/knowledge-bank/why-the-sense-of-belonging-is-crucial-to-teamwork/

Allen, K. A., Kern, M. L., Rozek, C. S., McInereney, D., & Slavich, G. M. (2021). Belonging: A review of conceptual issues, an integrative framework, and directions for future research. *Australian Journal of Psychology, 73*(1), 87–102. https://doi.org/10.1080/00049530.2021.1883409

American Association of Colleges of Nursing. (2024). *Domain 2: Person-centered care.* https://www.aacnnursing.org/essentials/tool-kit/domains-concepts/person-centered-care

Baumeister, R. F., & Leary, M.R. (1995). The need to belong: Desire for interpersonal attachments as a fundamental human motivation. *Psychological Bulletin, 117*(3), 497–529.

Cornell University. (2024). *Diversity and inclusion: Sense of belonging.* https://diversity.cornell.edu/belonging/sense-belonging#:~:text=Belonging%20is%20the %20feeling%20of,and%20their%20personal%20lives%20suffer

Davis, A. S., Kafka, A. M., Gonzalez-Morales, M. G., & Feitosa, J. (2022). Team belonging: Integrating teamwork and diversity training through emotions. *Small Group Research, 53*(1), 88–127. https://doi.org/10.1177/10464964211044813

Foust, D. (2024, March). *Peter Drucker never said, "culture eats strategy for breakfast."* Medium. https://medium.com/@deanfoust_94519/peter-drucker-never-said-culture-eats-strategy-for-breakfast-0fe87beeb357

Ganesh, K. (2024). *Inclusion examples in the workplace: Inspirations and tips to create an inclusive culture.* https://www.culturemonkey.io/employee-engagement/inclusion-examples/

Green, B. N., & Johnson, C. D. (2015). Interprofessional collaboration in research, education, and clinical practice: Working together for a better future. *Journal of Chiropractic Education, 29*(1), 1–10. https://doi.org/10.7899/JCE-14-36

He, G. (2024). *How to create a sense of belonging in the workplace.* https://teambuilding.com/blog/belonging-in-the-workplace

Interprofessional Education Collaborative. (2023). *IPEC core competencies for interprofessional collaborative practice: Version 3.* Interprofessional Education Collaborative. https://ipec.memberclicks.net/assets/core-competencies/IPEC_Core_Competencies_Version_3_2023.pdf

Johnson & Johnson. (2024). *Diversity, equity, and inclusion.* https://www.jnj.com/diversity-equity-inclusion

Keehn, M. T. (2024). *Collaborative practice definition & key features.* University of Chicago Illinois. https://uofi.app.box.com/s/v6mf0unudntjsah8qqy1punweuwpjfly

Kupershmidt, S., Bell, K., Boyd, A., Zipp, G., & Breitbach, A. (2024). Innovative model for promoting interprofessional dialogue and action across healthcare stakeholders: The ASAHP collaborative stakeholder engagement model. *Journal of Allied Health, 53*(1), 3–9a.

Maslow, A. H. (1962). *Toward a psychology of being.* Von Nostrand Reinhold.

Microsoft Alumni Network. (2024). *Microsoft Autism hiring program: Inclusive hiring for people with disabilities.* https://www.microsoftalumni.com/s/1769/19/interior.aspx?gid=2&pgid=1119&sid=1769

Ohio University. (2024). *Building bridges of support: Collaboration in the field of social work.* https://www.ohio.edu/news/2024/06/building-bridges-support-collaboration-field-social-work

Painter, C. V. (2013). Sense of belonging: Literature review, *Research and Evaluation.* https://www.canada.ca/content/dam/ircc/migration/ircc/english/pdf/research-stats/r48a-2012belonging-eng.pdf

Pakkanen, P., Haggman-Laitila, A., & Kangasniemi, M. (2022). Ethical issues identified in nurses' interprofessional collaboration in clinical practice: A meta-synthesis. *Journal of Interprofessional Care, 36*(5), 725–734. https://doi.org/10.1080/13561820.2021.1892612

Strayhorn, T. L. (2019). *College students' sense of belonging: A key to educational success for all students*. Routledge.

Strayhorn, T. L., & Johnson, J. (2023, May 30). Beyond enrollment: Addressing Black college students' sense of belonging through admissions and recruitment. *Medium*. https://medium.com/@terrell.strayhorn/beyond-enrollment-addressing-black-college-st  udents-sense-of-belonging-through-admissions-and-61189c9b7d2f

Tajfel, H., & Turner, J. C. (1979). An integrative theory of inter-group conflict. In W. G. Austin, & S. Worchel (Eds.), *The social psychology of inter-group relations* (pp. 33–47). Brooks/Cole.

Verlinden, N. (2024). *Diversity, equity, inclusion and belonging at work: A 2024 guide*. Academy to Innovate Human Resources. https://www.aihr.com/blog/diversity-equity-inclusion-belonging-deib/

Wei, H., Horns, P., Sears, S. F., Huang, K. Smith, C M., & Wei, T. (2022). A systematic meta-review of systematic reviews about interprofessional collaboration: Facilitators, barriers, and outcomes. *Journal of Interprofessional Care, 36*(5), 735–749. https://doi.org/10.1080/13561820.2021.1973975

World Health Organization. (2010). *Framework for action on interprofessional education & collaborative practice*. https://iris.who.int/bitstream/handle/10665/70185/WHO_HRH_HPN_10.3_eng.pdf?sequence=1

# 4 Partner Abuse in Domestic and Dating Relationships

## How Trauma Impacts the Brain, the Family, and Functioning

*Corinne D. Warrener*

## Introduction

Interpersonal violence can take many forms, including violence perpetrated by strangers or by someone close to the victim. It is an intentional use of violence or force against another individual or group (Mercy et al., 2017). This chapter focuses on a subset of interpersonal violence, partner abuse (also called intimate partner violence [IPV]), which can include many forms of violence or abusive behavior used against a current or past partner, spouse, or significant other. Partner abuse, broadly, includes domestic violence and dating violence. The element of a partner, spouse, or significant other being the perpetrator adds layers of betrayal and trauma to an already-complex situation. Abuse by a partner is done with intimate knowledge of fears, desires, likes/dislikes, and the most vulnerable parts of the victim (Stark, 2007). The implications for survivors are significant but also reach beyond the survivor to their families and loved ones and can impact legal, physical, mental, emotional, social, and financial outcomes (Centers for Disease Control [CDC], 2024; Wood et al., 2020).

## Power and Control

Partner abuse can assume many different forms. Partner abuse is recognized as a person attempting to exert power and control over the other through a pattern of behaviors (Office on Violence Against Women [OVW], 2023). Whether the relationship is marriage/cohabitation (i.e., domestic violence) or dating or whether an intimate relationship has ended, this dynamic is what drives abuse.

Evan Stark (2007) offered the most nuanced and descriptive analysis of power and control in intimate relationships, which he called "coercive control." He describes coercive control as "comprised of structural forms of deprivation, exploitation, and command that compel obedience indirectly by monopolizing vital resources, dictating preferred choices, microregulating a partner's behavior, limiting her options, and depriving her of supports needed to exercise independent judgement" (Stark, 2007, p. 229). Intimidation becomes a useful tool for an abuser because one need not use physical violence every time (or ever) but rather can use the threat of violence, destruction of property, harm to objects or people, or risk of losing one's home or financial security (Stark, 2007). Abusers learn through experimentation what works and how to prompt desired reactions (Stark, 2007). The desire is for power and control, and the behaviors are the method. The categories of abuse vary depending on the source, but the commonly discussed categories include physical, sexual, emotional/psychological, economic, and technological abuse (OVW, 2023).

DOI: 10.4324/9781003531258-6

A common misconception is that a specific behavior automatically indicates abuse. There are many problematic behaviors in relationships that can also be the result of stress, mental illness, addiction, incompatibility, or other factors. For example, cheating on a significant other could be the result of one of these other factors, or it could be part of a broader pattern of seeking power. Name-calling or yelling could be part of a difficult period in a relationship, or it could be part of a growing pattern of control and dehumanization. Physical and sexual violence, however, are not part of a healthy, respectful relationship.

Michael P. Johnson, a leading expert in the research of domestic violence, offers further nuance in understanding partner dynamics, distinguishing abuse as a distinct phenomenon separate from other forms of violence in intimate relationships (Johnson, 1995). Johnson (2008) presented four major types of relationship violence: (1) situational couple violence; (2) intimate terrorism; (3) violent resistance; and (4) mutual violent control (Johnson, 2008). Situational violence lacks that dynamic of control and is rather the result of the escalation of conflict. Intimate terrorism is characterized by the coercive control of one partner over another and is what we think of in traditional "domestic violence" situations. Violent resistance is where the victim reacts in response to a pattern of intimate terrorism. Mutual violent control denotes violence used by both partners. It is important to recognize the etiological differences in partner abuse, as there is evidence that the outcomes are different and that interventions to address the perpetrator need to be tailored to the specific nature of the abuse (Velonis, 2016). With intimate terrorism, victims are more likely to be injured and experience trauma symptoms (Johnson & Leone, 2005). Also, with intimate terrorism, the abuse is less likely to stop (Johnson & Leone, 2005).

Abuse often goes in cycles, switching between periods of (relative) calm, stress, or acts of violence. These cycles can vary in length of time, often with longer stretches of calm in the earlier periods of a relationship and then cycling through faster as the relationship progresses (NCADV, n.d.). This cycle of abuse to calm can be confusing for victims, making it harder for them to leave a relationship because sometimes the relationship feels good.

### Forms of Abuse

The term "partner abuse" can conjure images of a battered woman, but the reality of abuse is that it takes many forms: physical, sexual, financial/economic, emotional/verbal, and more. As noted previously, these behaviors are the way a partner manipulates the other person to maintain control in the relationship. The various forms of abuse could fill a book on their own, but the following text will provide an overview of common areas. The CDC has good resources for further reading on the types of abuse and related tactics (Breiding et al., 2015).

Physical abuse is hurting a partner through physical force, such as hitting, punching, kicking, shoving, strangling, choking, hair-pulling, or burning (note that this list is not comprehensive). It can also include the use of weapons or restraining a person (Breiding et al., 2015). About a third of women and one in four men will be victims of physical violence in their lifetime; women are at greater risk for severe injury (Black et al., 2011; Truman & Morgan, 2014). Almost half of the time, when a woman is murdered, it is by a current or former partner (Cooper & Smith, 2001).

Case example: Olivia and her husband, Matt, have been married for about four years, following a two-year period of dating and engagement. Olivia reports that when they were dating they did occasionally have more heated fights but that she didn't think it was anything to be concerned about. After they married, she found that disagreements more and more frequently turned into big fights with yelling and screaming. Over time, he started throwing objects when he would get really mad. She remembers the first time he pushed her as he stormed out of the room during a fight, about six months after they got married. She reports now that they have big fights about once every three months and that some of the common things he has done include pushing her into walls, pushing her onto the floor, and throwing objects at her face. If she tries to leave the room, he will block the doorway.

Questions for reflection: What questions might you want to ask about Olivia's history with her husband? Do you notice any red flags here?

Sexual violence refers to coercive or forced touching, sexual acts, or exposure to sexual events (Breiding et al., 2015). Contemporary interpretations include a multitude of areas beyond the more commonly accepted violations of rape, assault, and molestation. Other behaviors include exposing a partner to unwanted pornography, recording or taking nude pictures without consent, sharing/distributing sexual pictures/videos without consent, stealthing, tampering with birth control, or changing sexual activities during the act without gaining explicit consent (Breiding et al., 2015). In addition, there is another category of consensual traumatic sex, which refers to instances where an individual might consent to sex, but it occurs within a pattern of coercion or manipulation (Wasserman & McGuire, 2024).

Case example: Amber has a boyfriend, Troy, for about three years. She disclosed that she is struggling with their sexual relationship. She reports that earlier on in their relationship things were great but that over time he kept asking her to do things she wasn't comfortable with. She reports that even when she has told him she doesn't want to perform a certain sexual act, he will continue to pressure her by guilt-tripping her or talking about how previous girlfriends would do it. She says that on a couple of occasions he has tried to do these same acts and then said he "didn't remember" that she told him no before. She also disclosed that sometimes she will just go along with what he wants because she is afraid of how angry he gets or because he will ignore her for days afterward. She says he has never hit her. She says she loves him and that she wants to make him happy, but she wishes that he would listen when she says no to things that hurt her or that she doesn't like.

Questions for reflection: How might the trauma Amber is experiencing be presenting here? How would you move forward with Amber to explore her experiences and goals, while also keeping in mind the influence trauma might have on how she frames her experiences?

About 1 in 5 women report sexual violence in their lifetime (Leemis et al., 2022), and about 1 in 13 men report sexual violence by a partner in their lifetime (Leemis et al., 2022). In the overwhelming majority of cases, the perpetrator is known to the victim (80% of cases), and in many cases (about 1/3) the perpetrator is someone with whom the victim is currently or previously in a relationship (RAINN, 2024).

Sexual assault at the hands of a partner can have a lasting impact on the survivor. The reality is that most sexual assault happens at the hands of someone who is known to the victim. (For the context of this chapter, this section focuses only on sexual assault by a partner or significant other.) Survivors often experience short-term and long-term problems that include debilitating psychological and physical symptoms, including depression, post-traumatic stress disorder, sleep disturbance, sexual problems, and alcohol abuse (Ahrens et al., 2010; Gómez & Freyd, 2018; Jacques-Tiura et al., 2010; Overup et al., 2015; Zinzow et al., 2010). These problems can affect daily living and functioning, such as academic achievement (Jordan et al., 2014). Additionally, survivors of sexual violence in college are at increased risk for future victimization (Walsh et al., 2012).

Economic abuse refers to several areas, including control over finances or interfering with work, education, or the ability to earn income or maintain a job (NCADV, 2017).

While this is a newer area of exploration in partner abuse literature, evidence suggests that a large portion of victims experience economic abuse (Postmus et al., 2012). Abuse negatively impacts economic outcomes for survivors (Postmus et al., 2012; Warrener et al., 2013). In fact, abuse (with or without economic factors) has a sustained negative impact on survivors (Voth Schrag, 2015).

When it comes to technology, it can be a means of control but can also be a tool for protecting victims. In terms of control, perpetrators can monitor phones, computers, and other devices; this might include monitoring emails or other accounts. Phones can be used to threaten, monitor, or track (i.e., stalk) a partner. Conversely, victims can use technology to reach out for help and support or can track a perpetrator's movement to protect themselves (Boethius et al., 2022).

Religion and spirituality can be another means of control. Scripture, traditions, or cultural norms might be used to manipulate or punish the victim. This might involve children (such as how they are raised), neglecting care, asserting authority, using the religious community as manipulation, or isolating the victim (National Resource Center on Domestic Violence, n.d.). In some religious communities, gender norms put women in positions of vulnerability because they are expected to maintain peace in the home (Murugan, 2022). Victims in the orthodox Jewish community sometimes experience challenges in getting help because of shame and judgment resulting from the immense value placed on family (Murugan, 2022). At the same time, religion/spirituality can be a resource for victims who are looking for emotional/spiritual support or means for leaving the relationship (National Resource Center on Domestic Violence, n.d.).

Case example: Sarah married her husband about ten years ago, and she says their faith is a big part of their marriage. She describes her husband as a "good man" but goes on to say that they frequently have disagreements about how to manage their household and children. When she became pregnant with their first child, he demanded that she leave her job. She reluctantly agreed but only after stating that she wanted to return to work when their children went to school. They have two children, and the younger one will be going to kindergarten soon, so she would like to go back to work. She says that when she brought this up, her husband became so angry he threw a vase at her, which broke and cut her hand. He then left her to clean up the mess alone. She did not seek medical attention for the cut, though she thinks it might have needed stitches because it bled so much. She says that this argument, like many others, comes from her husband's ideas about what a wife "should" do in the family and how it would make him look bad if he let her work. Sarah says she tried talking with a pastor from her church, but he mostly told her she needs to respect her husband's role and tried to explain why she didn't need to work. Sarah does not want to lose her connections to the church community and is afraid of telling anyone else there but feels like she needs someone with a religious background to help her navigate what she is experiencing.

Questions for reflection: In what ways can religion be both a protective and a risk factor? How is that playing out here with Sarah? What were your initial reactions to hearing about the influence their religion has on their marriage? Are there any biases (positive or negative) that you need to explore for yourself?

Culture and immigration status are further factors that impact experiences of partner abuse (Warrener & Koivunen, 2014). If family is far away or in another country, immediate support (such as a place to stay) may not be feasible. In the Latino community, some forms of partner abuse, such as jealousy, are excused as machismo. Language can be a further barrier to finding or receiving services, first by learning about the services and then whether the agency has bilingual staff (Postmus et al., 2014). Abusers might threaten immigration status by saying they will take away passports or claim the individual will be deported if the victim calls the police (National Network to End Domestic Violence [NNEDV], 2017).

With so many behaviors that can be present in healthy, unhealthy, or abusive relationships, professionals need to proceed prudently when encountering relationship issues among clients. Human service professionals must gather information about the relationship, environment, supports, and history to gain a more accurate assessment of the individual or family (Warrener & Koivunen, 2014). A thorough assessment is critical in developing a plan for working with these individuals that prioritizes safety as paramount and presents realistic and client-centered goals.

## Violence, Trauma, and the Brain

Traumatic events impact the brain in the way it interprets the events, how memories are stored, and how those memories are recalled and processed after the event (Bremner, 2006). The three major areas that are impacted by trauma are the amygdala, hippocampus, and prefrontal cortex. Neurochemicals such as cortisol and norepinephrine play a significant role in how trauma and its memories are processed in the brain (Bremner, 2006). When a traumatic event occurs, the prefrontal cortex is impeded or shut down; this is where higher-order thinking is processed and makes sense of the many inputs the brain is receiving (Van der Kolk, 2015). As the fear response (sympathetic nervous system) takes over, people experience the fight, flight, freeze, or fawn responses. The fawn response, while less commonly known, is important to discuss in the context of partner abuse because victims may increase risk if they fight back (fight response), may not have the ability to leave (flight response), or may endure continued or escalating violence if they do nothing (freeze response). The fawn response is a way of attempting to soothe the perpetrator in the hopes that the threat will subside (Herman, 2015). This particular response occurs for people who have no perceived ability to leave or ameliorate the situation through other responses; it is unique to people who cannot escape a more long-term, chronically dangerous situation with another person.

As the higher-order thinking of the prefrontal cortex shuts down or is inhibited, memories are also impacted. Memories are typically stored in the hippocampus, and the amygdala attaches emotional significance (Bremner, 2006). During a traumatic event, memories may not be stored in chronological order. The basic brain processes are still working, so the victim might recall sensory-based memories of sight, sound, smell, touch, and taste (Bremner, 2006; Van der Kolk, 2015). This can complicate legal investigations because the victims may have disjointed memories that emphasize the senses rather than a logical, chronological recollection that emphasizes details.

Trauma can occur from one event or from multiple events over time. When talking about partner abuse, the very nature of an ongoing relationship connotes multiple or continued trauma. Over time, a victim of prolonged trauma from partner abuse may feel less like himself or herself, they may lose a base level of calm or security, and they adapt to living in a constant state of fear or stress (Herman, 2015). The depersonalization that occurs is due to parts of the brain shutting down and operating in a more primitive state that focuses on the basics for survival. The lack of context, emotion, and processing results in a disconnect from the experience and the human being part of oneself (Herman, 2015).

Case example: Maya divorced her husband several months ago and has stabilized her living situation and finances. She reports feeling "lost" now that things have settled, but she isn't sure why. When discussed further, Maya expresses that she often doesn't know what to do with herself outside of work if she isn't caring for her children, but they are busy with school and activities, leaving her with more free time than she is used to. She says that she used to spend every minute of her day trying to keep up with the demands of her abusive husband, from cooking and cleaning to managing his schedule and the rest of the house. She says that she doesn't even know what foods she likes anymore because she never got to choose when she was married. She reports not having any hobbies and says she hasn't had contact with friends in years because anything she did for herself inevitably resulted in a fight or violence, so she eventually gave up. She says that when she was younger she loved activities like walking and hiking and that she used to love making pottery. Now she feels isolated and isn't sure where to start.

Questions for reflection: What elements of depersonalization or numbing do you see here? How might Maya have got to this point? As you think through steps for her to take to reach her goals, how might trauma hinder her efforts?

Trauma can result in hyperarousal, flashbacks, nightmares, disproportionate response to startling stimuli, and intrusive thoughts (Herman, 2015). The brain can have difficulty distinguishing between safety and danger, resulting in behaviors or reactions that do not match the situation (e.g., they misconstrue people's behaviors as threatening when they are not or miss signs of danger when someone is aggressive) (Herman, 2015; Van der Kolk, 2015). Flashbacks are particularly pernicious because they can occur at any time and have no logical start and no clear end; they can occur while awake or asleep (Herman, 2015).

There is growing evidence that repeated trauma has cumulative effects (Sacchi et al., 2020). Notably, some research suggests that violence in childhood or physical violence in adulthood predicted the greatest severity of post-traumatic stress disorder (PTSD) in older adulthood (Ogle et al., 2014). Research on adverse childhood experiences has demonstrated that the more adverse encounters that a person engages in, the more likely poor health outcomes may occur later in life (Hughes et al., 2017; Kalmakis & Chandler, 2015; Nelson et al., 2020). While complex PTSD is not recognized by the *Diagnostic and Statistical Manual* (*DSM-5*), many practitioners and researchers reference the unique concerns for people who experience ongoing trauma (U.S. Department of Veterans Affairs, 2022).

In addition to the trauma resulting from partner abuse, further accumulation may result from racial, intergenerational, and historical trauma (U.S. Department of Veterans Affairs, 2024). Racial trauma results from the emotional stress of discrimination and race-related stress (U.S. Department of Veterans Affairs, 2024). Intergenerational trauma and historical trauma can also be passed down to children and provide yet another cumulative effect (DeAngelis, 2019). Historical trauma refers to events experienced by a group, such as survivors of the holocaust, Native Americans, because of the long history of colonization and oppression, or Black people who have survived generations of slavery, segregation, and violent racism. Trauma experienced by previous generations might be passed down through stories and messages to children and younger generations but also can be passed down physiologically through epigenetics (DeAngelis, 2019). This can also include families who experience multigenerational events of domestic violence or incest, where the behaviors are accepted and normalized for younger generations, despite the severe negative impacts (Reese et al., 2022).

Trauma is rooted in the brain, and as such many of the evidence-based treatments for trauma are rooted in regaining a mind–body–brain connection and shifting brainwaves (Van der Kolk, 2015). Effective treatments include Eye Movement Desensitization and Reprocessing (EMDR) therapy, yoga, and theater; van der Kolk recommends a combination of social engagement and regulating physical tensions to move people from the survival mode, increase their capacity to differentiate danger from safety, and regulate their body and response systems (Van der Kolk, 2015).

### Betrayal Trauma

Betrayal trauma as a theory was constructed by Jennifer Freyd and refers to betrayal by close others, such as relationship partners (Gómez & Freyd, 2019). Betrayal trauma gets to the crux of the issue with partner abuse: a partner is a trusted individual, and the abuser violates that trust. Within partner abuse, there is an ongoing dynamic whereby the trust is repeatedly violated, and the victim's sense of trust is obliterated. When there is a level of dependence on the abuser (whether financial or emotional), the victim may not be able to leave (Gómez & Freyd, 2019). When considered in the context of what is happening within the brain, the betrayal of an intimate partner through whatever form of abuse can have numerous, long-lasting negative impacts on the victim (Freyd, 1999).

### Partner Abuse in Married/Cohabitating Relationships

According to the CDC's National Intimate Partner and Sexual Violence Survey, over 40% of women report physical violence by a partner in their lifetime (Leemis et al., 2022). In a 12-month period, about 4.5% of women experience physical violence, and just over 3% report severe physical violence (Leemis et al., 2022). The rates of physical violence victimization are about the same for men, with over 40% reporting lifetime victimization, 5.5% reporting violence in the last year, and 3% reporting severe violence in the last year (Leemis et al., 2022). The reported rate of injury is higher for women (about 75%) than for men (about 48%). Reported PTSD symptoms, concern for safety, fear, and needing help from law enforcement are all higher for women than men (Leemis et al., 2022).

### Children and Domestic Violence

Research suggests that somewhere between 30% and 60% of cases where there is domestic violence or child abuse, the other form also exists (Jouriles et al., 2008). (This is outside of the debate over whether witnessing domestic violence is a form of child abuse.) Human professionals who come across clients experiencing either partner or child abuse must be aware of the possibility that the other form of abuse also occurs. Practitioners may be limited in their role as to how to prioritize or intervene for the adult, child, or family, but that should not preclude the assessment of all areas and subsequent planning and referrals that ensure protections for all victims. This may also necessitate referrals or coordination/consultation with other agencies.

The negative impact of childhood exposure to domestic violence is well-established. These impacts can be traced to exposure during pregnancy or in the early days of infancy (Carpenter & Stacks, 2009; Huang et al., 2010). High levels of stress during pregnancy can result in low birth weights and higher stress hormone levels in the infant postnatally (Carpenter & Stacks, 2009). Particularly in early childhood, there are negative impacts on attachment. This is thought to be the result of the mother's impaired functioning (e.g., depression, anxiety, stress) from the abuse, which then impacts the maternal–child relationship (Carpenter & Stacks, 2009).

Throughout childhood and adolescence, exposure has negative effects. Children in households where mothers experienced domestic violence in infancy exhibited both internalizing (e.g., poor mental health, difficulty in social relationships) and externalizing (e.g., bullying, delinquency) behavioral problems later in childhood (Huang et al., 2010, 2015). Interestingly, in cases where the mother (victim) was unmarried, children fared better, which could possibly be due to less exposure to domestic violence because the relationship ended (Yoo & Huang, 2012). Witnessing physical violence toward a caregiver can be traumatic for a child (Carpenter & Stacks, 2009), but the abuse does not need to be physical, as the effects are seen with other forms of abuse, such as economic abuse, also (Huang et al., 2015). Even when children or adolescents do not directly witness IPV, they still suffer. A study across several countries that examined both direct and indirect exposure to interparental conflict found negative consequences for children regardless of the type (Bradford et al., 2003). Overt conflict among parents is more likely to result in antisocial behavior, and covert conflict is more likely to result in depression (Bradford et al., 2003). Many of these results were repeated across countries and cultures from South Africa, Bangladesh, China, India, Bosnia, Germany, Palestine, Colombia, and the United States (Bradford et al., 2003).

The chronic stress of growing up in an environment where partner abuse is occurring can have both short-term and long-term effects. Children experiencing chronic stress from a household with partner abuse may develop a chronic state of hyperarousal (i.e., elevated stress hormones). This is associated with greater reactivity, emotional regulation, memory difficulties, difficulty interpreting emotions, and thinking/learning (Carpenter & Stacks, 2009). Children who experience the chronic stress and trauma of witnessing abuse and/ or child abuse may experience myriad mental health and physical health problems. They blame themselves, feel helpless, and have difficulty forming healthy relationships later (Herman, 2015). These children struggle with developing any sense of safety in the world and may experience dissociation, depersonalization, and derealization (Herman, 2015).

It is important for human service professionals not to blame victims or become focused on acting as judge and jury as to the validity of a victim's account. Trauma symptoms can present in varied and unusual ways and may deviate from how professionals *assume* a victim should act or appear. Professionals need to listen to the client first, understand how the brain might be affected by trauma, and proceed thoughtfully. Victims will not present the same way or on the same timeline, and what may be traumatic to one person may not result in trauma symptoms for another.

### Male Victims

Professionals who encounter victims of domestic violence need to be holistic in their assessment. Beyond the dynamics of control, there are many factors that impact safety and the client's functioning. Some women are often recognized as abuse victims, but men are often overlooked. Some men are not aware that they are victims of abuse or may feel there are no resources for help or they will be believed (Bates, 2019; Huntley et al., 2019; Lysova et al., 2020; Tsui et al., 2010). The abusive dynamics that men experience have many similarities to women's experiences, including physical and emotional abuse, manipulation, control, and sexual abuse (Machado et al., 2020). These men also experience profound emotional or psychological impacts, such as depression or suicidal thinking. At the same time, many men have discouraging experiences when seeking help through formal channels (Lysova et al., 2020; Tsui et al., 2010). They are not taken seriously or may be blamed for the abuse (i.e., perceived as the abuser), which may be in part due to the manipulation of the abusive partner (Machado et al., 2020).

## Victims with Disabilities

Another area of special consideration is for people with disabilities. People with disabilities are at greater risk of abuse, with the addition that, depending on the type of disability, it may also create further difficulties or barriers to leaving. Both mental and physical impairments increase risk (Hahn et al., 2014). Victims with disabilities might experience withholding of medications, medical treatment, or assistance devices. All other forms are also possible in these cases, from physical, sexual, verbal, to financial (NCADV, 2018). As is the case with other special populations (like men and LGBTQ+), victims with disabilities might have more difficulty finding resources that are familiar with the particularities of their situation and needs (NCADV, 2018).

## LGBTQ+

With the LGBTQ+ population, partner abuse can take on some unique dynamics or challenges. Abusers might use tactics such as telling the victim that no one will help them because of their gender or sexuality, threatening to "out" them, questioning or undermining gender or sexual identity, and reinforcing phobic perspectives like homophobia and transphobia (Human Right Campaign, 2022). This, coupled with societal discrimination and heterosexism, may make identifying partner abuse difficult for LGBTQ+ people, can make it hard to leave, and can make it harder to find welcoming resources (Human Rights Campaign, 2022).

Just as past trauma can have a cumulative effect, falling into multiple special categories of victim can complicate the abuse, trauma, leaving a relationship, and resiliency afterward. A gay man or woman of color may experience the abuse in the context of intersectional identities, along with the discrimination or struggles that come with it (Barrios et al., 2020). These nuances are important to consider when working with clients to better identify the client's needs and how best to serve them.

## Dating Violence

National data from the Centers for Disease Control's Youth Risk Behavior Surveillance System found that the rates of physical and sexual dating violence reported by high school students decreased between 2013 and 2019 (Puzzanchera, 2022), but it remains a problem. Female high school students reported higher rates of physical and sexual violence than male students, and LGBTQ+ people reported higher rates than their heterosexual peers (Puzzanchera, 2022). In analyzing vulnerable populations research, de Heer and Jones (2017) suggest that surveys are likely underestimating sexual victimization rates and experiences of vulnerable populations, such as LGBTQ+ people and Native Americans. Dating violence victims frequently have poor mental health outcomes, regardless of race, ethnicity, gender, or sexuality, or any other status (Barrick et al., 2013; Bossarte et al., 2009).

There is a link between childhood exposure to partner abuse and later dating violence. As might be expected, teenagers who witness partner abuse by their parents are more likely to experience dating violence victimization (Karlsson et al., 2016). There is also a growing body of research that indicates that exposure to partner abuse in the first few years of life also increases the likelihood of involvement in teen dating violence situations later on (Cheung & Huang, 2023).

Professionals in the human service field need to consider the ever-changing world of adolescents and young adults. The social world of adolescents is of enormous importance, and thus a major factor in how relationships are perceived and pursued. Race is an integral part of this developmental process, as a positive ethnic identity serves as a protective factor among Black adolescents (Henry & Zeytinoglu, 2012), and thus should be included in work with adolescents as part of discussions are healthy relationships. Care must be taken to disentangle race from class, where community violence and socioeconomic class can be risk factors for victimization (Black et al., 2015). While the community environment is sometimes tied to socioeconomic class and also race, these things are not one and the same. Racial or ethnic identity needs to be viewed not as a risk factor, but examined in its own right as a potential protective factor. Furthermore, an urban environment can have varying socioeconomic conditions. Ideally, prevention and intervention efforts should be tailored to the individual community's context and needs.

Another major consideration for dating violence is around help-seeking. Boys are less likely to talk to someone about dating violence than girls (Black et al., 2008), but very few adolescents will talk to an adult. Severity of the violence does not appear to be related to reporting, but if someone witnesses it that does prompt the victim to seek help (Black et al., 2008). This phenomenon suggests that young people need to be given language, resources, and knowledge on how to respond to friends or peers when they are approached by a victim. Navigating intimate relationships is new for adolescents, and they should be equipped with information about how to support each other and when to seek help from an adult or professional.

## Summary

The most significant lesson from this chapter is that trauma impacts the brain in ways that affect the victim both in the short term and long term. Memories and behavior may be unusual or abnormal. Trauma can be cumulative, even tracing back to prior generations of family or groups. The betrayal of an intimate partner can be traumatic on its own or may be magnified by a history of other traumas. Professionals who encounter clients with a history of victimization at the hands of a partner must rely on thorough, multidimensional assessments that consider history, culture, functioning, family, supports, and any and all areas that are impacting the individual(s) sitting in front of them.

## Questions for Reflection

1  Safety is paramount as a human service professional, but that may be complicated by concern for multiple people and concern for emotional well-being and re-traumatization. Thinking beyond the immediate of safety planning or emergencies, how would you promote safety for the victim and family members to foster long-term well-being?
2  Each area of partner abuse that has been covered here involves many factors that can influence risk and outcomes. How would you approach assessment and intervention with clients to ensure you are considering critical areas?
3  Trauma from partner abuse can significantly impact the brain. How might this manifest among people who have experienced violence, intimidation, or other forms of abuse at the hands of their partner? Consider affect, behavior, decision-making, functioning, or other areas.
4  Ethical dilemmas in this field can have major consequences for victims and their families. It is critical to first understand legal parameters. From there, consider the source of other influences: personal beliefs, employer priorities, safety concerns, and more. How and when do you allow these areas to influence your work? What can you do to manage your own biases?

## References

Ahrens, C. E., Stansell, J., & Jennings, A. (2010). To tell or not to tell: The impact of disclosure on sexual assault survivors' recovery. *Violence and Victims, 25,* 631–648.

Barrick, K., Krebs, C. P., & Lindquist, C. H. (2013). Intimate partner violence victimization among undergraduate women at Historically Black Colleges and Universities (HBCUs). *Violence Against Women, 19,* 1014. https://doi.org/10.1177/1077801213499243

Barrios, V. R., Khaw, L. B. L., Bermea, A., & Hardesty, J. L. (2020). Future direction in intimate partner violence research: An intersectionality framework for analyzing women's processes of leaving abusive relationships. *Journal of Interpersonal Violence, 36*(23–24), 1–26.

Bates, E. A. (2020). No one would ever believe me: An exploration of the impact of intimate partner violence victimization on men. *Psychology of Men & Masculinities, 21*(4), 497–507. https://doi.org/10.1037/men0000206

Black, B. M., Chido, L. M., Prebele, K. M., Weisz, A. N., Yoon, J. S., Delaney-Black, V., Kersnmith, P., & Lewandowski, L. (2015). Violence exposure and teen dating violence among African American youth. *Journal of Interpersonal Violence, 30*(12), 2174–2195. https://doi.org/10.1177/0886260514552271

Black, B. M., Tolman, R. M., Callahan, M., Saunders, D. G., & Weisz, A. N. (2008). When will adolescents tell someone about dating violence victimization? *Violence Against Women, 14*(7), 741–758.

Black, M. C., Basile, K. C., Breiding, M. J., Smith, S. G., Walters, M. L., Merrick, M. T., Chen, J., & Stevens, M. (2011). *The national intimate partner and sexual violence survey: 2010 summary report.* https://stacks.cdc.gov/view/cdc/11637

Boethius, S., Akerstrom, M., & Hyden, M. (2022). The double-edged sword—Abused women's experiences of digital technology. *European Journal of Social Work.* https://doi.org/10.1080/13691457.2022.2040437

Bossarte, R. M., Swahn, M. H., & Breidling, M. (2009). Racial, ethnic, and sex differences in associations between violence and self-reported health among US high school students. *Journal of School Health, 79,* 74–81.

Bradford, K., Barber, B. K., Olsen, J. A., Maughan, S. L., Erickson, L. D., Ward, D., & Stolz, H. E. (2003). A multi-national study of interparental conflict, parenting, and adolescent functioning. *Marriage and Family Review, 35*(3–4), 107–137. https://doi.org/10.1300/J002v35n03_07

Breiding, M. J., Basile, K. C., Smith, S. G., Black, M. C., & Mahendra, R. (2015). *Intimate partner violence surveillance uniform definitions and recommended data elements.* Version 2.0. Center for Disease Control and Prevention, National Center for Injury Prevention and Control. https://www.cdc.gov/intimate-partner-violence/about/index.html

Carpenter, G.L. & Stacks, A.M. (2009). Developmental effects of exposure to intimate partner violence in early childhood: A review of the literature. *Children and Youth Services Review, 31,* 831–839. https://doi.org/10.1016/j.childyouth.2009.03.005

Centers for Disease Control [CDC]. (2024). *Fast facts: Preventing intimate partner violence.* https://www.cdc.gov/intimate-partner-violence/about/index.html

Cheung, S. P., & Huang, C. C. (2023). Childhood exposure to intimate partner violence and teen dating violence. *Journal of Family Violence, 38,* 263–274. https://doi.org/10.1007/s10896-022-00377-7

Cooper, A., & Smith, E. L. (2001). *Homicide trends in the United States, 1980–2008.* https://www.bjs.gov/content/pub/pdf/htus8008.pdf.

DeAngelis, T. (2019). The legacy of trauma. *American Psychological Association, 50*(2), 36. https://www.apa.org/monitor/2019/02/legacy-trauma

De Heer, B., & Jones, L. (2017). Measuring sexual violence on campus: Climate surveys and vulnerable groups. *Journal of School Violence, 16*(2), 207–221. https://doi.org/10.1080/15388220.2017.1284444

Freyd, J. J. (1999). Blind to betrayal: New perspectives on memory for trauma. *The Harvard Mental Health Letter, 15*(12), 4–6.

Gómez, J. M., & Freyd, J. J. (2018). Psychological outcomes of within-group sexual violence: Evidence of cultural betrayal. *Journal of Immigrant and Minority Health, 20,* 1458–1467. https://doi.org/10.1007/s10903-017-0687-0

Gómez, J. M., & Freyd, J. J. (2019). Betrayal trauma. In J. J. Ponzetti (Ed.), *Macmillan encyclopedia of intimate and family relationships: An interdisciplinary approach* (pp. 79–82). Cengage Learning Inc.

Hahn, J. W., McCormick, M. C., Silverman, J. G., Robinson, E. B., & Koenen, K. C. (2014). Examining the impact of disability status on intimate partner violence victimization in a population sample. *Journal of Interpersonal Violence, 29,* 3063. https://doi.org/10.1177/0886260514534527

Henry, R. R., & Zeytinoglu, S. (2012). African Americans and teen dating violence. *The American Journal of Family Therapy, 40*(1), 20–32. https://doi.org/10.1080/01926187.2011.578033

Herman, J. (2015). *Trauma and recovery: The aftermath of violence—From domestic abuse to political terror.* Basic Books.

Huang, C. C., Vikse, J. H., Lu, S., & Yi, S. (2015). Children's exposure to intimate partner violence and early delinquency. *Journal of Family Violence, 30,* 953–965. https://doi.org/10.1007/s10896-015-9727-5

Huang, C., Wang, L. R., & Warrener, C. (2010). Effects of domestic violence on behavior problems of pre-school aged children: Do maternal mental health and parenting mediate the effects? *Children and Youth Services Review, 32*(10), 1317–1323.

Hughes, K., Bellis, M. A., Hardcastle, K. A., Sethi, D., Butchart, A., Mikton, C., Jones, L., Dunne, M. P. (2017). The effect of multiple adverse childhood experiences on health: A systematic review and meta-analysis. *The Lancet, 2*(8), e356–e366.

Human Rights Campaign. (2022). *Understanding intimate partner violence in the LGBTQ+ community.* https://www.hrc.org/resources/understanding-intimate-partner-vilence-in-the-lgbtq-community

Huntley, A., Potter, L., Williamson, E., Malpass, A., Szilassy, E., & Feder, G. (2019). Help seeking by male victims of domestic violence and abuse (DVA): A systematic review and qualitative evidence synthesis. *BMJ Open, 9,* 1–13. https://doi.org/10.1136/bmjopen-2018-021960

Jacques-Tiura, A. J., Tkatch, R., Abbey, A., & Wegner, R. (2010). Disclosure of sexual assault: Characteristics and implications for posttraumatic stress symptoms among African-American and Caucasian survivors, *National Institutes of Health, 11*(2), 174–192. https://doi.org/10.1080/15299730903502938

Johnson M. P. (1995). Patriarchal terrorism and common couple violence: Two forms of violence against women. *Journal of Marriage and Family, 57,* 283–294.

Johnson, M. P. (2008). *A typology of domestic violence: Intimate terrorism, violent resistance, and situational couple violence.* Northeastern University Press. ISBN: 9781555536947.

Johnson, M. P., & Leone, J. M. (2005). The differential effects of intimate terrorism and situation couple violence: Findings from the National Violence Against Women Survey. *Journal of Family Issues, 26.* 322. https://doi.org/10.1177/0192513X04270345

Jordan, C. E., Combs, J. L., & Smith, G. T. (2014). An exploration of sexual victimization and academic performance among college women. *Trauma, Violence, & Abuse, 15,* 191–200. https://doi.org/10.1177/1524838014520637

Jouriles, E. N., McDonald, R., Smith Slep, A. M., Heyman, R. E., & Garrido, E. (2008). Child abuse in the context of domestic violence: Prevalence, explanations, and practice implications. *Violence and Victims, 23*(2), 221–235.

Kalmakis, K. A., & Chandler, G. E. (2015). Health consequences of adverse childhood experiences: A systematic review. *Journal of the American Association of Nurse Practitioners, 27*(8), 457–465.

Karlsson, M. E., Temple, J. R., Weston, R., & Le, V. D. (2016). Witnessing interparental violence and acceptance of dating violence as predictors for teen dating violence victimization. *Violence Against Women, 22*(5), 625–646. https://doi.org/10.1177/1077801215605920

Leemis, R. W., Friar, N., Khatiwada, S., Chen, M. S., Kresnow, M. J., Smith, S. G., Caslin, S., & Basile, K. C. (2022). *The national intimate partner and sexual violence survey: 2016/2017 report on intimate partner violence.* National Center for Injury Prevention and Control, Centers for Disease Control and Prevention.

Lysova, A., Hanson, K., Dixon, L., Douglas, E. M., Hines, D. A., & Celi, E. M. (2022). Internal and External Barriers to Help Seeking: Voices of Men Who Experienced Abuse in the Intimate Relationships. *International journal of offender therapy and comparative criminology*, 66(5), 538–559. https://doi.org/10.1177/0306624X20919710

Machado, A., Hines, D., & Douglas, E. M. (2020). Male victims of female-perpetrated partner violence: A qualitative analysis of men's experiences, the impact of violence, and perceptions of their worth. *Psychology of Men & Masculinities*, 21(4), 612–621. https://doi.org/10.1037/men0000285

Mercy, J. A., Hillis, S. D., Butchart, A., Bellis, M. A., Ward, C. L., Fang, X., & Rosenberg, M. L. (2017). Interpersonal violence: Global impact and paths to prevention. In C. N. Mock, R. Nugent, & O. Kobusingye et al. (eds), *Injury Prevention and Environmental Health* (3rd ed., Chapter 5). The International Bank for Reconstruction and Development/The World Bank. https://www.ncbi.nlm.nih.gov/books/NBK525208/

Murugan, V. (2022). Intimate Partner Violence in an Orthodox Jewish Community in the United States: A Qualitative Exploration of Community Members' Perspectives. *Violence Against Women*, 29(6–7), 1368–1390. https://doi.org/10.1177/10778012221120444

National Coalition Against Domestic Violence [NCADV]. (2017). *Quick guide: Economic and financial abuse.* https://ncadv.org/blog/posts/quick-guide-economic-and-financial-abuse

National Coalition Against Domestic Violence [NCADV]. (2018). *Domestic violence and people with disabilities: What to know, why it matters, and how to help.* https://ncadv.org/blog/posts/domestic-violence-and-people-with-disabilities

National Coalition Against Domestic Violence [NCADV]. (n.d.). *Dynamics of abuse.* https://ncadv.org/dynamics-of-abuse

National Network to End Domestic Violence [NNEDV]. (2017). *Immigration policy.* https://nnedv.org/content/immigration-policy/

National Resource Center on Domestic Violence. (n.d.). *Overview: Faith, spirituality, religion, and domestic violence.* https://vawnet.org/sc/faith-based-and-multi-cultural-resources

Nelson, C. A., Scott, R. D., Bhutta, Z. A., Harris, N. B., Danese, A., & Samara, M. (2020). Adversity in childhood is linked to mental and physical health throughout life. *BMJ (Clinical research ed.)*, 371, m3048. https://doi.org/10.1136/bmj.m3048

Office on Violence Against Women (OVW). (2023). *Domestic Violence.* Department of Justice. https://www.justice.gov/ovw/domestic-violence

Ogle, C. M., Rubin, D. C., & Siegler, I. C. (2014). Cumulative exposure to traumatic events in older adults. *Aging Mental Health*, 18(3), 316–324. https://doi.org/10.1080/13607863.2013.832730

Overup, C. S., Dibello, A. M., Brunson, J. A., Acitelli, L. K., & Neighbors, C. (2015). Addictive Behaviors Drowning the pain: Intimate partner violence and drinking to cope prospectively predict problem drinking. *Addictive Behaviors*, 41, 152–161.

Postmus, J. L., McMahon, S., Silva-Martinez, E., & Warrener, C. D. (2014). Exploring the challenges faced by Latinas experiencing intimate partner violence. *Affilia*, 29, 462. https://doi.org/10.1177/0886109914522628

Postmus, J. L., Plummer, S. B., McMahon, S., Murshid, N. S., & Kim, M. S. (2012). Understanding economic abuse in the lives of survivors. *Journal of Interpersonal Violence*, 27, 411. https://doi.org/10.1177/0886260511421669

Puzzanchera, C. (2022). *Dating violence reported by high school students, 2019.* Office of Juvenile Justice and Delinquency Prevention. https://ojjdp.ojp.gov/library/publications/dating-violence-reported-high-school-students-2019

RAINN. (2024). *Perpetrators of sexual violence: Statistics.* https://www.rainn.org/statistics/perpetrators-sexual-violence

Reese, E. M., Barlow, M. J., Dillon, M., Villalon, S., Barnes, M. D., & Crandall, A. (2022). Intergenerational transmission of trauma: The mediating effects of family health. *International Journal of Environmental Research and Public Health*, 19(10), 5944. https://doi.org/10.3390/ijerph19105944

Sacchi, L., Merzhvynska, M., & Augsburger, M. (2020). Effects of cumulative trauma load on long-term trajectories of life satisfaction and health in a population-based study. *BMC Public Health, 20*, 1612. https://doi.org/10.1186/s12889-020-09663-9

Stark, E. (2007). *Coercive control: How men entrap women in personal life.* Oxford University Press.

Truman, J. L., & Morgan, R. E. (2014). *Nonfatal domestic violence, 2003–2012.* https://www.bjs.gov/content/pub/pdf/ndv0312.pdf

Tsui, V., Cheung, M., & Leung, P. (2010). Help-seeking among male victims of partner abuse: Men's hard times. *Journal of Community Psychology, 38*(6), 769–780.

U.S. Department of Veterans Affairs. (2022). *Complex PTSD.* PTSD: National Center for PTSD. https://www.ptsd.va.gov/professional/treat/essentials/complex_ptsd.asp#one

U.S. Department of Veterans Affairs. (2024). *Racial trauma.* PTSD: National Center for PTSD. https://www.ptsd.va.gov/understand/types/racial_trauma.asp

Van der Kolk, B. A. (2015). *The body keeps the score: Brain, mind, and body in the healing of trauma.* Viking.

Velonis, A. J. (2016). "He never did anything you typically think of as abuse": Experiences with violence in controlling and non-controlling relationships in a non-agency sample of women. *Violence Against Women, 22*(9), 1031–1054. https://doi.org/10.1177/1077801215618805

Voth Schrag, R. J. (2015). Economic abuse and later material hardship: Is depression a mediator? *Affilia, 30*(3), 341–351. https://doi.org/10.1177/0886109914541118

Walsh, K., Dilillo, D., & Messman-moore, T. L. (2012). Lifetime sexual victimization and poor risk perception: Does emotion dysregulation account for the links? *Journal of Interpersonal Violence, 27*(15), 3054–3071. https://doi.org/10.1177/0886260512441081

Warrener, C., & Koivunen, J. M. (2014). The complex nature of serving divorced and separated women: A qualitative analysis of needs and service provision. *Families in Society, 94*(4), 245–252.

Warrener, C., Koivunen, J., & Postmus, J. L. (2013). Economic self-sufficiency among divorced women: Impact of depression, abuse, and efficacy. *Journal of Divorce and Remarriage, 54*(2), 163–175.

Wasserman, J., & McGuire, K. (2024, January 29). *Unwanted consensual sex: The socially sanctioned indoctrination of submission.* Continuing education presentation, Rutgers, the State University of New Jersey, Zoom.

Wood, L., Voth Schrag, R., & Busch-Armendariz, N. (2020). Mental health and academic impacts of interpersonal violence among IHE-attending women. *Journal of American College Health, 68*(3), 286–293.

Yoo, J. A., & Huang, C. C. (2012). The effects of domestic violence on children's behavior problems: Assessing the moderating roles of poverty and marital status. *Children and Youth Services Review, 34*, 2464–2473.

Zinzow, H. M., Resnick, H. S., McCauley, J. L., Amstadter, A. B., Ruggiero, K. J., & Kilpatrick, D. G. (2010). The role of rape tactics in risk for posttraumatic stress disorder and major depression: Results from a national study. *Depression & Anxiety, 27*, 708–715.

# 5 The Power of Play

## Exploring the Efficacy of Play Therapy in Child Abuse Cases

*Michelle M. Pliske*

Maria entered the play therapy room for her first visit with her head down. Her dark hair fell to cover most of her face, and she never spoke directly to me. Maria looked around the room and proceeded to sit on the sofa. She seemed to wait. I introduced myself and the room, and then offered the room for exploration as she wanted.

> This is a room where you get to be you. You can do whatever you need or want to do and I'm here with you. You get to choose here, and you never have to do something you don't want to do. This room is ours and this time is yours.

Maria sat for several moments before glancing up. I smiled and gave her a nod of encouragement. Maria walked through the play therapy room, selecting a princess miniature and placing it in the sand. Maria created a bedroom scene using furniture from the dollhouse. She added a wooden door, bed, and small desk with a globe on top. A large dragon was placed outside the door. She systematically put the princess on the bed and moved the dragon to enter the room. The dragon slowly circled the room, with Maria making hissing sounds from the dragon and then whimpering sounds from the princess. Maria placed the dragon on top of the princess. She stared at the scene as it was displayed, staring at it as if she were staring into an abyss.

Maria, a seven-year-old Latina child, was referred by the local forensic interviewing team. Her interview had been inconclusive because she wouldn't answer the team's questions— she simply wouldn't speak to anyone at all. Maria had regressed in her development. Two years prior she was described as a happy child with spunk and spirit. Maria's mother, Sara, reported she was a shell of her former self. Sara's presentation during the initial assessment was one of deep reserve with mild hostility. Sara described receiving "no help for Maria." She didn't understand why the pediatrician had sent Maria to be interviewed at the hospital. Sara was unsure what was happening to her child, and no one explained to her what the problem was, nor could they provide any solutions. Maria had seen two other mental health providers. The first provider closed Maria's case at the onset of the treatment because she wouldn't answer questions or talk during the assessment. The provider concluded therapy wouldn't be helpful until she was older or became willing to communicate. The second provider charged exorbitant rates, with policies requiring weekly sessions, and did not accept health insurance for payment of services. Sara worked two jobs, and her commute to and from work was lengthy. She rode two buses, connected to the light rail system, and then rode another bus to get to her morning job at a restaurant. Sara returned home from her shift at the restaurant to sleep for a couple of hours before starting her second job cleaning offices at night. Sara's frustration over finding a provider was clearly articulated. The cost of care and finding support to get Maria to and from appointments was staggering.

DOI: 10.4324/9781003531258-7

## Pediatric Abuse and Trauma

Children arrive at therapy for an array of reasons linked to trauma. Some referrals to human service counseling professionals may be in response to a serious medical illness or accident, natural disaster, significant traumatic loss of a parent or loved one, physical or sexual abuse, or community violence or experiences related to bullying. Children may have experienced a single traumatic event (e.g., loss of home due to a wildfire, severe car accident), or they may seek help because of chronically stressful and adverse experiences over time (e.g., child sexual abuse, neglect, domestic violence). Long-term outcomes for children vary depending upon protective factors in places such as community and social supports or resources available to the child and the nature of the trauma or adverse experiences (Pliske et al., 2021). The paucity of mental health resources to meet the current demand for pediatric services is alarming the social service community. Data clearly demonstrates that pediatric behavioral health problems are increasing exponentially in the United States, with rising demand for services to address depression, anxiety, and trauma among children, an escalating trend expected to extend well beyond the effects of the COVID-19 pandemic (Chien et al., 2022). The trend is more troubling because the data also shows a steady decline in human service specialists who treat pediatric mental health conditions, despite federal legislation designed to expand access to behavioral healthcare (The Mental Health Parity and Addiction Equity Act of 2008; the Patient Protection and Affordable Care Act of 2010). Finally, the small pool of pediatric behavioral health providers across the United States who work within systems or independent practices is unaffordable for most families (Chien et al., 2022; Graaf et al., 2022), limiting available specialists even further for vulnerable populations.

Mental health professionals specializing in pediatrics face a complex set of challenges when they are tasked with assessment and intervention for pediatric abuse and trauma. These cases require more time and resources from the provider, compared to mental health professionals working with adult survivors of childhood abuse. Pediatric abuse and trauma cases require multisystemic intervention, taking considerable time, much of which is often unpaid for the rendering service professional. Providers must collaborate frequently with the family system (e.g., parent consultation and family therapy, phone calls, written communication). Collaboration is necessary with the child's school system, allied healthcare professionals (e.g., primary care provider, medical specialists depending upon injury, psychiatry), and often work extends into the judicial system. To excel in pediatrics, one needs specialized skills, in-depth knowledge, and extensive supervised training, commonly gained through postgraduate professional development, conferences, and certification. The time and cost to acquire specialized pediatric mental health training for counseling and social work professionals is a deterrent for providers who are not adequately compensated for their time, additional training, and use of play equipment. Pediatric mental health providers must work to develop a trauma framework to identify factors associated with early exposure to adversity or adverse childhood experiences (ACEs).

### Adverse Childhood Experiences

A child's capacity to express their full potential across social, relational, and cognitive domains is related to how the brain organizes the child's perception of challenge within their developmental experience (Perry & Hambrick, 2008; Solomon & Siegel, 2003). Studies in pediatric trauma identify several phenomena of post-traumatic stress-related symptoms unique to children. These include regressive behaviors to earlier developmental stages, nightmares that may generalize into less specific monsters or childhood fantasy, post-traumatic play in which children re-enact the trauma, daydreaming or dissociation, difficulties concentrating, academic underachievement, and a marked change in attitude about the future (Gil, 2017). Terr (1981) first coined the term "posttraumatic play" in pediatric populations following research with survivors of traumatic incidents, most notably the data acquired from the longitudinal study of children kidnapped in Chowchilla, California. Her clinical observations yielded a unique type of play. This play was repetitive, rigid, literal, and devoid of all pleasure and failed to produce the typical gains play provided children in problem-solving or the decreasing of anxiety states (Terr, 1992). Play typically offers a release for most children, but for some traumatized children it serves as a cage. Terr (1981) summarized, providers may see any or all of the following play behaviors:

*Repetition of play:* Play behaviors will become compulsive and unrelenting. The child often finds it difficult to stop playing through the trauma narrative.

*Literal quality of the play:* Play can provide children with an escape into metaphor. Pretending for children is buried in the metaphor, and the child may never realize that the protagonist of their story is really themselves. They are lost entirely within the metaphor of play and work through thoughts, emotions, and future scenarios within that play. Traumatized children can become stuck within their play, failing to translate their stories into fluid metaphors. The post-traumatic play does little to satisfy the child and will become monotonous, often grim, and overly specific. The play is literal and rigid.

*Play and trauma have an unconscious link:* Klein (1975) proposed theories for how play revealed the unconscious mind. Approaching play in a similar way to how we might interpret dreams suggested an opportunity to access the child's unconscious mind or provide an avenue for children to engage in free association. Trauma experiences can hold unconscious content associated with implicit memory networks. These memory networks have fragmented sensory and emotional states, such as imagery, sounds, and physical sensations, often disorganized or lacking a logical narrative, as one would ascertain from an explicit memory network.

*Play fails to relieve anxiety or states of stress:* The quality of play holds intensity and doesn't offer a release from emotions that typically comes within play. Children don't feel better after playing, and the play is largely devoid of positive emotions, humor, or any joy.

*Play may be dangerous:* Reenactments of relationships or trauma experiences within post-traumatic play can place the child or others at risk. Therapists need to have appropriate training prior to taking on pediatric trauma cases. Early career professionals should have clear guidance or supervision to support their professional growth. Providers will need to understand the process of therapeutic limit setting to support not only the child but also other children attending subsequent sessions (Ray, 2011). The provider or child should not be placed in a situation where one or the other could become injured in the play therapy process. Finally, the provider must continuously be aware of how dangerous play might alter or negatively affect the therapeutic relationship (Ray, 2011).

Traumatic early childhood experiences have been expanded over recent years to include trauma outside of familial settings (Finkelhor et al., 2015) and expanded further beyond the type of trauma and loss within familial settings to include bullying, incarceration of any type, parental loss, adoption, foster care involvement, immigration, or issues associated with oppression and racism (Pliske et al., 2021). Abuse, trauma, neglect, and other adversity reorganize the developing brain and create a range of serious emotional and behavioral issues, along with cognitive deficits that impact growth and learning (Panksepp & Biven, 2012; van der Kolk, 2014). ACEs are often dosage dependent; the greater the number of ACEs one acquires, the more likely one will develop serious physical and mental health complications later in life (Burke Harris, 2018). Peterson et al. (2023) identified current data as an estimated 160 million of the total 255 million U.S. adult population (63%) who have one or more ACEs. These ACEs are associated with an annual economic burden of $14.1 trillion ($183 billion in direct medical spending and $13.9 trillion in lost healthy life-years) (Peterson et al., 2023). This data relies heavily on victim reporting, and if we factor in community-based trauma (e.g., mass shooting events, natural disasters, gang violence), intangible costs increase as the overall estimated cost of child maltreatment escalates. The impact of trauma is further compounded by the conditions in which children live; those social determinants of health will influence the trajectory and outcome of care.

### Social Determinants of Health

Social determinants of health are most widely recognized as the conditions in which people are born, grow, work, live, and age and include the wider set of forces shaping the conditions of our daily life (World Health Organization, 2024). These forces include economic policies, social policies, and political systems. Health inequalities are connected to the following: income, social protections, education, unemployment, job insecurity, working life conditions, food insecurity, housing, basic amenities, the environmental stressors, early childhood development, social inclusion, discrimination, structural conflict, and access to affordable health services (World Health Organization, 2024).

We understand that where children live and grow influences their physical and emotional health. The conditions encompassed by the WHO's definition of social determinants of health are often predetermined based on an individual's or community's access to money, power, and resources, which are influenced by local and global policy choices (National Academies of Sciences, Engineering & Medicine, 2016). The cumulative impact of multi-system trauma results in a greater need to access healthcare, and children living in families with lower socioeconomic statuses who need mental healthcare already face difficulty finding available providers (Graaf et al., 2022). Parents experiencing economic hardship often sacrifice their own health needs, delaying or skipping necessary medical care because of financial stress. The best predictor for a child's success is a parent who can attend to their needs and co-regulate when faced with extreme stress and uncertainty. Social and economic policies which erode stability and safety for American children and their families further strain disenfranchised populations. Healthcare should be a human right. Access to healthcare for children, which is affordable, equitable, developmentally appropriate, culturally inclusive, and delivered by highly trained and specialized pediatric mental health providers, is a fundamental necessity to improve outcomes.

Maria's records from her previous mental health providers elucidated very little insight into her previous assessments or sessions. The first provider's records described Sara as unaware of and lacking insight into her daughter and described Maria as non-compliant with the assessment, concluding that Maria was a poor candidate for treatment. The second provider's records were sparse, lacking a treatment plan or a complete assessment. The progress notes from sessions were all the same, with no variation in wording or description. This provider described during a phone conversation that sessions were like "talking at a brick wall." The provider reported that the mother was uninvolved and lazy, rarely coming to the appointments herself. Maria was brought by a neighbor or grandmother, neither of whom spoke English. The provider stated Maria sat on the sofa "like a lump on a log" and said nothing. She reported asking Maria questions about why she wet the bed and tried to verbally pry out what happened to cause her current state. The provider stated she had coloring crayons for kids and a few fidget toys to play with during the session, but Maria never wanted to color or play with those items. The provider ended the call, stating, "She is such an unhappy child. I'm sure if her mother were a more involved parent she wouldn't need therapy."

Maria's mother appeared to be caught in a cycle of powerlessness and oppression. Examining the family's social determinants of health, Maria and Sara were facing multiple barriers. Maria lived in an unsafe neighborhood, as the family compromised safety for affordable housing. The neighborhood lacked access to greenspaces and outdoor play areas, resulting in a childhood which didn't offer the same accommodations as wealthier families who live on cooler tree-lined streets with parks to extend their living space. Sara worked constantly. She had to choose between working so that she and Maria could live or take time off to attend therapy appointments. Taking time off work risked the loss of employment, which threatened their entire existence. The second provider characterized Sara as uninvolved and lazy for not attending treatment with her child. The reality was that Sara worked hard to the point of physical and emotional exhaustion. These providers failed both Maria and Sara due to a lack of sociocultural insight and clinical expertise. Sara was clearly devoted to her child, found ways to budget for therapy copays (solutions which often meant she missed meals or cut back on personal necessities), and desperately wanted to understand what happened to change Maria so drastically.

### Play Therapy to Foster Emotional Expression and Trauma Processing

Play therapy is a developmentally appropriate form of mental health service delivery which offers children an environment of safety to express their emotions, thoughts, and ideas. Play can be described as a neural exercise enabling co-regulation of the physiological state to promote optimization of neurophysiological states for mental and physical health (Porges, 2024). Early views of play emphasized its use as building skills, assimilating information from the environment to develop new ideas or constructs about how the world works, and that it created a bridge between concrete and abstract thought. Maria Montessori posited that play, movement, and cognition were closely entwined; movement therefore enhanced thinking and learning, and, when children were given a sense of control, it improved emotional well-being (Lillard, 2007). Furthermore, when children were interested in what they were learning, the likelihood of success in learning increased. Hypotheses from evolutionary biologists and zoologists studying play across species argue that play enhanced juvenile connective tissues, nervous system functioning, and cardiovascular systems, providing motor development training for the organism (Toomey, 2024). Furthermore, these hypotheses offer play's ability to contribute to brain development as youth environments serve to shape the brain's function through synaptic pruning (nature's "waste not, want not" viewpoint on life) (Toomey, 2024). Play supports the brain in developing the knowledge of how much we can do and how well we can accomplish the task, gaming out risks or dangerous situations within imagination or through metaphor. Children can create possibilities for a future that has never existed through their play, problem-solving, or building strategies for how to regulate heightened emotions of stress within play sequences (Brown, 2010). Play and playfulness need not end during childhood. Adults who continue to engage in forms of play find a greater appreciation for life and a pathway toward supporting emotional regulation and problem-solving (Pliske et al., 2021). Once one experiences and appreciates play activities, a "satisfaction from it even when youth is gone" (Toomey, 2024, p. 27) will continue to be possible.

Virginia Axline (1974) furthered the conversation of play as therapy based upon the fact that play was the child's natural medium of self-expression. Play offered the opportunity for a child to express their feelings and problems just as adults did in traditional talk psychotherapy. Creating an environment specifically designed for children to engage in self-discovery, learn new tools for navigating stress, and regulate distress within relationships was the vehicle for health and recovery. Play offered children the opportunity to move through difficult content or revisit the experiences which brought them to therapy, and play environments also brought respite from the emotions and memories of their lived experiences. Play therapy can serve as an avenue to experience positive emotions, increasing the child's life satisfaction, coping skills, their view of self and others, and overall well-being, and create a deeper appreciation for being with another person (Kottman, 2014).

### Assessment and Treatment Planning

Children impacted by abuse and trauma require intentional planning for the assessment process. The initial visit should be a meeting with the child's parents independently to gather pertinent information about the child and the circumstances of the case. This ensures that the child is not being exposed to further traumatic details, events, or the parent's perspective of the child and their trauma encounter(s). The initial appointment with either a single parent or multiple caregivers allows for a detailed history of the child's development, family dynamics, parent histories, medical histories, educational functioning, abuse and trauma histories, risk inventories, and any current or future court involvement. This first session is the play therapist's moment to not only gather relevant biopsychosocial histories but also connect with the child's parent to form an alliance. Trust within multi-stressed families is not freely given. Children are embedded in their environments; therefore, it is crucial to forge a strong working relationship with the parent. This relationship and trust will serve as the conduit for psychoeducation and skill-building to be received and implemented, thereby amplifying the effect of therapy outside of the playroom.

The assessment process for trauma treatment must include gathering information about the child's strengths, already-established coping mechanisms, and how the child perceives themselves (capacity for self-empathy). Therapists explore parent concerns but also elicit information from the parent about what the parent views as positive qualities in their child. Parents who struggle to identify positive attributes or qualities about their child offer important insight to the play therapist about the child's worldview and the potentially established attachment patterns. It is imperative to engage in the analysis of history to identify the child's personal strategy for disconnection, meaning what behaviors does the child use to successfully disengage from others? These behavioral patterns are often the reason for referral. A child's behavior typically isn't without reason but rather has a clear purpose. That purpose may not be fully understood by the child (it is not uncommon for parents to perceive their child as purposefully lying or that they are manipulative); instead if a provider shifts their thinking of these behaviors toward that of a survival strategy, logical assumptions can be made regarding the child's method of self-preservation to overcome challenges. Understanding a child's behaviors involves the provider uncovering where the behaviors may have been learned, what purpose they serve, and how effective they are in meeting the child's needs.

Relational-cultural play therapy assessments identify potential sources of shame, environmental stressors, and negative images represented within the community or larger society that may be influencing the child's perception of self or influencing the parent's perception of the child and family. Systemic oppression, marginalization, and examination of the child's social determinants of health to include inequality allow a play therapy provider to begin building a treatment plan which incorporates larger macrosystem thought and engagement.

The play therapist is simultaneously assessing the parent's history during the assessment process. This is not to form a clinical opinion of the parent but rather to broaden the therapist's knowledge of the child's environment. A therapist needs the knowledge of the family system to provide clarity of the parental relationship, determine if tension or conflict exists, identify the nature or existence of coparenting, and assess parent attachment patterns. The provider assesses for parent-related stressors, which may involve extended family systems (lifespan developmental stressors or ongoing conflicts within larger family systems), work-related stress, and the impact of community- or macrolevel stressors on parent functioning. Family functioning depends on the nature of all individuals within the system and their relationships with one another (Bronfenbrenner, 1979). When parents are anxious and experiencing deep, complex psychosocial stressors, their cerebral cortex (the primary region for thinking, reasoning, and problem-solving) is flooded with anxiety and unable to properly function (Banks, 2015; Gilbert, 2006). When parents are unable to engage in logical problem-solving, anxiety can escalate. The parent's anxiety is perceived by their child, which, in turn, escalates the child's anxiety states. It is not uncommon for parents to cite their child's behaviors in the form of opposition, tantrums, defiance, lying, or manipulation. The root of these behaviors typically lies within anxiety, and a child is simply trying to meet a need which is vacant in their life.

Assessment of the macrolevel policies impacting the child stems from the assessment of the parent and family system. This approach can be thought of as giving context to what is bringing children and families through the door. Providers building a treatment plan utilizing relational-cultural theory to guide their practice will investigate the effects of intersectionality and the impact the larger culture imposes on the family (Jordan, 2018). It is imperative that the provider keep abreast of current rules, regulations, policy, prospective policy changes, and other community variables to know where the child will need advocacy. Treatment plans can offer advocacy at the larger system level through alliances with professional organizations, supporting coalitions working on social system reform in the area directly impacting the provider's clients, participating in leadership roles within a professional discipline, contributing expertise and knowledge through writing amicus briefs, short articles, or writing to legislators.

Maria participated in an extended play-based developmental assessment (Gil, 2011). When Maria created her first sandtray, my reflection to her was "you showed me a story about the princess and the dragon. I heard her make sounds and I wonder if she is ok." Maria whispered, "It hurts her" and put each toy carefully back where she found them. She spent the remaining session using the kitchen set and toy food, making meals for a puppet shaped like a queen. The first several sessions provided Maria with the time she needed to engage in play freely. This approach was designed to determine Maria's overall functioning, identify current clinical symptoms, recognize cultural variables and sources of shame or negative images which represent her social identities contributing to psychosocial stress and trauma impact, and assess her perception of parental support and guidance. Finally, I wanted to determine Maria's perceptions of her internal and external resources. Maria had been through multiple interviews with pediatricians, child protection workers, forensic interviewers, two mental health providers, and her mother. She had been questioned repeatedly. It was reasonable to assume this child was scared, disoriented, and confused.

Two providers had seen her and disappeared, placing Maria in a position where she may have felt distrustful toward another helping professional. I entered the process knowing her social identities and my own were divergent, coupled with the knowledge about rotating providers and interviewers, which led me to utilize a relational-cultural extended play-based assessment model. Providing Maria with an environment which was predictable, consistent, and supportive created a gateway for her to make sense of her world and what happened to her. During this assessment process, I learned that Maria wanted to care for and nurture others. She was protective of family, was deeply religious, believed rules were to be obeyed, and created lush garden landscapes for her characters to spend time in. Every space she created was invaded by the dragon. The dragon was clever, tricking all the adults in the land, was sneaky, and told terrible lies. The dragon claimed that no one would believe any story but his. He was powerful and could kill you.

### Developing Trust and Safety with Children

Play can be seen as a function whereby children explore the environment by taking risks. Dangers within creative and imaginative play are problem solved and survived, and connections of belonging and a sense of not having to navigate life alone are actualized through the therapeutic alliance. Providers may disagree on theory or which evidence-based practice is most effective, but all assert that the formation of a relationship is vital to the success of therapy. Simply stated, the relationship matters. This relationship is what will serve as the vehicle that supports a theory's success (or failure). Authenticity is a key component. A provider's confidence with a theory, understanding how the theory is implemented in session, and the ability to feel authentic within their chosen theory are fundamental components to the therapeutic outcome.

### Self-Expression through Metaphorical Play

Regardless of age, we think, speak, and experience our world through metaphors. Metaphors can help structure our thinking or make connections among ideas (Kottman & Meany-Walen, 2018). Children can express their perception of who they are and how they think and feel about their family members, community, and society through play. Traumatized children often tell the same story repeatedly. These stories may have negative perceptions or thoughts about their role and involvement in the traumatic experience. Play therapists evaluate session content, identifying when a reflection can assist with metaphor shifting or to reframe a thought using symbolic language, shifting how the child thinks or feels about specific people, events, relationships, circumstances, or themselves (Kottman & Meany-Walen, 2018). This approach can support a cognitive interweave, targeting post-traumatic symptoms, harnessing the power of metaphor to challenge negative thinking patterns about the trauma and their conceptualization of how the trauma unfolded.

### Therapeutic Art and Storytelling

Traumatized children can be offered a chance to express their emotions and story through therapeutic art and storytelling. Art can be an original creation by the child using a variety of art mediums, it can be created through existing images (e.g., Dixit cards) or by selecting miniatures to place in a sandtray. Expression through art combines psychological theories and therapeutic art techniques with an understanding of the creative process (Malchiodi,

1998). Many therapists find it challenging to patiently sit and bear witness to the creation of art, the careful selection of images or miniatures; however, refraining from filling the silence with comments or questions provides children the space they need for exploration and discovery. Asking a child why they drew a particular element, selecting a specific image card or miniature, is usually unproductive. Questioning disrupts the flow state, and most children feel compelled to answer the provider's questions out of obligation, training, or schematic experiences from school settings. Children may reach for a meaning or tell the therapist what they think the provider wants to hear to avoid displeasing their provider. When a child has completed their work, rather than "why" questions, the therapist can reflect upon what they see (e.g., "the roots of your tree extend to these people drawn below") instead of asking a direct question (e.g., "why are these people drawn down here below the tree?"). Simple reflections of what is visible without the therapist adding emotion, content, or meaning give the child an opportunity to define these elements for themselves and explore the work at their own pace. When approached from a simple description, the child will frequently add information about their creation. A provider can deepen the reflection on the work by wondering or proposing an idea out loud as if they are narrating their own thoughts. "I wonder what that person could be thinking, considering they are at the top of the tree." These techniques are more effective in eliciting a response from a child. They yield a more productive conversation about the work, and the child remains in control of how information is revealed.

Maria created many sandtrays with imagery but repeatedly returned to the scene she first laid out in the sand. The play held intensity, was repetitive, and fit the context of her life, unifying a theme (Ray, 2011). The princess would be in her bed, and the dragon would enter the room, the dragon made sounds, and the princess's sounds were consistently present, alternating between whimpering and gasping. I named what I saw, offering slight variations of the reflection to return control to Maria or to highlight she wasn't alone (emphasizing the therapeutic relationship). I wondered aloud what the story of the princess would look like if it weren't in the sand. The reflection was to provide Maria with an opening to tell the story in a new way, the goal being to give her room and prevent an excessive cycle of post-traumatic play, which can become toxic if left to continue indefinitely. Maria approached the dress-up clothes and selected a gown (for me), and she wore a dragon mask and tail. Maria placed pillows and blankets from the sofa on the floor. She got a small stool and placed a large stuffed ball shaped like the world on top of the stool. She told me it was time for bed and instructed me that I was to go to sleep. Marie pretended to open a door and come into the room. She whispered, "There you are. Right where I want you." I used a stage whisper, cupping my hand to my mouth, "I don't know what the princess should say." Maria looked at me and said, "You can't say anything at all. He will hurt mama if you do." Maria walked up to me, reached for my neck, and prepared to wrap her hands around it.

I set a limit on her play for safety. "We can pretend in here the dragon puts its hands on my neck. That way everyone stays safe in this room while we tell our story." Maria completed her scene, voicing for the dragon the entire time an awful series of lies and untruths. It was clear someone had hurt Maria physically and sexually, and that it had happened often. After the dragon left, staying in my role as the princess, I announced to the room that as a princess it was my right to tell my story. I had a court of knights and ladies in waiting who would listen to me, so I wasn't alone.

Maria decided to draw a picture during her next session. She drew a picture of a dragon, larger than life, and a small figure. She spent time carefully constructing her image, looking up every so often to see if I was there. Each time she looked up, I stated, "I'm here." After her drawing was completed, Maria pointed to the dragon. "He is a bad man." I nodded and repeated back her words and then added, "She looks small next to him, I can't help but wonder what she needs to feel bigger, safer." Maria looked at her image and stated, "She can't do anything." I examined the picture carefully. "He is much bigger than she is. I think she is doing something. She is surviving, but I still can't help and wonder what she needs." Maria responded, "She needs him to go away." I looked at Maria and offered, "I can see that. What if she told everyone what he did? What if she told and that telling made him smaller and weaker and that is how the princess defeats the dragon?" Maria appeared thoughtful and got up from the art table to make food for the puppet queen.

### Safety and Advocacy

Child abuse involves many people embedded within the system, all working toward a goal of safety. Child protection services (CPS), law enforcement, and the criminal justice system work together in response to an abuse allegation.

Maria arrived at her session and created her story of the princess and the dragon in the sand. She narrated the story, using her metaphor, to describe a queen at work to ensure the kingdom had enough money. The castle was expensive, and the princess needed to be a good girl and follow directions when she was being watched by the neighbor. The neighbor didn't stay in the castle but often left to go to her own castle at night. The neighbor had a pet dragon who came into Maria's castle at night and hurt the princess. She described physical abuse (being choked to the point of loss of consciousness) and repeated sexual abuse. Maria's description was clear, detailed, and identified a perpetrator. I placed several knights outside the sandtray. "These knights have sworn to serve and protect the princess. They will want to ask her questions. The princess can tell her knights what happens in her castle at night and identify the dragon."

I placed a call to CPS outlining the case, her disclosure, and my concerns for Maria's safety. Mandatory reporting falls under the Child Abuse Prevention and Treatment Act, which has been amended several times, reauthorized on June 25, 2003, as the Keeping Children and Families Safe Act. Reporting suspected abuse is a requirement for mental health providers by law. When the referral is made, CPS supervisory staff determines whether the report necessitates further involvement (Van Eys & Beneke, 2012). CPS will follow state policy and procedures and a structural decision-making process to determine if an assignment needs to be made or whether the referral is closed. M. Field (personal communication, November 7, 2023), a past child welfare supervising trainer, outlines three possible options for all calls that come into the child abuse hotline: (1) The information is documented, and a determination is made that the information does not meet statutory criteria to be assessed for child maltreatment or there is not an allegation of child maltreatment. (2) The call of concern does not meet the statutory requirement for assessment, and the family will be referred to a community service agency for support. (3) The information results in an allegation of child maltreatment, and it is assigned to a child protective service for full assessment.

Children may interact with CPS and law enforcement. Law enforcement works closely with the investigative team to determine the criminal allegations of the abuse case. Forensic interviewers are integral to the investigative process. They typically provide a developmentally appropriate, legally defensible, neutral fact-finding interview of the child involved with the allegation (Van Eys & Beneke, 2012). Suspected child abuse cases involve a medical examination to provide potential physical evidence and evaluate the overall health of the child. Child sexual abuse cases often are crimes that are unseen and usually perpetrated without any outside witnesses; therefore, evidence relies heavily on the child's testimony (Williams et al., 2022). Prosecutors often describe child sexual abuse cases with offenders who target children because the child does not comprehend the acts perpetrated. These perpetrators may spend time grooming the child to endure the sexual abuse. Therefore, the child's testimony may reflect confusion about the events, reflect feelings of shame or self-blame, become distorted by negative cognitions not uncommon to post-traumatic stress, or be delayed by fear of the consequences of a disclosure (Williams et al., 2022). Children may not disclose their abuse if the perpetrator makes threats to harm the child or another family member.

Child safety in abuse cases is paramount, and members of the system work collaboratively to reach this goal. The district attorney or prosecution will work with the child's mental health provider and can prepare that provider to testify at trial. Mental health providers cannot testify in criminal cases on the child's behalf, but they may be asked to testify about the disclosures a child made during the course of treatment (Van Eys & Beneke, 2012). Children may be assigned a family advocate or a guardian ad litem to support them throughout the process and serve to protect and represent the interests of the child who is incapable of representing themselves due to their status as a minor.

Maria disclosed the physical and sexual abuse to child protection workers, forensic interviewers, and the detectives assigned to her case. She provided a clear testimony during the court process, identifying her perpetrator as the son of their neighbor providing childcare who lived in the same apartment complex while Sara worked her second shift. When Maria fell asleep, the neighbor often went across the hall to her own apartment to read and watch television, thinking Maria was asleep for the night. This left Maria alone and vulnerable. She was systematically abused and threatened repeatedly. She remained silent out of fear that her mother would be harmed or angry with her because of her behavior. Maria created a new image in the sand following the trial. The princess was not alone and surrounded by help and protection. The dragon was dead and would never harm the princess again (Figure 5.1).

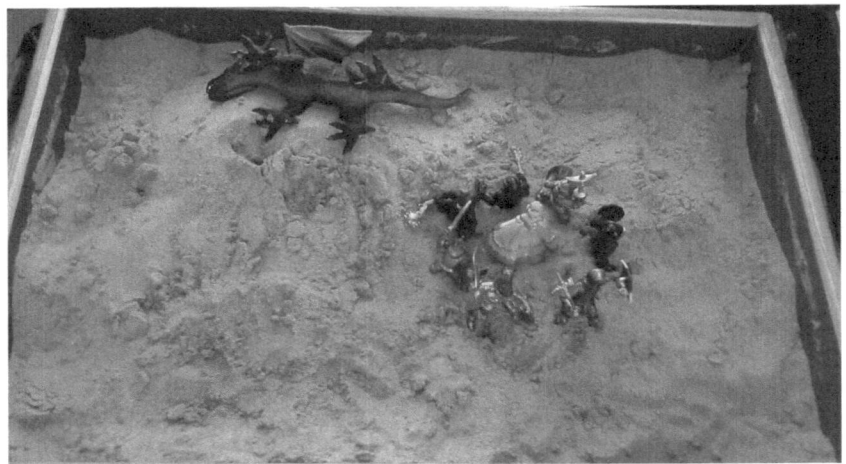

*Figure 5.1* Maria's final sandtray: safety and empowerment.

## Conclusion

Giving children access to play provides them with their right to understand the world. Access to healthcare systems for traumatized youth and families requires activism and action from social workers and human service professionals. Policy reform focused on mitigating social determinants of health to prevent compounding stressors for children affected by ACEs, alongside improving access to services that heal individual and community-inflicted wounds, must take priority. The complexity of factors and symptomatology as a result of trauma requires a slowed-down and intentional approach. The rushed medical model focused on brevity and speedy results falls short in pediatrics cases. The extended relational-cultural play-based developmental assessment forms a secure therapeutic relationship where a child experiences authenticity and mutual empathy, illuminating hope that support is accessible and new possibilities for life are possible.

## Reflective Questions for Consideration

1  What role does the therapeutic relationship have in the effectiveness of play therapy with traumatized youth?
2  How can play therapy be anti-oppressive and inclusive to meet the needs of a child and family system who have experienced trauma?
3  What are some challenges you might encounter when implementing play therapy techniques with traumatized youth, and how would you address them?
4  What emotions or reactions do you anticipate experiencing when working with traumatized children, and how will you manage them?
5  How can you ensure that you are practicing self-care as a therapist while working with traumatized youth?

## References

Axline, V. M. (1974). *Play therapy*. Ballantine Books.

Banks, A. (2015). *Wired to connect: The surprising link between brain science and strong, healthy relationships*. Tarcher Penguin.

Bronfenbrenner, U. (1979). *The ecology of human development: Experiments by nature and design*. Harvard University Press.

Brown, S. (2010). *Play: How it shapes the brain, opens the imagination, and invigorates the soul*. Avery.

Burke Harris, N. (2018). *The deepest well: Healing the long-term effects of childhood adversity*. Houghton Mifflin Harcourt.

Chien, A. T., Leyenaar, J., Tomaino, M., Woloshin, S., Leininger, L., Barnett, E. R., McLaren, J. L., & Meara, E. (2022). Difficulty obtaining behavioral health services for children: A national survey of multiphysician practices. *Annals of Family Medicine, 20*(1), 42–50.

Finkelhor, D., Shattuck, A., Turner, H., & Hamby, S. (2015). A revised inventory of adverse childhood experiences. *Child Abuse and Neglect, 45*, 13–21.

Gil, E. (2011). *Extended play based developmental assessment*. Self Esteem Shop.

Gil, E. (2017). *Posttraumatic play in children: What clinicians need to know*. Guilford Press.

Gilbert, R. M. (2006). *The eight concepts of Bowen theory: A new way of thinking about the individual and the group*. Leading Systems Press.

Graaf, G., Baiden, P., Keyes, L., & Boyd, G. (2022). Barriers to mental health services for parents and siblings of children with special health care needs. *Journal of Child and Family Studies, 31*, 881–895. https://doi.org/10.1007/s10826-022-02228-x

Jordan, J. V. (2018). *Relational-cultural therapy* (2nd ed.). American Psychological Association.

Klein, M. (1975). *The psychoanalysis of children.* Delacorte.

Kottman, T. (2014). Positive emotions. In C. E. Schaefer, & A. A. Drewes (Eds.), *The therapeutic powers of play: 20 core agents of change* (pp. 103–120). Wiley.

Kottman, T., & Meany-Walen, K. K. (2018). *Doing play therapy: From building the relationship to facilitating change.* Guilford Press.

Lillard, A. S. (2007). *Montessori: The science behind the genius.* Oxford University Press.

Malchiodi, C. A. (1998). *Understanding children's drawings.* Guilford Press.

National Academies of Sciences, Engineering & Medicine. (2016). *A framework for educating health professionals to address social determinants of health.* Board of Global Health. https://www.nap.edu/21923

Panksepp, J., & Biven, L. (2012). *The archaeology of mind: neuroevolutionary origins of human emotions.* Norton.

Perry, B. D., & Hambrick, E. P. (2008). The neurosequential model of therapeutics. Reclaiming *Children and Youth, 17*(3), 38–43.

Peterson, C., Aslam, M. V., Niolon, P. H., Bacon, S., Bellis, M. A., Mercy, J. A., Florence, C. (2023). Economic burden of health conditions associated with adverse childhood experiences among us adults. *JAMA, 6*(12), 1–11. https://doi.org/10.1001/jamanetworkopen.2023.46323

Pliske, M., Stauffer, S., & Werner-Lin, A. (2021). Healing from adverse childhood experiences through therapeutic powers of play: "I can do it with my hands." *International Journal of Play Therapy, 30*(4), 244–258. https://doi.org/10.1037/pla0000166

Porges, S. W. (2024). Forward: Play therapy through the lens of polyvagal theory. In P. Goodyear-Brown, & L. A. Yasenik (Eds.), *Polyvagal power in the playroom: A guide for play therapists* (pp. xii–xix). Routlege.

Ray, D. C. (2011). *Advanced play therapy: Essential conditions, knowledge, and skills for child practice.* Routledge.

Solomon, M. F., & Siegel, D. J. (2003). *Healing trauma: Attachment, mind, body and brain.* Norton.

Terr, L. (1981). "Forbidden games:" Post-traumatic child's play. *American Journal of Psychiatry, 148*(1), 10–20.

Terr, L. (1992). *Too scared to cry: Psychic trauma in childhood.* Basic Books.

Toomey, D. (2024). *Kingdom of play.* Scribner.

van der Kolk, B. (2014). *The body keeps the score: Brain, mind and body in the healing of trauma.* Penguin Press.

Van Eys, P., & Beneke, B. (2012). Navigating the system: The complexities of the multidisciplinary team in cases of child sexual abuse. In P. Goodyear-Brown (Ed.), *Handbook of child sexual abuse: Identification, assessment, and treatment* (pp. 71–97). Wiley & Sons.

Williams, L. M., Block, S. D., Johnson, H. M., Ramsey, M. G., & Winstead, A. P. (2022, April). Prosecution of child sexual abuse: Challenges in achieving justice. *Wellesley Centers for Women.* https://www.wcwonline.org/Fact-Sheets-Briefs/prosecution-of-child-sexual-abuse-challenges-in-achieving-justice

World Health Organization. (2024). *Social determinants of health: Overview.* https://www.who.int/health-topics/social-determinants-of-health#tab=tab_1

# 6 Digital Community Explorations

## How Can Incel Community Insights Inform Generalist Human Services Practice in the Digital Era?

*Cayetana Calderon-Smith*

## Introduction

Our modern digital era is a great experiment. New technologies—namely, our smartphones, devices, and digital media services—are embedded within many, if not most, domains of living (Rice & Sara, 2019). We currently *connect, communicate*, and *search* with tools that, until quite recently, were relegated to science fiction, specialist laboratories, or the imagination. Consequently, an opportunity exists to explore the emergent, person-scaled technological phenomena of the digital era. This chapter rises to the occasion by inviting Human Services practitioners into the fold.

A "zoom-in, zoom-out" approach scaffolds this broad, generalist endeavor. An initial "zoom-in" reviews the discrete member characteristics of a vulnerable-yet-feared online population, *Incels*. This chapter initially asks *How does a multidisciplinary literature operationalize and engage with Incels?*

A subsequent "zoom out" supports practice and praxis, as a discussion of digital entry pathways to Incel communities is re-deployed for generalist insight. In this section, two questions are asked: (1) *What identified digital phenomena are linked to Incelosphere engagement?* and (2) *Are these insights of relevance to other populations or people?*

Consequently, this chapter is exploratory, translational, theoretical, and non-pathologizing. This approach supports a nuanced discussion of digital-era topics that, across popular culture, are arguably rife with fear-mongering, anxiety, and conflict.

## 1. Let's "Zoom In" to Meet Incels: A Brief Introduction

*Incel* is a portmanteau of the words "involuntary" and "celibate." Members of this digital demographic congregate across independent, anonymous message boards and user-generated social media platforms with others who seek but cannot find a romantic partner. Discrete definitions of "Incel" vary across academic disciplines (Czerwinsky, 2024), as do the self-applied definitions held by Incels themselves (Speckhard et al., 2021).

Though the original Incel community emerged as a welcoming digital self-help space (Kassam, 2018), linkages are well documented between the Men's Rights movements of the 1960s as well as today's digital, loosely affiliated "Manosphere" communities that disseminate racist, homophobic, and sexist themes (Czerwinsky, 2024; Gheorghe, 2023; Vink et al., 2024). These diametrically opposed origins have sown a vitriolic yet paradoxically supportive network. Across forums, Incels vent, share grievances, develop digital alliances, and even offer support (Speckhard et al., 2021). According to some users, the toxic posts and inflammatory language of Incel communities are a false flag, as this engagement style is central to the group's humor and culture (Daly & Nichols, 2024). Consequently, at first

DOI: 10.4324/9781003531258-8

glance, users are afforded a wide spectrum of experiences ranging from *protective and supportive* to *risky and toxic.*

An important branch of Incel scholarship is, by virtue of necessity, housed within criminology, radicalization, and terrorism studies (for example, see Brzuszkiewicz, 2020; Hoffman et al., 2020), as almost 60 Incelosphere-related fatalities have been documented (Moonshot, 2020 in Whittaker et al., 2024). However, the categorization of Incels as a terrorist threat is debated, as those who commit acts of violence may be outliers or an "extreme minority" (Costello et al., 2024, p. 32).

Incel violence initially emerged as a risk of undetermined size and scope after fatal attacks in the United States and Canada, and the classification of Incel violence is debated. For example, a contemporary argument identifies a 1989 perpetrator as the *first* Incel (Bloom, 2022). A lack of consensus emerges across other acts of violence, as a 2014 perpetrator's Incel affiliation is identified in some but not all literature (for example, see Vink et al., 2024 and Speckhard et al., 2021, *both which document varying perspectives*). However, other acts of violence—driven by themes of female rejection, loneliness, and a sense of aggrieved entitlement to sexual partners—have been conclusively linked to Incelosphere engagement (Center on Extremism, 2020). This broad variance is discussed by DeCook and Kelly (2022) and, as demonstrated here, is partially driven by a debated retroactive scholarly classification of Incel-coded acts of violence. *(A review of Incel violence is outside the scope of this chapter; for risk-aware clinical training, see Marett, Wygant, and Daly's asynchronous training hosted by Palo Alto University).*

### Incel Mental Health

A highly relevant question quickly emerges: *To what degree are Incels a risk to the public and, additionally, to themselves?* A budding arm of scholarship harnesses interview or survey data to explore the lived experience of Incels *(for example, see* Daly & Nichols, 2024; Moskalenko et al., 2022; Sparks et al., 2023; Speckhard et al., 2021; Whittaker et al., 2024). In the literature, a discussion of prior methodological limitations is acknowledged (Daly & Reed, 2022; Hart & Huber, 2023; Sparks et al., 2022; Speckhard et al., 2021; Whittaker et al., 2024), as early Incel scholarly corpus relied upon analysis of public, anonymous posts or limited data sets, which—by virtue of the data—could not comprehensively document the breadth and scope of posters' lived experiences. Additional data now offer explanatory power, as a 2022 report finds one popular forum hosts 2.6 million visits a month, yet 406 "power users" account for almost 75% of forum content (Center for Countering Digital Hate, 2022). Consequently, these insights now introduce an emergent branch of phenomenological, qualitative inquiry, which welcomes Human Services providers into the fold.

An important contribution to Incel scholarship identifies three Incelosphere subtypes, inclusive of those with (1) *internalizing* concerns, (2) *externalizing* concerns, and (3) a *hopeful* presentation, proposed to be most amenable to intervention (Ellenberg et al., 2023). This *hoping* subtype—defined by those who believe they can "ascend" out of their current position—may be less captured by deterministic, Incelosphere narratives. Importantly, pathway analyses find poor mental health is one predictor of internalized or externalized harm (Costello et al., 2024), which supports findings that Incels use more problematic coping strategies than their non-Incel counterparts (Sparks et al., 2023).

Those with *internalizing* presentations may struggle with suicidal ideation, depression, and/or anxiety. This assertion is widely echoed across the literature (Broyd et al., 2023; Costello et al., 2024; Moskalenko et al., 2022; Sparks et al., 2023; Speckhard et al., 2021; Van

Brunt & Taylor, 2020). To date, the largest, anonymous, self-report web survey of Incels (*n* = 561) finds one in five respondents have contemplated suicide within a single, two-week period (Whittaker et al., 2024). Moreso, an anonymous, self-report web survey of 274 Incels, finds 95% report depression, 93% report anxiety, 74% report autism symptoms, and many report prior trauma (Moskalenko et al., 2022). Additional subclinical concerns—namely, social isolation and loneliness (Sparks et al., 2023)—are common.

Conversely, the *externalizing* presentation—the presentation most commonly depicted across popular media—may endorse or justify violence. Clinical providers may be inclined to perform risk assessments for individuals who fit within this sub-cluster. Importantly, radicalization scholarship provides additional nuance, as not all individuals transition from *opinion* to *action* (Moskalenko, 2023); this suggests not all Incels necessarily move from holding beliefs to acting on beliefs. These metaphorical waters are further muddied by an acknowledgment of Incels' discussions of violence; as previously mentioned, this rhetoric may proffer a form of in-group social capital (Daly & Nichols, 2024).

### Incels and Pornography

A small branch of Incel scholarship discusses Incels' pornography use. A noteworthy argument, housed within evolutionary psychology, theorizes that it may limit possible violence (Costello & Buss, 2023). These authors suggest digital spaces pacify young men by providing a counterfeit version of sex, which is theorized to negatively moderate possible externalized aggression. Indeed, in interviews, some Incels report pornography addictions, which may be partially experienced as *protective* or *promotive*, as pornography offers opportunities for discussion and bonding with other men and may replace deeply desired experiences of intimacy (Regehr, 2022). In contrast, digital violence is also documented: "*Tribs*," or videos depicting non-consensual ejaculation on photos of women, are found within greater Manosphere-aligned communities (Ging, 2019).

### Incel Beliefs

*What Incel beliefs exist?* This section's brief discussion of Incel beliefs is introductory and far from exhaustive. Beliefs may vary by person or community (Hart & Huber, 2023).

Most broadly, one well-established linguistic analysis of publicly available, anonymous forum posts identifies five supraordinate Incelosphere themes: (1) the existence of a "sexual marketplace," (2) the narrative that women are naturally evil, (3) the legitimization of masculinity constructs, (4) the experience of male oppression, and (5) the discussion of violence (O'Malley et al., 2022). When analyzed in tandem with additional scholarship, this chapter suggests the first aforementioned theme—the existence of a sexual marketplace—may hold special relevance. A 2024 study (McGlashan & Krendel, 2024) identifies Incelosphere-specific terms used *within* but not across other distinct Manosphere spaces. Of the top ten most common Incel-specific terms, a full half are associated with women and sexual status; the remainder are feeling-based communication terms (e.g., "tee tee") or direct references to mental health constructs. Importantly, these latter findings dovetail with mental health insights that are identified throughout the Incel scholarly corpus (*see discussion above, Incel Mental Health*).

A brief review of some common terminology (Moonshot, 2020; Squirrell, n.d.) is discussed to support reader comprehension. According to Incels, a small number of handsome men, *Chads*, enjoy unfettered sexual access to women, while *Normies* or *Betas*, that is, regular people, are only granted provisional access. Incels—at the bottom of this hierarchy—struggle to secure any sexual partners. *Lookism*, a central tenet, explains that appearance dictates life trajectory and romantic prospects. A related construct, *The Blackpill* argues appearance is genetic and immutable, but unlike *Lookism* (which is not expressly defined as deterministic or fixed), *The Blackpill* may argue any attempt at self-improvement is fruitless.

Though some Incels explain these beliefs are supportive (Daly & Reed, 2022), other scholarship argues the belief-holder is absolved of some responsibility for their circumstances (Regehr, 2022), and these belief systems may drive suicidal ideation (Moonshot, 2020). Here it is suggested Human Services clinicians working with Incels explore the functional value of these beliefs, as they may hold concurrent *protective/promotive*, *neutral*, or *risky* value.

### Incel Belief Classification

Incel beliefs may appear noteworthy. *How does a multidisciplinary literature engage with Incels' views?* Though discipline-spanning consensus does not exist, a suite of discrete positions may directly or indirectly support interventional pathways that delicately validate Incels' experience of grievance. The positions outlined in this section are simplified, generalized reviews; interested Human Services readers are urged to engage further to gain clarification and nuance.

Most notably, evolutionary psychology treats Incel positionality as a response to *sexual marketplace conditions* (*for example, see* Baselice, 2024; Costello & Buss, 2023; Lindner, 2023) in which some men struggle to find mates. Complimentary scholarship references *hegemonic masculinity*, which explores Incels' positionality in a hierarchal system that stratifies and subordinates non-dominant masculinities (*for example, see* Daly & Reed, 2022; Thorburn, 2023; Vallerga & Zurbriggen, 2022; *for seminal scholarship on hegemonic masculinity, see* Connell & Messerschmidt, 2005). These positions suggest Incels may be an identified population with constrained access and agency. Sensitive analysis is required, as collective grievances against feminism are documented across Incel populations (Ging, 2019).

An equally nuanced construct, housed in forensic psychiatry, introduces a new taxonomical term, *Extreme Overvalued Beliefs*. This term weaves together a century-old, nonviolent psychological construct, *Overvalued Ideas*, with contemporary radicalization, forensic and legal studies scholarship (Rahman et al., 2020). A narrative review links EOBs with Incel presentations (Broyd et al., 2023), defined as rigid, deeply held beliefs *not necessarily* accompanied by hallucinations, severe cognitive impairment, or severe mental disorders. Scholars subtly distinguish EOBs from delusions, as EOBs are held by *many individuals*, not just *one*, and can be fueled through online interaction (Rahman et al., 2020). The introduction of a term initially borne of violent acts may seem counterintuitive to this chapter's stated aims, yet this last insight—this statement that EOBs can be potentiated by online engagement—is a focal insight of clinical relevance discussed within the second section of this chapter.

### Incels and Therapy

Importantly, the aforementioned, discipline-spanning Incel taxonomies may partially shed light upon *why* Incels fare so poorly in therapy. For example, in Moskalenko et al.'s aforementioned 2022 study of 274 self-identified Incels, of the 51% who tried therapy, only 6% report it helped, and 15% report therapy worsened their symptoms (2022). An analysis of anonymous Incel suicide posts (Daly & Laskovtsov, 2021) identifies an inability to access mental health resources—driven by anticipatory shame or fear, or alternately, via poor responses from therapists or other providers—as a noteworthy antecedent to attempted or completed suicide. More broadly, masculinity constructs may play an additional role, as gender-driven barriers to clinical care are well documented (American Psychological Association, 2018).

A brief discussion of a common, evidence-based intervention supports this section's discussion of poor therapeutic outcomes for Incels. Cognitive-behavioral therapy, recommended within some scholarship (*for example*, Broyd et al., 2023; van Brunt & Taylor, 2020), may employ cognitive restructuring to support the development of new ways of seeing *self* and *world* (Davis et al., 2017). Crucially, this intervention may require the relinquishment of existing schemas or worldviews by updating beliefs. Here, it is argued that interventions which aim to directly restructure or update beliefs may interfere with the existing worldviews and social networks that—according to Incels themselves—are experienced as positive and supportive. Consequently, therapy in the service of belief restructuring or updating could be initially met with resistance and/or poor outcomes.

In contrast, clinical work with Overvalued Ideas explores the *values* held by the client but not their discrete *beliefs* (Veale, 2002). Aligned with this clinical approach, cognitive-behavioral interventions geared toward *delusions*—which, as referenced, are conceptually aligned yet distinct from Overvalued Ideas and EOBs—warrant mention. Treatment pathways suggest *normalizing*, a process that supports awareness of the functional value of beliefs, which, if confronted head-on, can impede alliance and therapy outcomes (Eisen et al., 2024). A complimentary discussion of Incel therapy interventions acknowledges the possible presence of distorted views (Costello & Thomas, 2024), as well as the value of supportive, alliance-driven approaches (Costello et al., 2024). In aggregate, these positions suggest clinicians (1) acknowledge their client's subjective lived experience while (2) carefully considering the optimal deployment of belief restructuring interventions. Therefore, this chapter underscores the importance of Human Services providers' deployment of empathic responses to identified Incel grievances.

### Let's "Zoom Out": How Do People Begin Identifying with Incel Communities, and Is This Applicable to Other Populations or People?

Thus far, a discussion of Incel communities and mental health has opened this chapter. Now, a "zoom-out" approach elicits a new set of questions: (1) *What identified digital phenomena are linked to Incelosphere engagement?* and (2) *Can these insights be re-deployed for other populations or people?*

A small arm of scholarship explores entries and exits associated with Incelosphere engagement (Brace et al., 2023; Burns & Boislard, 2024; Colliver et al., 2022; Osuna, 2024; Regehr, 2022; Thorburn, 2023). *Vulnerability* quickly emerges as a salient, networked theme. This vulnerability, it can be argued, is linked to discrete *digital engagement experiences*. Consequently, this insight elicits a timely, digital-era discussion of social media algorithms, digital echo chambers—defined as digital spaces that display and disseminate ideologically narrow content (Kitchens et al., 2020), and misapplied science principles/misinformation. This chapter "zooms out" with a bi-focal discussion of these phenomena across (1) Incel populations and (2) other populations and people.

As this section's theoretical, translational exploration begins, a key insight must be underlined, bolded, and italicized for emphasis: ***<u>Digital media effects may vary by person, population, age, vulnerability factors and other variables; contradictory findings exist. This body of literature is emergent.</u>*** For example, across the fields of *Media Effects Studies* and *Psychology*, the literature finds both positive/protective and risky/harmful relationships associated with well-being and digital media, and a veritable wealth of findings additionally demonstrate neutral/null or very small effects (Beyens et al., 2020; Hall, 2024; Kramer et al., 2014; Orben et al., 2024; Valkenburg et al., 2022). More so, as some popular public-facing texts conflate correlation and causation (Odgers, 2024), a review of the aforementioned scholarship is highly recommended.

### An Introduction to Incel Vulnerability

The corpus of Incel literature identifies a link between *perceived or experienced vulnerability* and *digital engagement experiences*. Vulnerability, however, is not formally defined as a psychological, psychosocial, or public health construct. Instead, it is thematically directly and indirectly identified on public message boards and within interviews or surveys.

Some young men in Manosphere spaces, for example, report dating struggles or a lack of sexual/life experience; this self-perceived social vulnerability may prompt an initial push to seek *online digital content* to understand or fix these concerns (Botto & Gottzén, 2023). Additional masculine inadequacies—also coded as vulnerabilities—may elicit exploratory, *open-ended digital searches* that ultimately lead insecure, answer-seeking browsers to digital Incel content (Thorburn, 2023). Subtle, relationally scaffolded vulnerabilities are also represented; some young men report feeling isolated, which is a hypothesized "gateway" to Incel communities (Lindner, 2023, p. 231).

*How can we better understand these vulnerabilities vis-à-vis digital engagement?* An exploratory discussion of *algorithms*, *echo chambers*, and *misapplied science principles/misinformation* introduces these areas of discussion. Admittedly, this chapter's referenced scholarship and concepts are far from exhaustive; instead, an attempt to pique the reader's interest and introduce a broad awareness of relevant digital phenomena is made.

### Algorithms and Incels

*How does Incelosphere literature treat algorithms?* Scholarly interest continues to gain traction, and algorithms are framed as digital discovery vehicles that may steer users toward radicalized Incel and Manosphere content (Colliver et al., 2022).

For example, digital Manosphere visitors have migrated, over time, from less-toxic to more-toxic digital spaces; Incel communities are referenced as one of these more-toxic destinations (Ribeiro et al., 2021). A related phenomenon, *outlinking*, explains that users' hyperlinks, found in comments and posts, can seed ideas across ideologically radicalized communities (Brace et al., 2023). External events, like the COVID-19 crisis, can further upregulate hyperlinking activity and may introduce larger numbers of casual web browsers to Incel content.

This subtle yet powerful "push" toward radicalized content is echoed across studies of YouTube recommendation algorithms, which find "some types of content are especially liable to send viewers down a conspiratorial rabbit hole" (Alfano et al., 2021, p. 837). And, though YouTube has admittedly attempted to enact change by updating its algorithms, these impacts are inadequate, as the dissemination of ideologically radicalized content is of global concern and is not localized to a sole platform (Colliver et al., 2022; Ribeiro et al., 2021).

*Does any literature document algorithmic harms or vulnerabilities* not *associated with Incels?* Our zoom-out approach continues in service of this question.

## Algorithms for Other People and Populations

To support population-level engagement for Human Services providers, this section initially focuses on algorithms and systemic racism, as racism is a construct not exclusively relegated to Incel communities; it appears to be broadly embedded within our digital ecosystems. A broad literature documents public health impacts of algorithms, specifically via bias within their underlying datasets. For example, algorithms can exhibit bias through under-representative data (Achiume, 2020; Chidambaram et al., 2024; Nazer et al., 2023; Noble, 2018), which is associated with unequal and discriminatory care outcomes, especially for people of color and underrepresented members of society.

A troubling yet important example of racism associated with algorithms identifies racially biased automated appointment scheduling, which can preferentially place people of color in "overflow" slots with longer wait times (Samorani et al., 2022). Additionally, algorithmically derived care management tools shorten care pathways for patients of color versus their white counterparts, thus eliciting inequitable care experiences (Obermeyer et al., 2019).

The impact of algorithms can additionally elicit mood and emotion shifts: a study conducted by Facebook demonstrates that content on user feeds can alter moods, thus resulting in *emotional contagion* (Kramer et al., 2014); this study subsequently received an Editorial Expression of Concern, as opt-out and informed consent practices were not conducted (Verma, 2014). Importantly, it is unknown if this seminal 2014 study still elicits identical outcomes today, as Facebook continuously updates its platform. Nevertheless, this insight prompts an interesting question: *To what degree do digital communities capture and reflect existing mood constructs, and to what degree are these same features reinforced—or even generated—within these spaces?* A brief discussion of echo chambers further highlights the nuance of this question.

## Echo Chambers and Incels

*What is an echo chamber, anyway?* The term is a conceptual metaphor designed to describe ideologically narrow spaces devoid of conflicting information (Kitchens et al., 2020). *Amplification*, which can be defined as the repeated digital recommendation of increasingly extreme content, can be found across platforms, like YouTube (Whittaker et al., 2021). Simply stated, the "like attracts like" principle explains how this may occur: as users engage with information encountered online, more and more of it is displayed: this may create a filter bubble in which ideologically or thematically diverse information is missing from digital feeds (Pariser, 2011), though filter bubbles are debated (Whittaker et al., 2021), and echo chambers may be a simplified explanation of a complex phenomenon that requires nuanced analysis (Kitchens et al., 2020).

Echo chambers—and by extension, filter bubbles—receive direct and/or indirect attention within Incel literature (Baele et al., 2019; Colliver et al., 2022; De Roos et al., 2024; Regehr, 2022), and a tandem discussion of belief formation supports additional insights. The repetition of *any* information can increase belief in *both fact and fiction* (Ecker et al., 2022; Fazio et al., 2019). Therefore, this phenomenon—namely, the proliferation of ideologically narrow, thematically repetitive content found within digital Incel communities—introduces a proposed mechanism by which Incels' beliefs could either *form* or *receive* digital reinforcement, as echo chamber-like digital spaces disseminate repetitive, homogenous content.

### Echo Chambers for Other People and Populations

Crucially, while Incel scholarship supports echo chamber effects, generalist perspectives vary. Some scholars argue that most people have "diverse media diets" (Arguedas et al., 2022), while others identify a social motivation mechanism by which users preferentially engage with ideologically aligned compatriots (Mosleh et al., 2025).

*Why, however, would the literature contain potentially contradictory information?* A suite of explanations has been proposed. First, the global measurement of echo chambers across platforms, users, and content is imprecise and incomplete; therefore, documented insights may not scale (Kitchens et al., 2020). Additionally, this research space requires a clear articulation of user-generated interaction versus platform-generated interaction, and this current lack of clarity may act as a confounding variable (Whittaker, 2020). Consequently, wide-ranging definitions, measurements, and results across the literature may be equally confounding, simply by virtue of their heterogeneity and lack of consensus. As this research domain is currently emergent, interested Human Services providers are urged to seek the latest scholarship associated with their special interests.

### Misapplied Science Principles and Incels

*Is misinformation a concern for Incels?* Misapplied science scholarship (Bachaud & Johns, 2023), deemed "evidence-based misogyny" (Rothermel, 2023), is self-published on The Incel Wiki. This collaborative document hosts over 1,400 distinct articles (Incels Wiki, 2024), replete with charts and layperson interpretations of peer-review scholarship. These assertions validate the lived experience of Incels, and this content arguably exists as a form community advocacy (Roser et al., 2023), as Incels are frequently mocked across digital spaces (Dynel, 2020). It may additionally act as an important reinforcement tool that supports Incel-coded beliefs, thus highlighting an additional digitally mediated Incel vulnerability.

### Misinformation for Other People and Populations

While the discussion of misinformation is driven by misapplied science principles in Incel communities, in service of Human Services practitioners' aims, this chapter's final section broadly focuses on health misinformation, a subject of contemporary relevance.

Health equity scholars succinctly raise a powerful misinformation alarm:

> A child who needlessly experiences disabilities caused by measles … and a patient with cancer who ceases chemotherapy in favour of a bogus alternative are … victims of misinformation that is being promulgated on social media and other internet platforms.
>
> (Perakslis & Califf, 2019)

Misinformation, therefore, is not exclusively an Incel-centric concern, nor is it exclusively relegated to social media platforms and user-generated content. An oft-cited 2015 review of Australian apps for bipolar disorder disseminates problematic app recommendations, some of which are downright dangerous (Nicholas et al., 2015). One app suggests drinking hard liquor at night to negatively moderate sleeplessness during a manic episode, while another offers dangerous and inaccurate psychoeducation material that claims bipolar disorder can be transferred to other individuals. Similar critique is voiced in the United States, as consumer health protections are a concern across disciplines and populations (Fowler & Roberts, 2022).

While these examples are extreme, they clearly articulate a suite of broad vulnerabilities faced by today's media users. Crucially, clinical providers and systems are equally at risk: In extreme cases, patients with underlying mental health concerns may struggle to parse fact from fiction, which may harm care relationships and may lead to clinician-led discontinuation of care (Wangler & Jansky, 2020). A term, "health information seeking behavior," explains that information searches can be supportive *or* problematic, and low e-literacy is a risk factor for problematic searches (Jia et al., 2021; Rice & Sara, 2019). For Human Services providers working with generalist and/or Incel populations, these insights suggest that psychoeducation and/or digital literacy education may be an important interventional avenue.

*Broad Summary*

Throughout this chapter's "zoom-in, zoom-out" approach, it is suggested that, among other factors, *discrete vulnerabilities* can intermingle with a suite of *digital engagement experiences*—namely engagement with algorithms, echo chambers, and misapplied science principles/misinformation—to interact with the well-being and/or mental health of populations and/or people. One vulnerable population, Incels, articulates the relevance of these digital factors. A subsequent exploration of these factors for other populations and people is discussed.

## Conclusion

The "great experiment" of our modern era elicits promise and challenge. As we continue to integrate new technologies into every facet of our lives, we concurrently navigate the complexities they bring. This chapter initially elicits a focused examination of Incel presentations for Human Services practitioners. It subsequently explores digital technologies' *relationship to* mental health and well-being by using Incelosphere engagement as a case study example. Moreover, this chapter's broader discussion of these themes highlights the necessity of a nuanced, person-scaled, population-aware approach to contemporary digital technology and mental health practice and praxis.

## Reflective Questions

1 This chapter recommends a nuanced and sensitive analysis of contemporary technology use for Human Services readers. In what additional ways could digital platform engagement elicit *protective, neutral/null,* or *risky* engagement for various people and populations of interest?
2 How might Human Services readers advocate on behalf of vulnerable users of contemporary digital technology and/or digital media?
3 This chapter suggests psychoeducation and digital literacy could be helpful interventional touchpoints. How might your professional practice or praxis accommodate this suggestion?

## References

Achiume, E.T. (2020). *Racial discrimination and emerging digital technologies: A human rights analysis: Report of the Special Rapporteur on Contemporary Forms of Racism, Racial Discrimination, Xenophobia and Related Intolerance.* United Nations Digital Library.

Alfano, M., Fard, A. E., Carter, J. A., Clutton, P., & Klein, C. (2021). Technologically scaffolded atypical cognition: The case of YouTube's recommender system. *Synthese, 199*, 835–858.

American Psychological Association. (2018). *APA GUIDELINES for psychological practice with boys and men.* https://www.apa.org/about/policy/boys-men-practice-guidelines.pdf

Arguedas, A. R., Robertson, C. T., Fletcher, R., & Nielsen, R. K. (2022, January 19). *Echo chambers, filter bubbles, and polarisation: A literature review.* Reuters Institute.

Bachaud, L., & Johns, S. E. (2023). The use and misuse of evolutionary psychology in online manosphere communities: The case of female mating strategies. *Evolutionary Human Sciences, 5*, e28.

Baele, S., Brace, L., & Ging, D. (2024). A diachronic cross-platforms analysis of violent extremist language in the incel online ecosystem. *Terrorism and Political Violence, 36*(3), 382–405.

Baselice, K. A. (2024). Analyzing Incels through the lens of evolutionary psychology. *Culture and Evolution, 20*(1), 42–58.

Beyens, I., Pouwels, J. L., van Driel, I. I., Keijsers, L., & Valkenburg, P. M. (2020). The effect of social media on well-being differs from adolescent to adolescent. *Scientific Reports, 10*(1), 10763.

Bloom, M. M. (2022). The First incel? The legacy of Marc Lépine. *The Journal of Intelligence, Conflict, and Warfare, 5*(1), 39–74.

Botto, M., & Gottzén, L. (2023). Swallowing and spitting out the red pill: Young men, vulnerability, and radicalization pathways in the Manosphere. *Journal of Gender Studies, 33*(5), 596–608.

Brace, L., Baele, S. J., & Ging, D. (2023). Where do 'mixed, unclear, and unstable' ideologies come from? A data-driven answer centred on the incelosphere. *Journal of Policing, Intelligence and Counter Terrorism, 19*(2), 103–124.

Broyd, J., Boniface, L., Parsons, D., Murphy, D., & Hafferty, J. D. (2023). Incels, violence and mental disorder: A narrative review with recommendations for best practice in risk assessment and clinical intervention. *BJPsych Advances, 29*(4), 254–264.

Brzuszkiewicz, S. (2020). *Incel radical milieu and external locus of control* (Vol. 1). International Centre for Counter-Terrorism (ICCT).

Burns, L. M., & Boislard, M. A. (2024). "I'm better than this": A qualitative analysis of the turning points leading to exiting inceldom. *Journal of Sex Research*, 1–17. Advance online publication.

Center for Countering Digital Hate. (2022). *The incelosphere: Exposing pathways into incel communities and the harms they pose to women and children.* Center for Countering Digital Hate. https://counterhate.com/research/incelosphere/

Center on Extremism. (2020, July 29). *Incels (Involuntary Celibates).* Anti-Defamation League.

Chidambaram, S., Jain, B., Jain, U., Mwavu, R., Baru, R., Thomas, B., Greaves, F., Jayakumar, S., Jain, P., Rojo, M., Battalino, M.R., Meara, J. G., Sounderajah, V., Celi, L.A & Darzi, A. (2024). An introduction to digital determinants of health. *PLOS Digital Health, 3*(1), e0000346.

Colliver, S., Popham, J., Henderson, S., Daly, S., & Pokrywa, L. (2022). *Tracing radicalization to the incel movement and its connection to loneliness.* Centre for Research on Security Practices, Wilfred Laurier University.

Connell, R. W., & Messerschmidt, J. W. (2005). Hegemonic masculinity: Rethinking the concept. *Gender & Society, 19*(6), 829–859.

Costello, W., & Buss, D. M. (2023). Why isn't there more incel violence? *Adaptive Human Behavior and Physiology, 9*(3), 252–259.

Costello, W., Daly, S. E., Sparks, B., & Thomas, A. G. (2024, September 6). *More than misogyny: The merit of a mental health perspective in incel research.* Osf.io. https://doi.org/10.31219/osf.io/92fhr

Costello, W., & Thomas, A. G. (2024, November 7). *Seeing through the black-pill: Incels are wrong about what people think of them.* Osf.io. https://doi.org/10.31219/osf.io/53mke

Czerwinsky, A. (2024). Misogynist incels gone mainstream: A critical review of the current directions in incel-focused research. *Crime, Media, Culture, 20*(2), 196–217.

Daly, S. E., & Laskovtsov, A. (2021). Goodbye, my friendcels": An analysis of incel suicide posts. *Journal of Qualitative Criminal Justice & Criminology, 11*(1). https://doi.org/10.21428/88de04a1. b7b8b295.

Daly, S. E., & Nichols, A. L. (2024). 'Incels are shit-post kings': Incels' perceptions of online forum content. *Journal of Crime and Justice, 47*(1), 4–26.

Daly, S. E., & Reed, S. M. (2022). "I think most of society hates us": A qualitative thematic analysis of interviews with incels. *Sex Roles, 86*(1), 14–33.

Davis, M., Witcraft, S., Baird, S., & Smits, J. (2017). Learning Principles in CBT. In S. G. Hofmann & G. J. G. Asmundson (Eds.), *The science of cognitive behavioral therapy* (pp. 51–76). Academic Press.

DeCook, J.R., & Kelly, M. (2022). Interrogating the "incel menace": The threat of male supremacy in terrorism studies. *Critical Studies on Terrorism, 15*(3), 706–726.

de Roos, M. S., Veldhuizen-Ochodničanová, L., & Hanna, A. (2024). The angry echo chamber: A study of extremist and emotional language changes in incel communities over time. *Journal of Interpersonal Violence, 39*(21–22), 4573–4597. https://doi.org/10.1177/08862605241239451

Dynel, M. (2020). Vigilante disparaging humour at r/IncelTears: Humour as critique of incel ideology. *Language & Communication, 74*, 1–14.

Ecker, U. K., Lewandowsky, S., Cook, J., Schmid, P., Fazio, L. K., Brashier, N., Kendeou, P., Vraga, E., & Amazeen, M. A. (2022). The psychological drivers of misinformation belief and its resistance to correction. *Nature Reviews Psychology, 1*(1), 13–29.

Eisen, K., Lean, M., & Hardy, K. (2024). Collaboration, not collusion: Befriending and normalizing. In K. V. Hardy & D. Turkington (Eds.), *Decoding Delusions* (pp. 163–178). Essay, American Psychiatric Association Publishing.

Ellenberg, M., Speckhard, A., & Kruglanski, A. W. (2023). Beyond violent extremism: A 3N perspective of inceldom. *Psychology of Men & Masculinities, 25*(3), 290–299.

Fazio, L. K., Rand, D. G., & Pennycook, G. (2019). Repetition increases perceived truth equally for plausible and implausible statements. *Psychonomic Bulletin & Review, 26*(5), 1705–1710.

Fowler, L. R., & Roberts, J. L. (2022). Mind the App. *Annals of Health Law and Life Sciences, 31*(2), 143–166.

Gheorghe, R. M. (2023). "Just be white (JBW)": Incels, race and the violence of whiteness. *Affilia, 39*(1), 59–77. https://doi.org/10.1177/08861099221144275

Ging, D. (2019). Alphas, betas, and incels: Theorizing the masculinities of the manosphere. *Men and Masculinities, 22*(4), 638–657.

Hall, J. A. (2024). Ten myths about the effect of social media use on well-being. *Journal of Medical Internet Research, 26*, e59585.

Hart, G., & Huber, A. R. (2023). Five things we need to learn about incel extremism: Issues, challenges and avenues for fresh research. *Studies in Conflict & Terrorism*, 1–17.

Hoffman, B., Ware, J., & Shapiro, E. (2020). Assessing the threat of incel violence. *Studies in Conflict & Terrorism, 43*(7), 565–587.

Incel Wiki. (2024, June 21). *Incel wiki, the encyclopedia of Incel Culture.*

Jia, X., Pang, Y., & Liu, L. S. (2021, December). Online health information seeking behavior: A systematic review. *Healthcare, 9*(12), 1740.

Kassam, A. (2018, April 25). *Woman behind "incel" says angry men hijacked her word "as a weapon of war." The Guardian.*

Kitchens, B., Johnson, S. L., & Gray, P. (2020). Understanding echo chambers and filter bubbles: The impact of social media on diversification and partisan shifts in news consumption. *MIS Quarterly, 44*(4), 1619–1649.

Kramer, A. D., Guillory, J. E., & Hancock, J. T. (2014). Experimental evidence of massive-scale emotional contagion through social networks. *Proceedings of the National Academy of Sciences, 111*(24), 8788–8790.

Lindner, M. (2023). The sense in senseless violence: Male reproductive strategy and the modern sexual marketplace as contributors to violent extremism. *Adaptive Human Behavior and Physiology, 9*(3), 217–251.

McGlashan, M., & Krendel, A. (2024). Keywords of the manosphere. *International Journal of Corpus Linguistics, 29*(1), 87–115.

Moonshot. (2020, June). *Incels: A guide to symbols and terminology.*

Moskalenko, S. (2023). The evolution of hybrid radicalization: From small group to mass phenomenon. In N. Stockman (Ed.), *Routledge handbook of transnational terrorism* (pp. 132–142). Routledge.

Moskalenko, S., González, J. F. G., Kates, N., & Morton, J. (2022). Incel ideology, radicalization and mental health: A survey study. *The Journal of Intelligence, Conflict, and Warfare, 4*(3), 1–29.

Mosleh, M., Martel, C., & Rand, D. G. (2025). Psychological underpinnings of partisan bias in tie formation on social media. *Journal of Experimental Psychology: General, 154*(2), 378–390.

Nazer, L. H., Zatarah, R., Waldrip, S., Ke, J. X. C., Moukheiber, M., Khanna, A. K., Hicklen, R.S., Moukheiber, L., Moukheiber, D., Ma, H & & Mathur, P. (2023). Bias in artificial intelligence algorithms and recommendations for mitigation. *PLOS Digital Health, 2*(6), e0000278.

Nicholas, J., Larsen, M. E., Proudfoot, J., & Christensen, H. (2015). Mobile apps for bipolar disorder: A systematic review of features and content quality. *Journal of Medical Internet Research, 17*(8), e198.

Noble, S. U. (2018). *Algorithms of oppression: How search engines reinforce racism.* New York University Press.

Obermeyer, Z., Powers, B., Vogeli, C., & Mullainathan, S. (2019). Dissecting racial bias in an algorithm used to manage the health of populations. *Science, 366*(6464), 447–453.

Odgers, C. L. (2024). The great rewiring: Is social media really behind an epidemic of teenage mental illness? *Nature, 628*(8006), 29–30.

O'Malley, R. L., Holt, K., & Holt, T. J. (2022). An exploration of the involuntary celibate (incel) subculture online. *Journal of Interpersonal Violence, 37*(7–8), NP4981–NP5008.

Orben, A., Meier, A., Dalgleish, T., & Blakemore, S. J. (2024). Mechanisms linking social media use to adolescent mental health vulnerability. *Nature Reviews Psychology, 3*, 407–423.

Osuna, A. I. (2024). Leaving the incel community: A content analysis. *Sexuality & Culture, 28*(2), 749–770.

Pariser, E. (2011). *The filter bubble: How the new personalized web is changing what we read and how we think.* Penguin.

Perakslis, E., & Califf, R. M. (2019). Employ cybersecurity techniques against the threat of medical misinformation. *JAMA, 322*(3), 207–208.

Rahman, T., Hartz, S. M., Xiong, W., Meloy, J. R., Janofsky, J., Harry, B., & Resnick, P. J. (2020). Extreme overvalued beliefs. *Journal of the American Academy of Psychiatry and the Law, 48*(3), 319–326.

Regehr, K. (2022). In(cel)doctrination: How technologically facilitated misogyny moves violence off screens and on to streets. *New Media & Society, 24*(1), 138–155.

Ribeiro, M. H., Blackburn, J., Bradlyn, B., De Cristofaro, E., Stringhini, G., Long, S., Greenberg, S., & Zannettou, S. (2021). The evolution of the manosphere across the web. In *Proceedings of the International AAAI Conference on Web and Social Media, Virtual Location15*, 196–207. Palo Alto, California, USA: AAAI Press.

Rice, L., & Sara, R. (2019). Updating the determinants of health model in the information age. *Health Promotion International, 34*(6), 1241–1249. https://doi.org/10.1093/heapro/day064

Roser, M., Chalker, C., & Squirrell, T. (2023). *Spitting out the blackpill: Evaluating how incels present themselves in their own words on the incel wiki* (pp. 1–23). Institute for Strategic Dialogue.

Rothermel, A. K. (2023). The role of evidence-based misogyny in antifeminist online communities of the "manosphere". *Big Data and Society, 10*(1), 1–6.

Samorani, M., Harris, S. L., Blount, L. G., Lu, H., & Santoro, M. A. (2022). Overbooked and overlooked: Machine learning and racial bias in medical appointment scheduling. *Manufacturing & Service Operations Management, 24*(6), 2825–2842.

Sparks, B., Zidenberg, A. M., & Olver, M. E. (2022). Involuntary celibacy: A review of incel ideology and experiences with dating, rejection, and associated mental health and emotional sequelae. *Current Psychiatry Reports, 24*(12), 731–740.

Sparks, B., Zidenberg, A. M., & Olver, M. E. (2023). One is the loneliest number: Involuntary celibacy (incel), mental health, and loneliness. *Current Psychology, 43*(1), 392–406.

Speckhard, A., Ellenberg, M., Morton, J., & Ash, A. (2021). Involuntary celibates' experiences of and grievance over sexual exclusion and the potential threat of violence among those active in an online incel forum. *Journal of Strategic Security, 14*(2), 89–121.

Squirrell, T. (n.d.). *A definitive guide to Incels part two: The A-Z incel dictionary*. Tim Squirrell, PhD. https://archive.ph/7DXOX

Thorburn, J. (2023). Exiting the manosphere. A gendered analysis of radicalization, diversion and deradicalization narratives from r/incelexit and r/exredpill. *Studies in Conflict & Terrorism, 24*(4), 1–25.

Valkenburg, P. M., Meier, A., & Beyens, I. (2022). Social media use and its impact on adolescent mental health: An umbrella review of the evidence. *Current Opinion in Psychology, 44*, 58–68.

Vallerga, M., & Zurbriggen, E. L. (2022). Hegemonic masculinities in the 'manosphere': A thematic analysis of beliefs about men and women on The Red Pill and Incel. *Analyses of Social Issues and Public Policy, 22*(2), 602–625.

Van Brunt, B., & Taylor, C. (2020). *Understanding and treating incels: Case studies, guidance, and treatment of violence risk in the involuntary celibate community*. Routledge.

Veale, D. (2002). Over-valued ideas: A conceptual analysis. *Behaviour Research and Therapy, 40*(4), 383–400.

Verma, I. M. (2014). Editorial expression of concern: Experimental evidence of massive-scale emotional contagion through social networks. *Proceedings of the National Academy of Sciences of the United States of America, 111*(29), 10779–10779.

Vink, D., Abbas, T., Veilleux-Lepage, Y., & McNeil-Willson, R. (2024). "Because they are women in a man's world": A critical discourse analysis of incel violent extremists and the stories they tell. *Terrorism and Political Violence, 36*(6), 723–739.

Wangler, J., & Jansky, M. (2020). General practitioners' challenges and strategies in dealing with Internet-related health anxieties—Results of a qualitative study among primary care physicians in Germany. *Wiener Medizinische Wochenschrift, 170*(13), 329–339.

Whittaker, J. (2020). Online echo chambers and violent extremism. In S. M. Khasru (Ed.), *The digital age, cyber space, and social media: The challenges of security & radicalization* (1st ed., Vol. 1, pp. 129–150). IPAG.

Whittaker, J., Costello, W., & Thomas, A. G. (2024). *Independent report Predicting harm among incels (involuntary celibates): The roles of mental health, ideological belief and social networking*.

Whittaker, J., Looney, S., Reed, A., & Votta, F. (2021). Recommender systems and the amplification of extremist content. *Internet Policy Review, 10*(2), 1-29.

# 7 Connected Recovery™

## Therapeutic Navigation of Problematic and Out-of-Control Sexual Behavior*

*Laney Knowlton*

### Foundational Background

Esther Perel (2017) states, "There is one simple act of transgression that can rob a couple of their relationship, their happiness, their very identity: an affair. Yet this extremely common act is poorly understood" (p. xiii). Infidelity and betrayal are worldwide issues, highlighted by Rokach and Chan (2023), who state that around the globe, infidelity is the most common reason relationships end. Warach et al. (2018) state that studies have shown that one-fifth to one-quarter of American marriages deal with infidelity and that the rate of infidelity expands to up to 65% if betrayal within non-married relationships is included. Understanding how to treat infidelity is particularly important for mental health professionals, as over half of couples who present for therapy list infidelity as the presenting concern. Infidelity is one of the most challenging issues for clinicians to treat (Warach & Josephs, 2021), and most therapists have very little, if any, training around treating infidelity (Rokach & Chan, 2023).

The field of infidelity treatment is very fragmented. Perel (2017) states, "Among therapists ... balanced, unbiased dialogue is rare" (p. 6). The majority of treatment providers and treatment approaches relating to infidelity and treatment of those struggling to heal from issues related to infidelity are based on one of four camps: sex therapy, sex "addiction" treatment, betrayal trauma treatment, and relational counseling (commonly referred to as "couples counseling," but "relational counseling" is a more inclusive term). Each of these areas of study has valuable pieces of information and should be considered in treatment. Additionally, treatment needs to be culturally informed, as opinions on the topic differ significantly between various cultures, groups, and countries. Perel (2017) corroborates that statement, sharing that the responses she gets when talking about infidelity differ dramatically depending on social norms, cultural mores, and belief systems.

Problematic sexual behaviors (PSBs), like other problematic behaviors, occur on a continuum (see Figure 7.1). While resources are needed for any issues that cause conflict or pain for individuals or relationships, there is a dramatic differentiation between the two ends of the continuum. Historically, both academia and the clinical community have struggled to agree on an official definition of out-of-control sexual behavior. This has increased confusion and hindered both research and development of effective treatment (Borgogna et al., 2022). Kowalewska and Lew-Starowicz (2021) explore the various phrases used to delineate this

---

* (Adapted from Connected Recovery™ Continuing Outpatient Treatment Curriculum: Comprehensive Treatment of Problematic Sexual Behaviors (PSB) and Betrayal Trauma by Laney Knowlton, 2024, and Healing from Betrayal, Infidelity, and Problematic Sexual Behaviors: A Guide to Individual and Relational Recovery by Laney Knowlton, 2023)

DOI: 10.4324/9781003531258-9

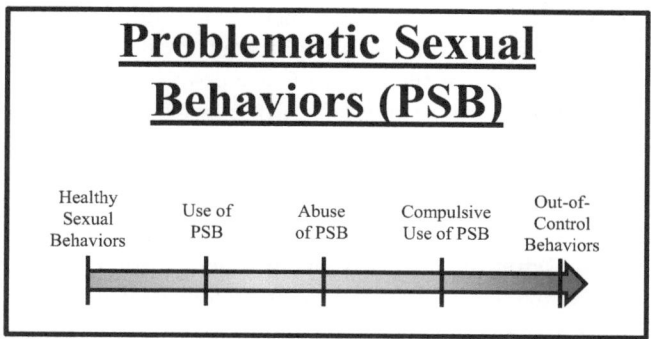

*Figure 7.1* PSB Continuum—continuum of problematic sexual behaviors (PSB).

issue over the three decades since its conceptualization. The list includes "compulsive sexual behaviors, sexual addiction or sexual dependence, (nonparaphilic) hypersexuality, sexual impulsivity, satyriasis and nymphomania, [and] out-of-control sexual behavior" (p. 17). Attempts to define PSB have ranged from the earliest reference of the topic as "pathological sexuality" to including the topic in personality disorders under sexual deviations and to the issues related to problematic levels of sexual behavior as psychosexual disorders, sexual disorders, and impulse control disorders. Kowalewska and Lew-Starowicz explain why the topic was not included in the *DSM-5*, stating that the primary concerns were a lack of empirical data and the potential misapplication of the diagnosis. They felt that the definitions proposed did not provide enough detail to distinguish between healthy sexual behaviors and unhealthy sexual behaviors. The lack of inclusion of some definition of PSB in the *DSM-5* led to increased study on the topic to explore it empirically, so an accurate definition could be created.

The current diagnosis related to PSB at a compulsive level is "Compulsive Sexual Behavior Disorder" (CSBD), included in the ICD-11 under Impulse Control Disorders. According to the ICD-11 (World Health Organization, 2024), CSBD is characterized by a persistent failure to control intense, repetitive sexual impulses, resulting in behavior that becomes central to the individual's life, often to the neglect of health, personal care, or other responsibilities. It is a pattern of behaviors over time (six months or longer) that continues despite multiple attempts to stop and causes significant distress or impairment. These behaviors cannot be explained by bipolar disorder, obsessive-compulsive disorder, personality disorders, paraphilic disorders, the effects of substances or medications, substance use disorders, and neurocognitive impairments. Often beginning in pre-adolescence or adolescence, the disorder is associated with high rates of childhood trauma, particularly sexual abuse, and frequently co-occurs with other mental disorders. It is crucial to distinguish between genuine impaired control and distress arising from internal or external moral judgments. Both CSBD and value-based distress can cause a behavior to be problematic for an individual or relationship, but treatment for CSBD often needs to include additional support to break the behavioral patterns.

### Understanding PSB and Betrayal Trauma

*PSB* is an umbrella term that includes any sexual or romantic behavior that is problematic to the individual and those connected to them. This definition is most closely aligned with

Bill Herring's PSB framework (2017), which considers the individual and relational impact of behaviors rather than focusing on pathology. Rather than focusing on complicated and lengthy assessments to determine if the behaviors are problematic, Herring (2017) asks five questions: "'Are you keeping your promises?'; 'Are you ok with what you're doing?'; 'Are you in control of yourself?'; 'Is everything ok?'; and 'Are you protecting others?'" These questions focus on "five distinct, but overlapping categories: (1) commitment violations, (2) values conflicts, (3) diminished self-control, (4) negative consequences, and (5) lack of sexual responsibility." The focus on individual and relational impact of the behaviors allows the model to be useful for those of varying genders, orientations, and cultures. This approach is non-pathologizing and does not focus on labels (Siegel, 2019), while providing a framework that helps individuals and relationships get help when needed.

*Betrayal trauma* in primary relationships is a potential response to the violation of a relational contract in a romantic relationship (Pandey & Vaish, 2022). Pandey and Vaish define an act of betrayal as a behavior that conflicts with the relational boundaries and makes the person who was betrayed question the emotional safety of the relationship. Betrayal trauma develops when the emotional and psychological impact of a violation of the relational contract creates an "attachment injury" (Pandey & Vaish) or unprocessed and painful events that have dysregulated an individual's nervous system (Lepak & Carson, 2022). The term "attachment injury" refers to a significant breach of trust that causes someone to doubt they can securely rely on the other person for emotional support and connection (Warach & Josephs, 2021). Warach and Josephs state: "Betrayed adult romantic partners are in a similar relational position to the child that suffers disorganized attachment. In both situations, the attachment injury derives from the same person that was previously trusted and relied upon for emotional security" (pp. 72–73). Rokach and Chan (2023) state: "The traumatic reactions caused by infidelity emulate behaviors and attitudes seen in a disorganized attachment style as immense emotional, psychological and cognitive dysregulation is evident" (p. 4).

Betrayal in primary relationships can impact those who have been betrayed on multiple levels, including emotionally, physically, mentally, and relationally (Warach & Josephs, 2021). Each individual's experience of relational contract violations is complex and differs based on multiple factors, both individual and relational (Lonergan et al., 2021). Research differs regarding the percentage of those who have been betrayed who experience clinically significant attachment wounds as a result. Lonergan et al. (2021) state that research suggests that 30–60% of those who experience betrayal in their primary relationships develop betrayal trauma at a clinically significant level. Steffens and Rennie (2006) found that 69.6% of those who experienced betrayal in primary relationships met all the criteria for PTSD with the exception of the first element, which applies to being exposed to actual or threatened death, injury, or violence. Hollenbeck and Steffens (2024) stated that 84% of those who experienced betrayal in their primary relationships reported that the anger they felt was stronger than anything else they've experienced, and two-thirds of them felt stuck in that anger.

### Treating PSB and Betrayal Trauma

The Connected Recovery™ model connects concepts and tools from current models in the field, including the treatment of PSBs, betrayal trauma, relational work through an emotionally focused therapy (EFT) lens, and sex therapy, providing a comprehensive, sex-positive treatment model that applies to both people who struggle with PSB and people who have experienced betrayal. This model applies to all genders, sexual orientations, relational orientations, and relational status. It divides recovery into three phases: early, middle, and late recovery. Early recovery (Repair) focuses on establishing truth and creating emotional safety, middle recovery (Reconnect) deepens connection and empathy, and late recovery (Restore) centers on healthy sexuality. This model creates a common language that creates the potential for connection and transparency throughout the process with a betrayal-sensitive lens. This model also helps remove shame from the recovery process.

The language used by clinicians creates a foundation that lets clients know you see them as human beings rather than defining them by what they've done or what's happened to them. It also helps clinicians shift away from pathological ideology. Rather than using terms like "sex addict" or "cheater," "betrayed" or "betrayed partner," use language like "those who are struggling with PSB" or "those healing from betrayal." This doesn't mean dismissing the client's understanding of the issue or telling them they can't use wording they connect to. Arguing about language is rarely, if ever, helpful, no matter what the reason behind the argument is (Siegel, 2019). Clients stuck in patterns of problematic behavior or recovering from betrayal are much more than just those patterns or that experience. They are first and foremost people, worthy of being loved and loving others.

As previously stated, PSB is an umbrella term. Due to the individual nature of sexuality, the definition of what defines a behavior as problematic is highly individual. "Healthy sexual behaviors" will differ for each person and each relationship. Healthy sexual behaviors are behaviors that align with an individual's moral values, the commitments they've made to themselves or others, don't harm them or others emotionally or psychologically, don't put their life or someone else's life at risk, and don't violate others. Using the above definition, sexual behaviors become problematic when they are not in alignment with the individual's moral values, cause individuals to break commitments they've made, harm themselves or others emotionally or psychologically, put their life or someone else's life at risk, or violate others.

*Format for Therapy*

Three different types of counseling are helpful when treating PSB and betrayal. These include individual therapy, relational counseling, and group therapy. Individual therapy provides space for clients to process through their experience and determine the best path for them as they move forward. For those recovering from PSB and betrayal, each person should have their own individual therapist; one therapist should not fill this role for multiple partners. The trauma and lack of trust make it very difficult for one therapist to be able to work individually with more than one party involved.

If the parties plan to continue their relationship, relational counseling is an essential part of the process. The term "relational counseling" is more inclusive than the term "couples counseling," as not all relationships are monogamous. If possible, cotherapy is recommended for couples. Cotherapy refers to therapy with both of the individual therapists and both of the clients. Please note, if the relationship includes more than two individuals, one therapist is usually more effective due to the number of people needed to make cotherapy work. Cotherapy allows continued support for each partner throughout the session. It also helps to decrease miscommunication and any deception. It is initially more costly but tends to shorten the process in the long term. If cotherapy is not possible or if relational counseling is preferred, a third clinician should be utilized rather than having one of the individual therapists fill the role.

Group therapy for both those struggling with PSB and those healing from betrayal is often very helpful. It provides a support network, which can be challenging to develop following PSB and betrayal due to the stigma connected to PSB and betrayal. The most common recommendations are to end the relationship or just "get over it," neither of which gives the parties involved the chance to sort through the emotions and do the work to heal. Group therapy can help clients develop hope for themselves and potentially for their relationship, give them the knowledge that they are not alone in their journey, help with the identification and rectification of relational patterns and dynamics, and provide connection and release of pain.

When treating PSB and betrayal, general relational patterns and dynamics cannot be the focus of treatment until the betrayal has been addressed. This does not mean that dysfunctional patterns are not part of the equation. Every relationship (romantic relationships, friendships, parent–child, siblings, etc.) is a connection between two people. Each of those people is human. As human beings, we each have things we've learned, experiences we've gone through, and personality traits we have. These contribute to the way we connect to others. Some of those traits and approaches are functional, meaning they increase our ability to connect to ourselves and others. Some are dysfunctional, meaning they disconnect us from ourselves and others. Those we connect to tend to have about the same level of function/dysfunction as we do. This does not include escape patterns or abuse.

Escape patterns, meaning behaviors used to escape or numb emotions in incongruent ways, and abuse are dysfunctional, meaning they cause disconnection, but they also cause a lack of safety beyond regular levels of dysfunction. No level of dysfunction warrants being abused or justifies escape patterns. Al-Anon tells those connected to alcoholics, "You didn't cause it, you can't control it, and you can't cure it." This concept is important for both those who have betrayed and those who have been betrayed to understand. Foundations for escape patterns often start in childhood or adolescence. Turning to escape responses isn't safe for either the person escaping or those connected to them. Escapes don't meet the individual's needs and are not congruent with who we want to be. We'll talk about this in more detail later in this chapter.

In any relationship, we need to work on decreasing dysfunctional patterns and behaviors to improve connection. We can't work on those within the relationship until the escape patterns or abusive behaviors have been addressed. Escape patterns or abusive behaviors are like a heavy ball on the end of a chain, whipping around and knocking both the person who is escaping and the person connected to them over, often causing significant pain and damage. Living in that environment that includes escape cycles can cause the development of significant trauma responses (we'll talk more about those later). Esther Perel (2017) describes the pain of betrayal, stating:

> The revelation of an affair is eviscerating. If you really want to gut a relationship, to tear out the very heart of it, infidelity is a sure bet. It is betrayal on so many levels: deceit, abandonment, rejection, humiliation—all the things love promised to protect us from. When the one you relied upon is the one who has lied to your face, treated you as unworthy of basic respect, the world you thought you lived in is turned upside down. The story of your life is so fractured you can't piece it together.
>
> (p. 56)

Because of the damage escape patterns and abuse cause, the earliest work in recovery focuses on creating safety. Those who have been betrayed start by creating safety for themselves because relying on the person who has betrayed them and lied to them isn't safe. Those struggling with PSB start by learning to stop their behaviors and create safety for themselves. By the same token, in cases where there is abuse, the person perpetuating the abuse needs to stop their behaviors and create safety for themselves and those connected to them, and the person being abused needs to start by creating safety for themselves, so their safety isn't based on the person who has abused them protecting them because that isn't safe to rely on yet. Early recovery is about creating safety and stopping the escape patterns and ineffective and unhelpful responses to those behaviors. Once we've taken those steps and built healthier and more helpful patterns, we can work on the dysfunctional patterns in the relationship and work to deepen our connection to ourselves and others. That work happens in the middle and late recovery.

*Early Recovery*

Early recovery works to establish emotional safety individually and relationally through exploration of the truth. This phase of recovery considers escape cycles and trauma cycles, includes disclosing behaviors and making amends for the damage that has been done, and changing basic relational dynamics to incorporate consent, relational accountability, and containment, to create a foundation upon which connection can be built.

*Connection to Self and Others*

Connection to self and others is essential to recovery. This begins with hope, with the belief that each individual matters and healing is possible. For those who have betrayed, the message they need to hear often sounds like: "You aren't a monster. You got here for a reason. You don't have to stay here. There is hope. You matter." Those who have been betrayed often need to hear something like: "You aren't so broken you can't heal. You aren't crazy. You're right that you need safety and it's ok to want that. It's possible to feel peace and joy again. I believe you."

Incorporating group therapy can often provide a supportive connection to others. If group therapy is not an option or if the individual does not feel comfortable with it, work with them to help them build their support system. I recommend a minimum of five people they can talk to and process with. Connection to self is just as important and is often overlooked. Recovery is not just processing what happened; it's also becoming more whole and finding or rediscovering yourself. One exercise that may be helpful is considering "bucket-fillers," or things that bring them joy. I recommend spending five minutes each day doing something that brings them joy, and once a week doing something that takes at least an hour that brings them joy. Have them focus on things that are related to their senses. I've had clients who stopped to watched the sunrise or sunset, got a corn dog at Sonic, treated themselves to their favorite specialized coffee or drink, stopped and watched bugs on the sidewalk, bought hand soap in their favorite scent, kept Dove chocolates in their desk or purse, watched birds eating fish, had soft blankets stored in their offices or homes, listened to recorded sounds of the ocean or rainstorms, or had playlists of their favorite songs divided by emotion or situation. Support of others and connection to self-help provide a counterweight to the pain of processing through the experience.

*Trauma and Escape Cycles*

Exploration of both trauma and escape cycles helps identify unhealthy and painful patterns so that change can happen. Additionally, as every person has trauma cycles, considering

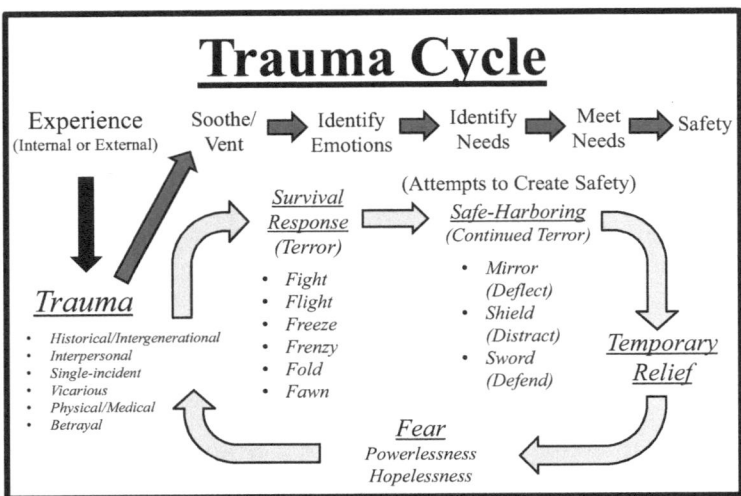

*Figure 7.2* Trauma cycle—my trauma cycle worksheet.
(© 2022 Laney Knowlton. All Rights Reserved. ConnectedRecoveryTraining.com)

both trauma and escape cycles helps to give those who have been betrayed context through which they can start to see their partner's escape cycles more clearly, which better equips them to create safety for themselves and provides potential for empathy, which is only possible when safety exists.

Starting on the left side of Figure 7.2 with "Experience (Internal/External)." Bad things happen to us. We're taught unhealthy coping skills because we live in a human world. The combination of these two factors produces painful emotions and experiences. When that pain is unresolved, it becomes trauma. Sometimes the trauma builds up gradually. One small thing after another, and eventually it gets to be too much. Other times, a very painful situation or experience might be traumatic enough that it's immediately too much to deal with. Either way, when we hit a point where it's too much, our mind and body automatically respond by shifting into survival mode.

Survival mode shifts us into functioning reactively. Survival responses work for life-or-death situations. Unless the situation is a life-or-death situation, our initial survival response doesn't resolve the situation. In cases where survival responses don't resolve the situation and we get stuck spinning in those responses, we move to safe-harboring behaviors. Safe-harboring behaviors fall into three general categories: mirror, shield, and sword (see Figure 7.3). Safe-harboring behaviors are survival responses that continue beyond the first instinctual response. When our survival responses aren't effective and we don't have the tools to reground ourselves and stop spinning, we can get trapped in our survival responses and attempt to create safety in any way we can. All three types of safe-harboring only work short term. These responses are often incongruent with who we want to be, don't actually create safety, and cause disconnection from ourselves and others.

We're now going to focus on escape cycles (see Figure 7.4). Everyone has times when they need to take a break or escape from life, but not everyone has escape cycles. Escape cycles are when we give up on ourselves and say, "screw it" and shift to numbing the pain rather than trying to deal with it. Escape cycles can escalate into compulsive or out-of-control cycles, but they don't start that way. Escape behaviors start with use, can move to abuse,

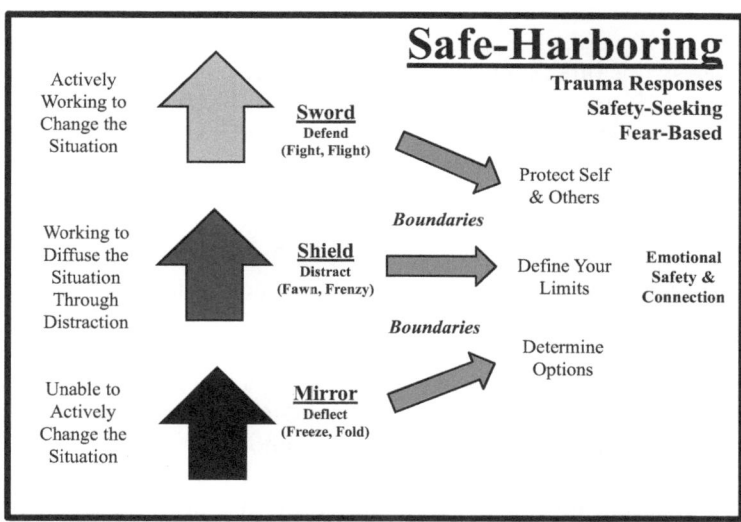

*Figure 7.3* Safe harboring—levels of safe-harboring responses.

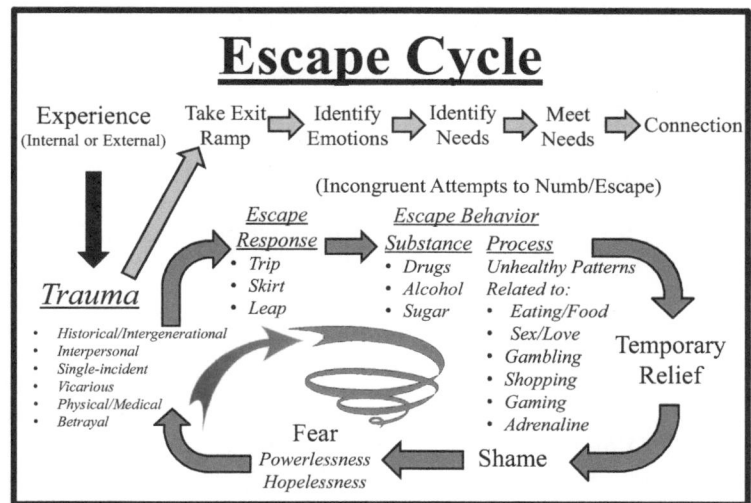

*Figure 7.4* Escape cycle—my escape cycle worksheet.

then can escalate to compulsive use, and become out of control when we get stuck in them and can no longer get out on our own. Escape cycles start as trauma cycles. As we talked about earlier, trauma cycles are attempts to create safety. Escape cycles develop when we give up on trying to create safety and instead try to numb or escape the pain. This can feel like it helps short term as the pain stops, but it numbs all emotions, including emotions like peace and joy, and the behaviors have to escalate to provide the same level of numbing, so it turns into a spiral rather than a spin.

*Disclosure*

Disclosure of betrayal is often an important part of recovery. There are professionals who argue that disclosure is unnecessary and even unhelpful. There is almost no research on the topic of disclosing infidelity (Curtis et al., 2021). Curtis et al. state: "Treating undisclosed infidelity as abuse that causes trauma is necessary to understand the devastating effects of such as offense, and, as such, will help counselors convey the necessary empathy needed when working with clients" (p. 4). This is supported by Siegel's statement that "nonconsensual sexual activity is sexual abuse" (2019, p. 225). Barraca and Polanski (2021) reviewed that data from a previous study (Marín et al., 2014) and found that disclosure of infidelity significantly increased the chances of a relationship continuing as opposed to relationships with undisclosed infidelity, as only 20% of couples with undisclosed infidelity were still together after five years and 57% of those with disclosed infidelity were still together. Additionally, they found that levels of relational satisfaction and stability among couples with disclosed infidelity were similar to couples with no infidelity.

It is important to utilize a non-shaming approach to disclosure. The goals for disclosure are to share the truth, rebuild trust and connection, and decrease shame. This does not mean blaming the person who has been betrayed, nor does it eliminate or decrease responsibility for the person who has betrayed. It is essential for the person who has betrayed to take accountability for what they did and work with those they have betrayed to help process the experience and rebuild a foundation of trust and safety.

There are several models of disclosure. The Connected Recovery model includes four "letters": What and How, Why, Impact, and Amends. These four steps walk individuals and relationships through a detailed apology for the betrayal. The What and How letter explains what happened and the steps taken to hide it. The Why letter explores how the individual got to a point where they betrayed themselves and others. The Impact letter is written by the person who has been betrayed and describes the pain they felt. The Amends letter reflects the pain expressed in the Impact letter and explains the steps taken to repair the damage done and the steps being taken so it won't be repeated. I highly recommend more in-depth training if you plan to facilitate disclosures.

*Stages of Grief*

The process of early recovery can be summarized as moving through the stages of grief. The stages of grief describe the journey from the initial discovery of a loss, through the ensuing pain, and ultimately to finding a way to move forward. In this case, the loss is trust and emotional security. The Connected Recovery model includes six stages of grief rather than the traditional five stages, and several of the stages are labeled differently. At the beginning, there is a whole lot of shock and very little acceptance. At the end, there is a whole lot of acceptance and very little shock. The rest is a mess of all six stages. The six stages of grief are detailed below.

The first stage of grief is traditionally referred to as "denial"; however, it is better understood as emotional shock. The word denial often connotes deliberate avoidance of an issue or emotion. This stage of grief is not deliberate avoidance. It is our mind's way of filtering the pain, so we survive it. The second stage of grief is anger. Anger is the energy behind the emotion. As a general emotion, anger tells us that something is wrong, and either we are being hurt or someone else is being hurt. It helps us know that there is damage that needs to be healed or changes that need to be made. It gives us the power to move forward and make changes so we can heal and minimize the chance of being hurt again. The traditional model of grief calls the third stage of grief "depression." It's more than depression. It's the raw emotions connected to the experience. It's the pain, the anguish, the despair, the ache. This stage of grief helps you process the experience. It honors the loss of what you had or possibly what you thought you had. It expresses the depth of the loss.

The fourth stage of grief is bargaining. It basically means trying to figure out how to change the story, so it has a different ending, so you don't have to hurt. It sounds like "if only …" or "what if …." The point of this stage of grief is to figure out what changes we can make in the future. The fifth stage of grief is not included in the traditional model of grief. It's making meaning. This stage is about taking our power back. It helps us figure out how we are going to use what we are going through or have gone through to change us and/or the world. The final stage of grief is acceptance. This doesn't mean "I'm ok with this." It means "this is what it is, and this is how I'm moving forward." It happens as the shock wears off, as the anger is used to provide energy to make changes, as the pain is felt and processed, as bargaining helps figure out changes to be made and as we take our power and/or our life back. Life will never be exactly the same again. Some things are lost for good. Some things are gained throughout the healing process. Acceptance is shifting to seeing life as it is now and moving forward with it.

### Middle Recovery

Once the pain of what happened is processed and emotional safety is recreated, the work of recovery shifts to focusing on developing empathy for self and others and strengthening connection. These steps are similar to traditional relational counseling in that they consider relational patterns, using understanding of emotions and needs to shift those patterns into more functional and healthy configurations. Often, exploration of family-of-origin trauma and attachment styles is helpful. Sharing is done at a deeper level as the connection is strengthened.

Connection to others is a biological imperative for human beings (Bowlby, 1982). Trauma and interpersonal trust both have a significant impact on attachment (Schröder et al., 2019). Gabbay and Lafontaine (2017) explain that, as individuals shift into adulthood, attachment figures change from parental units to romantic partners, but the foundational need for connection, support, and security continues. Zeifman (2019) highlights that the connection within romantic relationships can differ across cultures as the goal for primary relationships differs across cultures, along with differences in expectations and support structure. However, connection is healing, and lack of connection is damaging, regardless of cultural background.

EFT is a commonly used model of relational counseling. The underlying premise of EFT is explained as the belief that attachment is vital for each person and feeling loved and supported is critical for secure attachment (Greenman et al., 2019). The end goal of this model is secure attachment. The core of EFT is understanding needs through emotions. The concept of needs can be understood through Maslow's Hierarchy of Needs. Maslow's seminal study on Human Motivation (1943) introduced the idea of the Hierarchy of Needs, stating that basic needs must be met before more advanced needs can be considered. He divides needs into five categories: "physiological, safety, love, esteem, and self-actualization" (p. 394). Following this framework, once safety is developed, the focus is love and esteem.

Middle recovery helps balance between internally and externally focused connection, expanding on the concept introduced in early recovery of connection to self and connection to others. Part of that process is identifying our limits, setting boundaries, and learning to enforce those boundaries. Processing through emotions and needs gives us the information we need to know what our limits are and to understand the impact interactions have on us. Communicating those boundaries is the next step. Utilizing EFT to communicate starts with exploring the core of the message so the message can be expressed at the deepest level. The underlying message is the reason for the conversation, which is usually a bid for connection because the relationship matters. State that foundational message at the beginning of the dialogue, followed by the concern or pain point. If possible, work together to come up with a solution. If a collaborative resolution doesn't work, determine the steps needed to honor your limits.

Compassion for self and empathy for others are the primary goals of middle recovery. Self-compassion is patience and kindness toward ourselves when we are imperfect. Empathy is understanding the pain someone is going through by connecting that hurt to an emotion you have experienced. Both involve sitting in the pain rather than trying to fix it, minimize it, or distract from it. Sitting in the pain allows space for the emotions to be processed through and resolved, deepening the connection to ourselves and others.

### Late Recovery

With a foundation of emotional safety created through truth, upon which empathy and connection have been built, recovery can shift to the deepest level of connection to self and others, healthy sexuality. Healing from PSB and betrayal cannot solely include cessation of unhealthy or disengaging behaviors and exploration of the pain caused by them; it must also integrate healthy behaviors. This stage of recovery starts with defining healthy sexuality and moves on to processing any sexual trauma. Areas of sexual connection are reclaimed or redefined as needed, as sexual connection is deepened. This work addresses the deepest levels of trauma and happens after a significant amount of safety and connection has been built. This does not mean that sexual connection is not mentioned earlier in the recovery process; it should be discussed throughout the journey. However, an in-depth, focused examination of this area of connection helps ensure that the deepest levels of healing are reached.

The main objective of sex therapy is to achieve enduring and fulfilling sexual function. Sex therapy addresses physiological factors, psychological issues, relational dynamics, and psychosexual skills. White et al. (2023) emphasize that a sex-positive approach focuses on open-mindedness and communication rather than judgment around sexual orientations, interactions, and preferences. They highlight that it is about providing space for open communication and consideration, encouraging each individual to embrace their sexual needs and interests. This approach does not advocate for increased frequency or activity, nor does it endorse decreasing frequency or activity. Additionally, it does not avoid discussing the consequences of various sexual activities or choices, but rather provides a framework where consequences are discussed and factored into the equation. Emotional health, physical health, and sexual health are all considered. Open communication about sexual connection with self and partners is essential for both individual and relational satisfaction.

Healthy sexuality is a connection to yourself and your body and the ability to share that connection in ways that are safe for you and others. It is an individual and relational process that looks different for each person and each relationship. As Emily Nagoski says, a healthy sex life is about confidence and joy. "Confidence is knowing what's true. Joy is loving what's true" (Nagoski, 2016). Nagoski goes on to state that loving what's true includes loving our limitations, our struggles, our quirks. It includes knowing what turns us on and what turns us off. Healthy sexuality is about knowing who you really are and loving yourself.

Processing any sexual trauma is an essential step. Often trauma treatment modalities, such as EMDR, psychodrama, or somatic experiencing, can be helpful. Additionally, utilizing Internal Family Systems (IFS), a type of therapy that helps process trauma to connect with parts of us that are sexual or parts of us that have been traumatized can play a significant role. Once the trauma is processed, we need to get to know ourselves. The boundaries each person is comfortable using to explore themselves and their needs and desires will be different and need to be honored.

Sexual success includes experiences that build and strengthen a connection to self and partner(s). Each person needs to have control over their own body and what they choose to do with it or not do with it. Boundaries and needs should be communicated throughout the experience, allowing each person to stay congruent with themselves. Emotional safety needs to be maintained for each person involved throughout the process. Note that this list does not include any specific sexual or physical act. Sexual connection is highly personal and can include whatever each person connects to. Strong recovery includes the ability to have a deep connection to self and others in ways that are most meaningful for each person.

## Questions for Reflection

1  What would constitute PSB or betrayal for you?
2  What role might cultural differences, relational orientation, or sexual orientation play in the definition of PSB and betrayal?
3  Do you see trauma cycles in yourself? What about escape cycles? What, if any, new connections did you make about your patterns related to trauma and escape cycles?
4  What steps might be helpful for you to take to expand your knowledge around identifying and treating PSB and betrayal?
5  What personal biases do you have that might impact your ability to connect with clients' definitions of PSB and betrayal? What steps might be helpful to address those biases?

## References

Barraca, J., & Polanski, T. (2021). Infidelity treatment from an integrative behavioral couple therapy perspective: Explanatory model and intervention strategies. *Journal of Marital and Family Therapy, 47*(4), 909–924.

Borgogna, N. C., Garos, S., Meyer, C. L., Trussell, M. R., & Kraus, S. W. (2022). A review of behavioral interventions for compulsive sexual behavior disorder. *Current Addiction Reports, 9*(3), 99–108. https://doi.org/10.1007/s40429-022-00422-x

Bowlby, J. (1982). Attachment and loss: Retrospect and prospect. *American Journal of Orthopsychiatry, 52*(4), 664–678. https://doi.org/10.1111/j.1939-0025.1982.tb01456.x

Curtis, R., Likis-Werle, E., & Shelton, T. (2021). Counseling clients who have experienced undisclosed infidelity. *The Family Journal: Counseling and Therapy for Couples and Families, 29*(4), 457–464.

Gabbay, N., & Lafontaine, M.-F. (2017). Understanding the relationship between attachment, caregiving, and Same sex intimate partner violence. *Journal of Family Violence, 32*(3), 291–304. https://doi.org/10.1007/s10896-016-9897-9

Greenman, P. S., Johnson, S. M., & Wiebe, S. (2019). Emotionally focused therapy for couples: At the heart of science and practice. In B. H. Fiese, M. Celano, K. D. Deater-Deckard, E. N. Jouriles, & M. A. Whisman (Eds.), *APA handbook of contemporary family psychology: Family therapy and training* (Vol. 3, pp. 291–305). American Psychological Association. https://doi.org/10.1037/0000101-018

Herring, B. (2017). A framework for categorizing chronically problematic sexual behavior. *Sexual Addiction & Compulsivity*, 24(4), 242–247. https://doi.org/10.1080/10720162.2017.1394947

Hollenbeck, C., & Steffens, B. (2024). Betrayal trauma anger: Clinical implications for therapeutic treatment based on the sexually betrayed partner's experience related to anger after intimate betrayal. *Journal of Sex & Marital Therapy*, 50(4), 456–467. https://doi.org/10.1080/00926 23X.2024.2306940

Knowlton, L. (2023). *Facing hope*. Self-Published, Amazon. ISBN: 9798387356735.

Knowlton, L. (2024). *Connected recovery™ continuing outpatient treatment curriculum: comprehensive treatment of problematic sexual behaviors (PSB) and betrayal trauma* [Doctoral Project, Modern Sex Therapy Institutes].

Kowalewska, E., & Lew-Starowicz, M. (2021). Compulsive Sexual Behavior Disorder—The evolution of a new diagnosis introduced to the ICD-11, current evidence and ongoing research challenges. *Wiedza Medyczna*, 3(1), 17–23.

Lepak, M., & Carson, G. (2022). Presence psychotherapy: A novel integrated trauma treatment model for thorough memory reconsolidation. *Journal of Psychotherapy Integration*, 32(4), 426–442.

Lonergan, M., Brunet, A., Rivest-Beauregard, M., & Groleau, D. (2021). Is romantic partner betrayal a form of traumatic experience? A qualitative study. *Stress and Health*, 37(1), 19–31. https://doi.org/10.1002/smi.2968

Marín, R., Christensen, A., & Atkins, D. (2014). Infidelity and behavioral couple therapy: Relationship outcomes over 5 years following therapy. *Couple and Family Psychology: Research and Practice*, 3(1), 1–12. https://doi.org/10.1037/cfp0000012

Maslow, A. H. (1943). A theory of human motivation. *Psychological Review*, 50(4), 370–396. https://doi.org/10.1037/h0054346

Nagoski, E. (2016). Confidence and joy are the keys to a great sex life. *TEDx University of Nevada*. https://www.youtube.com/watch?v=HILY0wWBlBM

Pandey, R., & Vaish, A. (2022). Betrayal trauma. *International Journal of Technical Research & Science*, 8(1), 9–12. https://doi.org/:10.30780/IJTRS.V07.I01.003

Perel, E. (2017). *The state of affairs: Rethinking infidelity: by Esther Perel*. Harper Collins.

Rokach, A., & Chan, S. (2023). Love and infidelity: Causes and consequences. *International Journal of Environmental Research and Public Health*, 20(5).

Schröder, M., Lüdtke, J., Fux, E., Izat, Y., Bolten, M., Gloger-Tippelt, G., Suess, G. J., & Schmid, M. (2019). Attachment disorder and attachment theory - Two sides of one medal or two different coins? *Comprehensive Psychiatry*, 95, 152139. https://doi.org/10.1016/j.comppsych.2019.152139

Siegel, R. (2019). Therapists who address O.C.S.B., In J. C. Wadley & R Siegel (Eds.), *The Art of Sex Therapy Supervision* (pp. 221–253). Routlage.

Steffens, B., & Rennie, R. (2006). The traumatic nature of disclosure for wives of sexual addicts. *Journal of Sexual Health & Compulsivity*, 13(2–3), 247–267.

Warach, B., & Josephs, L. (2021). The aftershocks of infidelity: A review of infidelity-based attachment trauma. *Sexual and Relationship Therapy*, 36(1), 68–90. https://doi.org/10.1080/14681994.2019.1577961

Warach, B., Josephs, L., & Gorman, B. S. (2018). Pathways to infidelity: The roles of self-serving bias and betrayal trauma. *Journal of Sex & Marital Therapy*, 44(5), 497–512. https://doi.org/10.1080/0092623x.2017.1416434

White, A., Boehm, M., Glackin, E., & Bleakley, A. (2023). How sexual information sources are related to emerging adults' sex-positive scripts and sexual communication. *Sexuality & Culture*, 27(4)1–22.

World Health Organization. (2024). 6C72 Compulsive sexual behaviour disorder. In *International statistical classification of diseases and related health problems* (11th ed.). https://icd.who.int/browse/2024-01/mms/en#1630268048

Zeifman, D. M. (2019). Attachment theory grows up: A developmental approach to pair bonds. *Current Opinion in Psychology*, 25, 139–143. https://doi.org/10.1016/j.copsyc.2018.06.001

# Section II

# Leading Conversations about Public Health and Human Services

# 8  The Intersection of Public Health and Human Services

*Neil E. Duchac, Jill S. Minor, and Jonah N. Duchac*

## The Intersection between Public Health and Human Services

Inevitably, over time, mental health and public health cross treatment paths to include medical interventions and practices with those of the mental health community, to include social work, counseling, and psychology, to name a few professions. Often during this intersecting work, it can be challenging to know what protocol to follow and, at times, who is responsible for specific services. This chapter discusses the historical context of this intersection and how impacted professionals at times seem to operate in isolation from one another.

Sparkman-Key and Reiter (2016) surveyed members within the National Organization of Human Services to assess professional positions within the field. It was noted that many participants concluded that they were a part of more than one specific profession. Some specific professions included counseling, social work, and psychology. Other fields that were identified included special education, the medical field, emergency medical technicians, members of the correctional community, and addictions. The majority of those surveyed (80%) were female, and the majority of those providing services were from the southern and midwestern parts of the United States. The actual type of work that each human service professional was involved in was quite varied based on the geographical location and needs of the given area.

## Public Health

Public health has its origins as an environmentally based profession focused on sanitation, environmental concerns, and communicable disease (Rosen, 2015). As the science of the public health profession progressed, this venture led to a focus on medical issues and the genesis of various diseases with a primary goal of prevention. In the United States, the public health service was developed in 1913 as a mechanism to effect individual change by altering individual environments (Centers for Disease and Control, 2014). This perspective later evolved from changing the environment after the fact to trying to alter the individual in a more proactive manner (Fairchild et al., 2010).

The public health officer utilized his authority to control community infections and individuals with communicable diseases. Although this authority still rests in the public health department, it is today utilized in a different way. Efforts are made to gain the participation of the individual through their understanding of this need for care in order that infections within the community may be controlled. Now a broader program of services exists, including some programs of medical care for families and community groups. Formerly, public

DOI: 10.4324/9781003531258-11

health was concerned not only with environmental hygiene but also with other causes of ill health in the population (Rice, 1959).

Public health now attempts to relate its programs and services to the needs of the people rather than to have people fit the established program. Warne and Bane Frizzell (2014), among so many other authors, recognize the need to not only focus on social and environmental issues, access to services, and navigate cultural/governmental relationships. In so doing, it recognized that one must work with people where they are. Progress may be made in the health field, and people understand and desire to create change. Public health shares with clinical medicine and social work common concerns: there is the same need to understand the individual, illness, and the factors which contribute to or handicap prevention; the same desire to understand individuals within the context of family and community dynamics; the same necessity of knowing and coordinating community services to help meet the needs of individuals and groups; the same emphasis on comprehensive evaluation of the problem and the multidisciplinary nature of treatment; and the same goal of rehabilitation and prevention of ill health and disability (Gorin, 2001). There exists a connection between physical health, emotional health, and mental health and the various professions.

The mental health profession is fragmented, inadequate, and biased, with a global/societal mental health stigma impacting the resources and services to those who suffer from mental health concerns (Henderson et al., 2013; IOM, 2003). These factors engender a complex landscape for the public health and mental health practitioner to reduce the burden of mental illness. This chapter serves to further discuss the relationship between public health, social work, and mental health counseling, as well as models of advocacy related to each. Additionally provided is a discussion of the medical and mental treatment models to ameliorate the burden of mental health treatment.

### History of Public Health

The origins of public health date back to 1798 in the United States, when the federal government established a Marine Hospital Service to provide services to seamen (CDC, 2011). After seeing increased activity with various disorders requiring quarantine, the federal government changed the name of this hospital to the Public Health and Marine Hospital in 1902. In 1879, the National Board of Health was established. This board was the first organized attempt at medical research by the federal government (NIH, 2014). Later, in 1912, the name was changed to Public Health Service. In 1917, services were transferred from the federal government to state and local health boards. During World War I, the focus of the Public Health Service was venereal diseases (CDC, 2011). Following World War I, the role of public health in the United States began to expand to include a focus on preventive measures and education and on crippled children. In 1930, the National Institute of Health was established, and, in 1939, Public Health Services were combined with welfare services, the precursor to the Department of Health and Human Services. Following World War II, the focus again shifted to crippled children and building hospital buildings and tangible resources. In 1946, the Centers for Disease Control and Prevention was established, Medicare and Medicaid practices were added to the Public Health in 1965, and the Environmental Protection Agency and the Occupational Health and Safety Administration were added in 1970 (CDC, 2011).

According to the Centers for Disease Control and Prevention (2014), the 20th century was important to the field of public health in that people in the United States gained an average of nearly 20 years of additional life expectancy. Also noted are the ten greatest impacts made during the 20th century: advances in immunizations, workplace safety, motor vehicle safety, control of infectious diseases, increased safety in foods, a reduction in heart disease and stroke occurrences, fluoridating water, recognizing the risks of tobacco, family planning, and recognizing future trends in mental health.

Although public health predates social work, both fields evolved into their contemporary forms during the early 20th century. Social work drew its inspiration primarily from the community-oriented settlement house component, which was promulgated by activists. One such activist, Jane Addams, used interventions to address poverty, overcrowding, immigration, and child labor and, second, the charity organization component, which used casework to help individuals overcome poverty and avoid dependence on society for assistance (Ruth & Marshall, 2017).

The absence of specific mental health treatment modalities and information germane to advocacy efforts further suggests the disconnect existing between the mental health and public health communities. Moreover, future trends of mental health such as social determinants of mental health call for a more collaborative public health approach in that the major pathways of mental health outcomes (e.g., depression, anxiety, alcohol dependence) have multiple pathways influenced across societal factors, including, but not limited to, political, social, economic, and environmental factors that span across the life course and interact between the individual and the macrolevel of society (WHO & Calouste Gulbenkian Foundation, 2014).

## Stigma and History of Mental Health

Mental health has often suffered from a negative stigma, dating back to the ancient Greeks prior to 450 B.C. (Burger, 2011). During this time, the philosopher Hippocrates established mental health labels for individuals, including terms such as melancholy and mania. Though not discussing the origins of mental health concerns from a brain perspective, he believed that all ailments were related in some manner to a physiological origin (Burger, 2011).

Historically, the negative stigma of mental health continued through the Middle Ages, and the church, as an initial response, set up human services programs to aid those with perceived mental illness (Burger, 2011). The church in the early part of the Middle Ages felt a compelling obligation to help those considered to be less fortunate (Burger, 2011). During the latter stages of the Middle Ages, the view of the church changed somewhat, and the focus changed from establishing human service refugees to excluding people viewed as non-believers. This shift in paradigms caused more alienation to occur and, in a sense, furthered the stigma. In the United States, those who were considered less fortunate from socioeconomic and mental health viewpoints were placed in settlement houses, with the idea that they could work to the extent possible and be taken care of as needed. During the late 19th and early 20th centuries, there was an influx of those with perceived mental illness into mental health institutions. During this time, there was a social reform view that human services, up through the 1940s, were contributing to the establishment of a welfare state to provide services to those impacted by mental illness (Burger, 2011). According to a report by the World Health Organization (WHO) (Henderson et al., 2013), more than 70% of adolescents and adults with mental illness do not receive any mental health treatment. Globally, stigmatizing attitudes toward mental illness persist among the public and have been associated with the reluctance to seek help (Henderson et al., 2013).

## Human Services

Shally-Jensen (2015) describes human services as offering a direct and applied approach in supporting positive human development, with services being offered to individuals and communities. This desire to support the development of others offers a diverse population of clients, encompassing all ages, as well as possessing a wide range of issues. Often, it is not one single problem that the client is experiencing but instead a culmination of several that may classify the client into several client populations. Groups can range greatly from children in abusive situations to veterans who have a mental condition (Shally-Jensen, 2015).

## Blending of Public Health and Human Services

The Surgeon General of the United States in 1999 called upon the public health community and the mental health community to become integrated, citing that over the course of an individual's lifetime, approximately 46% of the population will suffer some type of mental illness, with approximately 26% of adults over the age of 18 suffering from a diagnosable mental health disorder (CDC). The recognition that there is a coaction between physical health and mental or emotional health has become more widespread (Schneiderman & Speers, 2010). As a result, the Centers for Disease Control and Prevention issued an executive summary calling for the integration of the public health and mental health communities to be completed by the end of 2015 (CDC, 2014). Though positive progress has been made, public health and mental health have not been fully integrated as of 2024.

Social work in healthcare settings includes numerous sub-disciplines, such as public health, behavioral health, oncology, nephrology, and palliative care. Most health social workers serve in direct roles such as counseling, health education, and crisis intervention, thus circumventing the stigma many experienced when seeking mental health services (Gorin, 2001). The rise of urbanization and industrialization created health problems that became impossible to ignore (Haines, 1991). Although members of the upper class could escape the overcrowded cities by moving to rural areas, members of the emerging urban middle class did not enjoy this luxury (Baltzell, 1964). They "paid taxes, supported cleanliness and public education, recognized and abhorred corruption, and, as home owners, had an investment in their cities" (Garrett, 2000, p. 284). The middle class took the lead in advocating a wide range of reforms, including the enactment of health and safety regulations.

The CDC (2014) discussed that the public health community has approached mental illness through the years, utilizing both a medical and surveillance model. There has been a focus on elements of public health, such as epidemiology as well as examination of specific risk factors affecting mental illness. As a result, there has been a development of prevention methods that are based upon the public health community as a whole and not specifically related to individuals who are impacted by the specific illness. Additionally, the public health community focused on examining policies impacting the mental health communities and attempts to present evidence-based research regarding mental health information that may be integrated into the hospitals that serve as treatment communities (CDC, 2011). The public health community began to recognize the resources utilized and how they were impacted by those with mental illnesses. The integration of mental health and public health is necessary for the benefit of the public and to support the multiple stakeholders that exist in each individual system (CDC, 2011; Jones & Tang, 2016; Schneiderman & Speers, 2010; World Health Organization and Calouste Gulbenkian Foundation, 2014).

In the early 1900s, with advances in medical research, more diseases were found to be caused by microorganisms, so public health stopped tying illness to environmental factors and tied it more to microorganisms (Gorin, 2001). A chasm between preventive health and curative health continued to develop, and medical research chose to focus more on the curative aspect. This advance in medical research changed the focus of their work from curative as the absence of disease and instead focused more on the goal of curing the disease (Gorin, 2001).

Social workers have a clear interest in addressing the crisis in public health. They have long been advocates for powerless and disenfranchised people. They also call attention to the connection between inequality and health. In a WHO report, a need was described for the inclusion of social justice in mental health: "A focus on social justice may provide an important corrective to what has been seen as a growing over-emphasis on individual pathology" (p. iv). Social workers who consciously incorporate social justice into their practice do so in a manner that attempts to address immediate crisis and emotional pain.

The public health paradigm is in alignment with social justice because it is understood as having universal commitments to bring about as much health as possible in a community, whether physical or mental (Ashcroft, 2014). It also seeks to be vigilant for evidence of inequalities related to those in privileged social groups and to intervene to reduce these inequalities as much as possible. Social work has been historically linked with the public health paradigm since the 1920s, when the profession expanded to meet the needs of public health's burgeoning preventive programs.

The role of social work practice is to focus on those directly affected by physical and emotional disorders—or, more importantly, those "at risk" of acquiring physical and emotional disorders. The task of social work practice is therefore to encourage individualized intervention strategies that are in alignment with the therapeutic view of social work (Ashcroft, 2014). From this perspective, social work primarily engages in preventive strategies directed at curbing harmful individual behaviors and identifying potential risks through the use of risk assessments. It addresses the preventive element of community mental illness by recognizing those individuals and situations of potential risk, while also working to treat and cure the symptoms and illnesses already being experienced by those within that community.

Elder and Silvers (2009) discussed the need for mental health practitioners and medical practitioners to work together on developing an integrated model of both public and mental health. Their article noted the disproportion of psychology professionals in a primary care medical treatment facility. With a ratio of two psychologists to nearly 10,000 patients, the need to have additional practitioners was recognized to aid in the treatment of conditions that appear to be mental health-based but may impact the medical side (Elder & Silvers, 2009). As part of the discussion, it was recommended that mental health practitioners receive some formal training in health psychology or behavioral and primary care medicine as a way of benefiting the patients who are seen by both the mental public health and mental health practitioners.

On the contrary, Semansky et al. (2012) conducted a study examining the interrelationship between mental health and public health, as the state of New Mexico sought to serve several mentally ill adults in New Mexico under the guise of non-profit public health, compared to for-profit mental health providers. This study provided much insight into the differences, noting that non-profit agencies relied more heavily on unlicensed mental health providers who required supervision and continued training. Second, they noted that there were fewer independently licensed individuals because there were not enough state-provided dollars to support these staff. Third, it was determined that funding for the non-profits was typically provided by state-funded dollars, while for-profits focused more on accruing insurance money for support.

Carver and Morrison (2005) conducted a qualitative study in England where they examined the perceptions of health advocates who worked on psychiatric in-patient units. The authors discovered that key relational differences existed in terms of both education and communication between public health and mental health advocates. Second, they examined factors which were perceived to help and hinder the advocacy process. Carver and Morrison revealed several themes: an increased need for advocacy training, the need for good interpersonal skills, a motivation to serve as a helper, and the ability to be non-judgmental. Also noted was the need for support and supervision and that there was an emotional impact caused by working as an advocate. Finally, advocacy in practice was examined by Carver and Morrison (2005), with primary factors noted being (1) that advocacy be independent of the healthcare that is being provided and (2) a need to respect the viewpoints of the mental health professional while approaching the mental health professional in a non-confrontational manner. Much of what was determined by this study would hold true today in the United States in terms of needing to improve communication between public health and mental health professionals. Additionally, though more collaboration is being seen, there is still some practice of mental health that occurs independently of public health professionals.

Yung et al. (2005) conducted a study that examined the relationship between public health psychiatrists and clinicians and private sector psychiatrists and clinicians. The participants in this study answered a survey asking about the relationship between these two sectors. Also discussed were methods of enhancing these relationships. Of note, several areas were identified as areas of concern. The first noted area of concern was communication between the public and private sectors. Second, a presumed barrier to a successful relationship was confusion about the various roles and whether the public and the private sector were to perform similar or different functions. Third, different treatment approaches were noted as a barrier to enhancing the relationship between the public and private sectors. This article also discussed how few referrals were made between the differing sectors because of the presumed differences in populations that were treated and because of a lack of knowledge about the areas of expertise that each sector's professionals possessed (Yung et al., 2005).

Similar to the Yung et al. (2005) study, Chaudry et al. (2000) examined the relationship between nurses in the public health sector and the mental health sector in Ohio. Presented was the idea that there was a lack of an integrated system where public health and mental health successfully co-existed, allowing for a sharing of available resources versus competition because of not knowing what was available. Another interesting aspect discussed by this study was the mandate for both sectors to provide services to disadvantaged groups of people. The study concluded typically that the organizations that were the most vocal were able to provide the services, while the other organizations fell by the wayside. This caused them to be non-compliant with this mandate and created relationship problems between the public health and mental health communities. Compliance is considered to be vital.

In a study by Williams et al. (2023), the effects of a campaign by the U.S. Department of Health and Human Services to help increase vaccination awareness during the COVID-19 pandemic are examined. The *We Can Do This* campaign aimed to help educate the public on the vaccine to raise both awareness and confidence, with the goal being to increasing the likelihood of members of the public receiving the first dose of the vaccine. The campaign utilized a mixture of television, print, digital, radio, and out-of-home channels to help educate the public. Williams et al. found a large uptick of 125% in terms of the likelihood of one seeking a first dose of the COVID-19 vaccination.

Advocacy is defined as the representation of a person for the attainment of needed services (Burger, 2011). Myers and Sweeney (2004) discuss advocacy as one of the fundamental essences of the field of mental health as it relates to assisting someone, emphasizing how advocacy as an action seems to conjure up ideas of protest and unrest, resulting in picket lines and going door to door as a mechanism of change. Advocacy is important because it helps people to be their best and includes elements that can be expanded to other fields of study, such as social justice and multiculturalism (Myers, 2014). It is believed that this tradition can be expanded in consultation with the field of public health, social work, and counseling.

## Advocacy Theory

Burger (2011) addressed the significance and impact of advocacy theory, specifically in three areas related to the human services field: community organizing, community outreach, and case management. Advocacy in the field of counseling takes on different forms and involves a multitude of people and professions. However, the areas, as noted above, are consistent throughout the helping profession. This section elaborates on each of these areas and how they are specifically related to advocacy efforts.

In the early part of the 20th century, emphasis on continuity of care, examination of contacts, and specific protection from infections were seen as important in the control of tuberculosis and the venereal diseases (Burger, 2011). This demonstrated perfectly the need for advocacy as well as preventive services. It became clear that patients, families, and community groups needed help, both through health education and through social work efforts, in utilizing medical resources. Before the 1960s, most social work in public health focused on secondary prevention; however, interest in primary prevention gradually intensified as it was studied more and in different arenas (Burger, 2011).

Krupa and Carter (2012) conducted a study that examined community organizing as it related to those who are mentally ill and seeking employment. Initially considered was the idea that those with mental illness had a more difficult time finding employment because they were considered part of a marginalized population working less stable jobs for minimum wage salaries when compared to others not experiencing a mental illness. Examined was the utilization of a provisional model of community organizing that focused on the mentally ill and the potential employers as the stakeholders. Education of potential employers and access to employment services were considered two key elements of this community organization approach. Key emphases in this study focused on defining employment for the mentally ill as a community need, establishing a community commitment to reduce the concern, and formulating a strategy of engagement and seeking active participation (Krupa & Carter, 2012). Overall, the final results of this study suggested that the notion of community organizing was successful in terms of garnering support and also in terms of having people from the community participate (Krupa & Carter, 2012).

A second element of Advocacy Theory is outreach (Burger, 2011). Community outreach refers to reaching those individuals in need of particular services in order of the most significant need (Day & Davis, 2006). Day and Davis (2006) conducted a study which examined community outreach for children impacted by mental illness. The idea behind their study was that outreach was becoming more necessary for children based on a decrease in functionality, as a result of an increase in family problems, poor educational attainment, and decreased social functioning. Outreach as it relates to this study called for an interaction between primary care providers, including primary care physicians; specialty providers, which could include occupational or speech therapists; and mental health professionals. Interacting and reaching out to other professionals was purported to allow for a reduction in the need for mental health services (Day & Davis, 2006). Overall, this study demonstrated that utilizing an outreach perspective led to a reduction in the need for mental health services in the short term and at the one-year mark that reduction was still present for the experimental group compared with the control group (Day & Davis, 2006).

Case management is a third element of Advocacy (Burger, 2011). Keegan (1998) wrote about the benefits of case management as they pertain to nurse practitioners and the increase of nurse practitioners working in consultation with primary treatment providers in treating mental health issues. In this instance, case managers were used to establish a plan of care and to aid the patient in following through with the needed treatment. In this article, it was suggested that nurse practitioners bridge a widening gap that a lack of primary care physicians was causing in terms of treatment and being able to reach more individuals. Another role where the case management would be helpful was in making home visits for those who are unable to be seen in an office or practice setting.

In the practice of social work case management, new emphasis on prevention has developed, such as work with persons who are not asking for help, but where the social worker's skill in observation indicates that there are emergent problems, often in such an early state that the patient himself is not yet ready to ask for help and other members of the team may not recognize the need (Ruth et al., 2015). Public health now attempts to relate its programs and services to the needs of the people rather than to have people fit the established program. In so doing, it recognized that one must work with people where they are, and that only by an understanding and a desire on the people's part to do something about their needs will real progress be made in the health field. The concept of health, too, has been broadened to include, as the World Health Organization defined it, "that state of physical, mental, and social well-being" (Ruth et al., 2015, p. 17).

Kondrat and Early (2010) examined case management as it related to the therapeutic or working alliance with those who are mentally ill and receiving case management. They determined that case managers were more successful in establishing such a working relationship. Second, it was determined that case managers could be trained to collaborate with their clients on establishing goals. Third, it was suggested by this study that case management and a working relationship could aid in reducing the sense of stigma attached to mental illness (Kondrat & Early, 2010). Three other variables noted in this study were the ideas that the general public discriminates against those with mental illness, self-esteem and quality of life are typically seen as being lower for those with mental illness, and current methods of changing stereotypes related to mental illness have not been successful (Kondrat & Early, 2010).

### Wellness Model

A more recent development in mental health treatment that is seemingly more aligned with the varying constructs of the treatment of health, with a focus not specifically on illness or the absence of illness, is the Wellness Model (Myers & Sweeney, 2008). Myers and Sweeney (2008) discussed the significance of wellness to the field of mental health and, in a larger sense, public health, by focusing on the wellness of the client and what accomplishes and maintains a level of wellness. The model focuses on strength, developmental growth, and remediating dysfunction, leading to personal optimization.

Foster (2010) discussed the need for mental health professionals to adopt the Wellness Model as a mechanism to help students and professionals to be successful, linking this model to future professional success and positive decision-making for both students who are doing well and those who are struggling. The Wellness Theory calls for practicing professionals to serve as both practitioners and educators to teach therapeutic techniques, with an emphasis on health and a holistic approach to health involving exercise, eating appropriately, and living a healthy, stress-reduced life. Finnerty and Jencius (2011) support the significance of developing a wellness model, specifying self-care for the practitioner in addition to the client, as it takes the form of a creative self, physical self, and social self. Considering the various elements related to maintaining wellness in training mental health professionals, Yager and Tovar-Blank (2007) indicate that these elements are applicable to mental health practitioners in the field and the development and maintenance of wellness in practice. The presented elements include introducing wellness directly into practice, associating self-growth and awareness, modeling wellness, noting that perfection is not the desired outcome, presenting wellness as a lifestyle, encouraging personal counseling as a mechanism of support, reviewing different wellness perspectives, promoting wellness through instructed courses, developing innovative ways to reinforce wellness, and exposing students to a more positive humanistic perspective.

For the past number of years, social work has turned its focus to a holistic approach (Ruth et al., 2015). This approach allows for the focus to include wider aspects of the client, including physical, mental, emotional, and spiritual. It calls for the social worker to acknowledge these components of the client, to assess each component, and to include them in the treatment plan as necessary. This vision, being more well-rounded than in previous years, allows for a more ethical approach toward the definition of wellness (Ruth et al., 2015).

King (2012) conducted an analysis of the ethical codes for each of the professional areas of mental health, including counseling, psychology, social work, and family therapy. He concluded that wellness was a vital aspect of the American Counseling Association's code of ethics and that Advocacy and Social Justice were considered to be important aspects with regard to the National Association of Social Workers' Code of Ethics.

## Conclusion

This chapter provides a literature review germane to the intersection of public health, social work, and mental health professions. It includes a historical context for social work, public and mental health, as well as advocacy related to each. The Human Services Model and Humanistic Model are presented in that they include theoretical frameworks that are specific to mental health prevention and intervention efforts. The Medical and Wellness Models and the Expectancy Model are also considered in this chapter. Lastly, Advocacy Theory and its connection to public health, social work, and mental health are discussed. The need for interprofessional collaboration and learning is highlighted and emphasized throughout this summary.

The integration of public health and social work can help progress research forward in ways that are not possible outside of this synthesis. As demonstrated through the recent COVID-19 pandemic, when both elements are considered in a more holistic way, methods can be utilized to help the general populace (Williams et al., 2023). As such, this remains a strong area for further research to help increase shared knowledge, as well as opening the door to possible areas of research within each of the individual fields.

It must be noted that public health and social work are vast areas of research. There are limitations to consider as well as opportunities for future research. Some limitations could include narrowing a population, geographical limitations, socioeconomic limitations, and gender or ethnic limitations. Opportunities to consider include the intersection of public health and social work, mental health, disparities, and social disparities. In looking at this review, there are areas where the fields of mental health, social work, and public health could not be fully covered. Regardless of the efforts made, something is inevitably missed in reviewing the germane literature. Additionally, significant milestones may be viewed differently. Further, the literature available in some areas was not as current as one might have hoped, suggesting that not a lot of research is being conducted in this area. From a future research perspective, conducting a qualitative analysis with treatment providers from the mental health disciplines and the public health community would prove interesting and expand knowledge for the fields, respectively.

## Reflective Questions for Consideration

1  How do public health and human services intersect?
2  What elements of public health most influence the field of human services?
3  What models reflect or influence the intersection of human services and public health?

## References

Ashcroft, R. (2014). An evaluation of the public health paradigm: A view of social work. *Social Work in Public Health*, 29, 606–615.

Baltzell, E. D. (1964). *The Protestant establishment: Aristocracy caste in America*. Vintage Books.

Bender, J. L., Wiljer, D., Sawka, A. M., Tsang, Alkazaz, N., & Brierley, J. D. (2016). Thyroid cancer survivors' perceptions of survivorship care follow-up options: A cross-sectional, mixed-methods survey. *Support Care Cancer, 24*, 2007–2015.

Burger, W. R. (2011). *Human services in contemporary America*. Cengage Learning.

Carver, N., & Morrison, J. (2005). Advocacy in practice: The experiences of independent advocates on UK mental health wards. *Journal of Psychiatric and Mental Health Nursing* [serial online], *12*(1),- 75–84. Retrieved from PsycINFO, Ipswich, MA.

Centers for Disease and Control. (2011). *Surgeon General's report on mental health*. Substance Abuse and Mental Health Services Administration. https://store.samhsa.gov/product/Mental-Health-A-Report-of-the-Surgeon-General-Full-Report/SG-RPT

Centers for Disease and Control (February, 2014). Mental health overview. https://www.cdc.gov/mentalhealth/

Cesta, T. (2017). *What's old is new again: The history of case management*. Case Management Insider. https://www.reliasmedia.com/articles/141367-whats-old-is-new-again-the-history-of-case-management

Chaudry, R., Polivka, B., & Kennedy, C. (2000). Public health nursing directors' perceptions regarding interagency collaboration with community mental health agencies. *Public Health Nursing*, 17(2), 75–84.

Day, C., & Davis, H. (2006). The effectiveness and quality of routine child and adolescent mental health care outreach clinics. *British Journal of Clinical Psychology, 45*(4), 439–452. https://doi.org/10.1348/014466505X79986

Elder, M. Q., & Silvers, S. A. (2009). The integration of psychology into primary care: Personal perspectives and lessons learned. *Psychological Services*, 6(1), 68–73. https://doi.org/10.1037/a0014006

Fairchild A., Rosner D., Colgrove J., Bayer, R., & Fried L. (2010). The Exodus of public health: What history can tell us about the future. *American Journal of Public Health* [serial online], 100(1), 54–63. Retrieved from CINAHL with Full Text, Ipswich, MA.

Finnerty, P. S., & Jencius, M. (2011). Building a personal model of wellness. *Counseling Today*, 53(7), 28–29.

Foster, T. (2010). Encouraging student wellness: An expanded role for counselor educators. *Journal of Counselor Preparation & Supervision*, 2(1), 10–22.

Garrett, L. (2000). *Betrayal of trust: The collapse of global public health*. Hyperion.

Gonzalez, M. J., & Gelman, C. R. (2015). Clinical social work practice in the twenty-first century: A changing landscape. *Clinical Social Work Journal*, 43(3), 257–262.

Gorin, S. H. (2001). The crisis of public health: Implications for social workers. *Health and Social Work*, 26(1), 49–53.

Henderson, C., Evans-Lacko, S., & Thornicroft, G. (2013). Mental illness stigma, help seeking, and public health programs. *American Journal of Public Health*, 103(5), 777–780. https://doi.org/10.2102/AJPH.2012.301056

Jones, D. E., & Tang, M. (2016). Health inequality: What counselors need to know to act. *Vistas, 60*. https://ccuniversity.academia.edu/DavidJones

Keegan, J. (1998). Community-based mental health care: Bridging the gap between community care and primary care. *Australian & New Zealand Journal of Mental Health Nursing*, 7(3), 95–102.

Kerson, T. S., & McCoyd, J. L. M. (2013). In response to need: An analysis of social work roles over time. *Social Work*, 58(4), 333–343.

King, J. H. (2012). *How ethical codes define counselor professional identity* [Order No. 3505737, Capella University. ProQuest Dissertations and Theses]. 215-n/a.

Kondrat, D. C., & Early, T. J. (2010). An exploration of the working alliance in mental health case management. *Social Work Research*, 34(4), 201–211. https://doi.org/10.1093/swr/34.4.201

Kottler, J. A. (2010). *On being a therapist* (4th ed.). Jossey-Bass. ISBN: 978047056547.

Krupa, T., & Carter, G. (2012). Enabling careers, autonomy, and prosperity: Using community organizing and building approaches to improve the educational outcomes of people with mental illness. *Social Work*, 43(1), 105–112.

Myers, J. E., & Sweeney, T. J. (2004). Advocacy for the counseling profession: Results of a national survey. *Journal of Counseling & Development*, 82(4), 466–471.

Myers, J. E., & Sweeney, T. J. (2008). Wellness counseling: The evidence base for practice. *Journal of Counseling & Development*, 86(4), 482–493.

National Institute for Occupational Safety and Health. (2012). *Alice b*. Hamilton awards. https://www.cdc.gov/niosh/awards/hamilton/hamhist.html

Olthuis, J. V., Wozney, L., Asmundson, G. J. G., Cramm, H., Lingley-Pottie, P., & McGrath, P. J. (2016). Distance-delivered interventions for PTSD: A systematic review and meta-analysis. *Journal of Anxiety Disorders, 44*, 9–26.

Putnam-Hornstein, E., Schneiderman, J. U., Cleves, M. A., Magruder, J., & Krous, H. F. (2014). A prospective study of sudden unexpected infant death after reported maltreatment. *The Journal of Pediatrics, 164*(1), 142–148.

Rice, E. P. (1959). Social work in public health. *Social Work*, January, 81–88.

Rosen, G. (2015). *A history of public health* (Rev. expanded ed.). John Hopkins University Press.

Ruth, B. J., & Marshall, J. W. (2017). A history of social work in public health. *American Journal of Public Health*, Supplement 3, 107(53), 236–243.

Ruth, B. J., Marshall, J. W., Velasquez, E. E. M., & Bachman, S. S. (2015). Teaching note—Educating public health social work professionals: Results from an MSW/ MPH programs outcomes study. *Journal of Social Work Education, 51*, 186–194.

Schneiderman, N., & Speers, M. (2010). Behavioral science, social science, and public health in the 21st century. In N. Schneiderman, M. A. Speers, J. M. Silva, H. Tomes, & J. H. Gentry (Eds.), *Integrating behavioral and social sciences with public health* (10th ed., pp. 3–28). American Psychological Association.

Semansky, R., Hodgkin, D., & Willging, C. (2012). Preparing for a public sector mental health reform in New Mexico: The experience of agencies serving adults with serious mental illness. *Community Mental Health Journal, 48*(3), 264–269. https://doi.org/10.1007/s10597-011-9418-5

Shally-Jensen, M. (Ed.). (2015). *Careers in human services* (1st ed.). Salem Press.

Warne, D., & Bane Frizzell, L. (2014). American Indian health policy: Historical trends and contemporary issues. *American Journal of Public Health, 104*(S3), s263–s267. https://doi-org.library.capella.edu/10.2105/AJPH.2013.301682

Williams, S. N., Dienes, K., Jaheed, J., Wardman, J. K., & Petts, J. (2023). Effectiveness of communications in enhancing adherence to public health behavioural interventions: A COVID-19 evidence review. *Philosophical Transactions of the Royal Society A: Mathematical, Physical & Engineering Sciences, 381*(2257), 1–27. https://doi.org/10.1098/rsta.2023.0129

World Health Organization & Calouste Gulbenkian Foundation. (2014). *Social determinants of mental health*. World Health Organization.

Yager, G. G., & Tovar-Blank, Z. G. (2007). Wellness and counselor education. *Journal of Humanistic Counseling, Education & Development, 46*(2), 142–153.

Yung, A., Gill, L., Sommerville, E., Dowling, B., Simon, K., Pirkis, J., Livingston, J., Schwietzer, I., Tanaghow, A., Herman, H., Trauer, T., Grigg, M., & Burgess, P. (2005). Public and private psychiatry: Can they work together and is it worth the effort? *Australian & New Zealand Journal of Psychiatry, 39*(1/2), 67–73. https://doi.org/10.1111/j.1440-1614.2005.01511.x

# 9 One Health and Human Services
## A Course in Land–Based Care Work

*Melina McConatha and Nikki DiGregorio*

## Land-Based Care Work

Human services is a broad area of study relating to care, community, and well-being. Interdisciplinary by nature, the field is uniquely informed by multiple ways of knowing care in and outside of academia. Care, similar to love, is as it does; it is defined by its will to extend itself (hooks, 1984). For the purpose of this chapter, we define care work as a process of supporting people and communities in regenerative, sustainable, and liberated ways (Piepzna-Samarasinha, 2018). Human service workers typically study care through physical, psychological, emotional, and developmental human needs. A healthy environment is required to meet these needs, but the field has yet to incorporate an ecological lens in our study.

This chapter explains the benefit of a One Health framework to reshape traditional education in how we care for each other and ourselves. One Health, as promoted by the World Health Organization (WHO), is a global initiative that advocates for well-being from an interconnected web of human health, environmental health, and animal health. This holistic lens links the health of multiple species, water, air, and land as part of an ecological community concept of well-being. A regenerative and sustainable framework that can be integrated in ways that we care for each other through local and global community care. To integrate a One Health initiative into the field, we must understand the current health and well-being of intentionally marginalized and silenced communities, for the formal study of care work cannot be teased out from systems of commodification, hierarchy, and control of people and planet. These systems shape our relationships with each other and the natural world.

Techniques such as deep listening provide space for other forms of care—a decolonized and liberated care for ourselves and the land. Narratives used here in this research frame an opportunity for human service work in what we call land-based care. For the purpose of this chapter and research, we define land-based care as work that aims to advocate for the health and well-being of an interconnected web of life in shared land. As activists and scholars, we see endless possibilities for service as humans in the formal study of how we care for our biodiverse community and land. In order to conceptualize a path forward, we must address the current context.

Colonization introduced concepts of ownership in land, people, and our natural world. Colonizers created an infrastructure for the oppression of people and other living beings (Glenn, 2015; Wolfe, 2006). The study of care in the academy has been historically whitewashed, with the majority of public health policy and practice in social services rooted in white supremacist ideologies (O'Connell, 2013; Pearce, 2022; Weaver, 2020). Still today,

DOI: 10.4324/9781003531258-12

the study of care for each other and the land we share is shaped by white supremacy, colonization, and the capitalist system.

Capitalism often dictates many of the service needs in the field of human services through imbalanced distribution models of resources needed to survive. In the current United States, a small percentage of the population hoards the majority of the people's natural resources on stolen land. Human services workers have historically been agents of the state used to allocate poorly distributed natural resources such as food, water, and shelter.

Our health and well-being are determined by our relationship with the land. How we care for the land mirrors how we care for ourselves. Healthy food systems, safe shelter, clean water, and fresh air are all necessary for sustainable and regenerative human development. Yet the exploitation of people and planet can persist only when we ignore our relationship with the control and commodification of these natural resources. Without accountability and repair, human service work will continue to unintentionally maintain and even reproduce systems of oppression.

Despite the complex history of failing systems of care, people have been doing land-based care work in creative and revolutionary ways across time and place. We envision a field that centers this kind of work, a form of collective service by humans that centers care on shared land, a form of care that is accountable and connected to the ecosystems that we work and live—a network of care that considers plants, animals, water, and air as part of the community and, in turn, works for the health of the whole, not a select few.

By highlighting possibilities of care outside of a human-centered lens, here we suggest a One Health and Human Service curriculum of study that puts the responsibility of land-based care into the field. We suggest a human service course that considers the care for our natural world not separate from our own. A curriculum that teaches how to listen and learn about land-based care outside of antiquated capitalist and colonized frameworks.

### Voices of the Global Majority

Indigenous people have been doing this work long before the first courses of study in the field of human services. This work is by no means new, and while the historical work of land-based care from indigenous, Black, and Brown scholars is not within the scope of this chapter, we suggest a decolonized curriculum informed (see Shahid et al., 2021) by the current narratives of Indigenous, Black, and Brown people—people of the global majority. Informed by both a One Health initiative and the digital narratives of communities with long traditions of land-based care, we suggest a course of study led by people who have cared for land throughout time and place.

Through a collection of social media posts, primarily Black voices, we highlight land-based care work already being done outside of colonized academic spaces. These narratives provided a guiding framework for what we call a One Health and Human Services course at the first degree granting Historically Black College (HBCU). The course, piloted at Lincoln University, introduces One Health research initiatives that have historically been based in predominantly white research institutions (see Appendix A). The exclusion and underrepresentation of HBCUs, Tribal Colleges, and Hispanic Serving Institutions is symbolic of a legacy of institutional and systemic racism in One Health education. The lack of representation suggests One Health research has been historically whitewashed, and data on ecological health and well-being is one dimensional and lacks the wisdom of communities with much more experience in land-based care practice.

Despite being the global majority, Black, Brown, and Indigenous communities experience disproportionate rates of environmental injustice and preventable obstacles in access to clean water, food sovereignty, and overall health (Njoku, 2021). Current academic literature in human services has failed to effectively share ways these communities continue to radically care for themselves and their environment despite these findings. One Health scholars suggest that new narratives, representation from the global majority, and the interconnected ecological care must shape a culturally responsive global plan of action in the field of human services (One Health High-Level Expert Panel, 2022).

These digital narratives were selected on social media platforms based on HBCU students' algorithms and feeds in digital spaces. Posts and stories were recorded and coded for common themes (Braun & Clarke, 2006; Patton, 2014). Student led, the themes provided guidance in a curriculum specific to the learning objectives in a One Health and Human Services course. These themes included a framework for land-based care work, which works for (1) decolonization, (2) accountability and reparations, and the need for (3) deep listening practices. A sampling of the land-based care narratives that informed our work is shared throughout this chapter.

We envision land-based care as a transitional process that ultimately aims to restore philosophical worldviews, self-determination, and sovereignty of the global majority—a decolonized non-hierarchical lens to collective land-based care. Reciprocity rather than exploitation is part of this land-based care. Also, to center land in care work, we must try to understand the current health of our ecosystems. Theories and practices that work for accountability and restorative relationships to dismantle colonial power and control structures in human health were used in this project. In this chapter we also share our prompts in the process of deep listening—a tool for decolonization and ecological liberation (Sosta, 2022). The prompts shared also provided an opportunity for accountability and reflection in our own writing. We reflect on our role as land-based care workers, witnesses, and oppressors in one space.

## Applications for a Land-Based Theory

To move toward the integration of land-based care in the field, theory helps give structure and provides a common language. Noting the importance of theory in the organization and sharing of knowledge, multiple theories guide our work. Care work cannot be neatly fit into disciplinary categories. To address complex problems, theoretical frameworks must be informed by diverse lived experiences. Tenets of ecological systems theory, queer science, social ecology, and decolonial feminist frameworks enable us to not only critique but to promote generative thinking. Here we outline opportunities in ecological systems thinking, specifically to integrate a One Health initiative into a classroom. Ecological systems theories remain a common tool for people studying care, humans, and their relationships with the world. Ecological systems theories (e.g., Bronfenbrenner, 1977) outline human health and well-being in development through nested systems of relationships in the environment. Often utilized within the social sciences, ecological systems theory looks to understand the interplay between the developing person and their environment. Bronfenbrenner's ecological model of human development is regarded as a response to the limited scope of research in the 1970s that emphasized the complexity of environmental factors and their impact on human development. Overlapping during a period of growth and formalization for human services as an academic field (Fine, 2018), the theory suggested that human health, growth, and development should be studied in the context of the environment (Bronfenbrenner,

1994). However, without representation from Indigenous, Black, and Brown people, the theory continues to represent the colonial voice. A settler view removes the person from the land and, in turn, ignores indigenous knowledge systems of interconnected care. Without these voices, the true health of the land and, in turn, ourselves is hidden, unseen, and unspoken.

The theory in its intention emphasizes the complex layers of environmental influence, which include the (1) microsystem of direct interactions; (2) the mesosystem, which highlights the interconnections between these microsystems, such as the relationship between family, local community, and education; (3) the exosystem that outlines the broader social systems that indirectly affect people; the (4) macrosystem representing the cultural, societal, and institutional systems, which encompass norms, values, and laws that influence all other ecological systems; lastly, the (5) chronosystem, which applies the lens of time, considering both life transitions and socio-historical events that impact human development (Bronfenbrenner, 1986). According to Bronfenbrenner (1979), these layers collectively shape human experiences and development.

From this common framework, we look to decenter the human and examine care from the land. In doing so, we seek to uncover ways to support the health and well-being of people from the context of place—a practice common in Indigenous knowledge systems. For example, in the study of care, as HBCU students at Lincoln University, we reflect on how we care for ourselves in the context of the land. We examine our relationship with land in each of the following systems:

- Microsystems: the health of the people, plants, animals, water, air, and soil we interact with most. This includes the health of animals and plants in our food webs, natural resources in our transformation and shelter systems, and the air and water we need to survive every day.
- Mesosystems: here we examine the relationship exchanges in our immediate systems outside of ourselves. For example, we can explore how our education system shapes these same food webs, natural resources, and air and water.
- Exosystem looks at the policies and structures, specifically at the university. For example, we might note that a for-profit organization controls the majority of our sustainability efforts due to outsourcing policy and practices.
- Chronosystem explores time as it relates to different layers of the environment with a focus on changes and transitions.

Applying these concepts utilizing a land-centered approach prompts us to recognize injustices and has the potential to illuminate more holistic means of addressing them. Microsystems examine social norms and philosophical world views that shape how land, labor, and resources on campus are currently being commodified and exploited in an extractive colonized capitalist educational system. Our current education system was funded by stolen land and labor. For example, land grant university status provides a leading position for funding opportunities in research, which was determined by the Morrill Act, a wealth transfer disguised as a donation. This transfer involved government land grabs from Indigenous people to create endowments for universities. Chronosystems capture the passage of time and record of memory. Lincoln was founded as a space of resistance to a society that intentionally marginalized the Black community—created on land and in space, surrounded by nature by intention. Its location was meant to remind us of our connection with the natural world.

Ecological systems theory provides helpful guidance to understanding development as a complex, multidimensional, multidirectional, nonlinear, ongoing process that is affected by numerous relationships, ranging from one's immediate relationships to broader levels of cultural, economic, political, and social context (Darling, 2007). A timely and necessary land-based adaptation of ecological systems theory requires de-centering the human to shift focus to our interconnected nature. As pleasure activist Adrienne Maree Brown shares, "The natural world is up to a lot of things, and we are natural. So anything that's happening out there can happen in us."

This lens looks to reframe health and growth from a more regenerative and sustainable lens. This perspective, rooted in indigenous and decolonized frameworks, warrants hope for a shift in how we care for each other and ourselves. The mission of human service work includes recognizing the capacity for human growth and change; advocating for justice; supporting physical, mental, emotional, and spiritual health; and promoting collaboration and accountability (National Organization for Human Services, 2024). In this One Health and Human Service course, we conceptualize human growth in the context of the current climate crisis from a less linear framework, suggesting reparative and regenerative forms of health, collaboration, and accountability for our entire ecological system.

## One Health and Human Services Curriculum

As noted, the One Health Initiative is a global initiative of care practices relating to the interconnected health of biodiverse plants, animals, people, and land. A community health model, One Health, provides a useful foundation for land-based collective care. More specifically, One Health research informs data on well-being in the age of the climate crisis (WHO, 2017). It is a global initiative that works with the WHO, the Food and Agriculture Organization of the United Nations, the United Nations Environment Programme, and the World Organisation for Animal Health. This approach mirrors the mission of the U.S. Department of Health and Human Services (HHS, 2023) by advocating for the well-being of people through interconnected food systems, clean water access, the humane treatment of animals, and the protection of shared and common land.

To initiate this movement these student-driven tenants frame a One Health curriculum in land-based care work. Using thematic digital narrative analysis to analyze Instagram stories and identify recurring themes, students focused on the content of these digital posts to outline learning objectives in land-based care. Themes that emerge from the narratives (Riessman, 2008) also provided a reflective land-based practice. The One Health and Human Services classroom three learning (or unlearning) objectives, simplified, include:

1  Unlearning the settler colonial framework of power, control, hierarchy, and commodification of people, animals, natural resources, and land. This begins with a non-hierarchical model of care.
2  Engage in care work that seeks to reclaim and repair human connection with land through local and global change. Transformative care work should maintain an ultimate objective of Land Back and collective liberation. Red Ma'at Collective of Black, indigenous, and radicalized femmes best capture this objective in genuine change in the context of colonization:
3  Practice deep listening as an indigenous process of care work to build and repair interconnected and natural relationships in our ecological system (Ungunmerr et al., 2022).

Engage in the practice of deep listening to educate yourself from multiple lived experiences, especially the voices of intentionally marginalized communities. Deep listening will help unlearn false narratives of well-being. The practice aims for accountability for human service workers in failing and oppressive systems of care. Deep listening, as a form of witness, can provide a process for solidarity and the honoring of memory in the life and death of much of the natural world.

Utilizing a participatory action research (PAR) design throughout the process, a pilot project consisting of deep listening sessions was also conducted with the large land-based systems of care, like the National Forest Service and the Environmental Protection Agency, and smaller local not-for-profits like Natural Lands Trust and Longwood Gardens. PAR is "based on reflection, data collection, and action that aims to improve health and reduce health inequities through involving the people who, in turn, take actions to improve their own health" (Baum et al., 2006, p. 854). As participatory action researchers, the process of data collection must also include hands-on work in our own communities with organizations doing land-based care.

In alignment with the recommendations made by the One Health High-Level Expert Panel (2022), we suggest the practice of deep listening to assess the health of our natural world. The Indigenous concept of deep listening is a practice of learning and working in a community in the right relationship with the land. It requires self-reflection (Atkinson, 2009) in the context of the interconnected web of life. Deep listening has been used as a tool for indigenous communities in creating and transforming relationships with the land (Ungunmerr, 2017).

Deep listening is also a process necessary in the act of storytelling. Storytelling has long been used as a tool for preserving and passing on knowledge through recorded lived experiences (Abbott, 2002). Storytelling affords important agencies for underrepresented communities by centering the lived experiences of individuals, as told from their own perspectives. Narrative approaches such as storytelling have been employed in numerous works detailing experiences outside of hegemonic, dominant, and cisheteronormative parameters (Bradway, 2021). Indigenous scholars suggest storytelling to decolonize research methods and transform care work (Tuhiwai Smith, 2012). A contemporary form of storytelling, the digital narrative is accessible to many more people than traditional academic scholarship.

## Land-Based Care in Practice: Deep Listening Pilot

The pilot project's deep listening sessions provided prompts for local organizations that students designated as land-based care. An interesting, but not surprising, finding was that we found the majority of public and not-for-profit land-based care organizations to be predominantly white. With this observation, HBCU students tailored listening session prompts, especially for predominantly white spaces, to reflect on privilege and reparations needed for genuine change in land-based care. Drawing upon the literature exploring the "insider–outsider" paradoxes, we acknowledge the demand of participating Black students and scholars to navigate this project without compromising personal identity and values, while interacting with others (Yeo & Dopson, 2018).

This work contributes to efforts to disrupt conventional ways of conducting research (Pollack & Eldridge, 2015). The prompts developed by Black students for white organizations were shared on posters with visual artwork created by Favianna Rodriguez, an Oakland-based interdisciplinary artist, cultural strategist working in climate action and racial equity. The deep listening prompts shared below illustrate the reflexive practice in sessions:

---

### Deep Listening Prompts for Historically White Open-Space Organizations
### A Reflective Practice for Open Space and Public Land

What are the narratives that are represented in your historical and cultural preservation efforts? Do you have cultural markers relating to the experiences of Black and Brown communities on this land?

What kind of visibility do Black and Brown communities currently have on this open space? Do you have initiative efforts to contribute to the representation, recreation, leadership, and relationships of diverse cultures on this land?

What is the racial composition of your boards, local governing agency, and administrative entities?

Do you hold listening sessions for groups with racial identities other than your own at your organization? How? When? Why?

Do you bring in local representatives of Black and Brown communities and compensate them?

Does your organization work toward reparative justice on open spaces and public land?

Do you practice culturally responsive and sustaining efforts in Land Back movements?

We value your feedback:

Pilot Facilitation Project by Lincoln University
Funded by the National Science Foundation
Chinemere Ihejirika, Makyia Jones, and Melina McConatha, PhD
Original artwork (not displayed) by Favianna Rodriguez

These prompts were shared with multiple organizations through small, short listening sessions led by HBCU students. The prompts were also integrated through the writing process of this chapter for accountability and reflection in our own writing. We reflect on our role as land-based care workers, witnesses, and oppressors in one space. As part of the academy, it is impossible to tease out the complex nature of how we live our own lives on stolen land. From property ownership to land grant university status-stolen land has provided platforms to do this work, and we aim to acknowledge, be accountable, and repair relationships in this process.

## Future Research in Land-Based Care

Given its broad and interdisciplinary background, the human service field has a unique opportunity to focus on the study of care in the context of an ecological community. Yet, due to the inextricable links between service delivery, care work, and the current systems of control, it is futile to try and parse them apart. However, a fundamental shift in educational approaches could provide the necessary catalyst to help break the cycle of environmental injustices for people and the planet. A human service field that centers collective care and ecological health is the path forward. One Health scholars suggest that, in an aggregate fashion, new narratives that engage the voices of the global majority and center the interconnected ecological care of the community must drive a culturally responsive global plan of action in the field of Human Services (One Health High-Level Expert Panel, 2022). This proposed One Health and Human Services course of study, informed by the adoption of a land-based ecological systems theory, provides an adaptive framework from which to move onward.

Driven by community-level data and deep listening sessions, as well as the preliminary findings from our pilot project, this course provides an opportunity for emergent strategies in land-based care (Maree Brown, 2017) in land-based collective care. These changes would provide the foundation for continual progression toward the development of ecological health models within the social sciences. Land-based education provides a platform for opportunities in human service for animal advocacy, multi-species community work, and humane education (Bretzlaff-Holstein, 2018). Future research from land-based models may foster an ecological consciousness (see García-Carrión et al., 2019; Thompson & Gullone, 2003).

Additionally, the proposed One Health and Human Services curriculum would involve education around PAR and advocacy. This is of particular interest given that the implementation of policy through networks of cooperating human service care workers is common in the United States (Provan & Milward, 2001). Given the public face of human service work, including, but not limited to, supporting individuals and communities, addressing needs, quality-of-life concerns, and promoting self-sufficiency, the field finds itself well-positioned to integrate the tenets of One Health and promote awareness of the need for land-based care. A more comprehensive approach to health is at the core of the proposed course of study. Fundamentally, community-driven land-based education guides us in developing ecological education in human service curricula and the social sciences more broadly.

Furthermore, a One Health and Human Services curriculum must be informed by sustainable philosophies in alignment with Indigenous, Black, and Brown narratives. Collectively, these voices help guide land-based care practice. It is through the collective liberation of these communities and our natural world that human service scholars can support meaningful and intentional change. Much of today's global conflict is tied to land and the control of natural resources. By caring for the land and unlearning frameworks of control, commodification, and hierarchy, we can interrupt the cycle of environmental injustice. Through this process, we learn how to collectively work for the liberation of all living beings. Dr. Jaiya John (*We Birth Freedom at Dawn*), a freedom worker, reminds us:

> Perhaps your greatest challenge each day is not to stand up against the forces of oppression, but to resist the ever encroaching tendency to feel that you are too small to stop the forces of oppression. Remember, if your soul and its actions are sourced from Love and from your ancestors of kindred spirit, not only are you not small, you are immense infinity. When you are rooted in the sanctity of collective life and liberation, your soul size is legendary.

We encourage our readers to reflect for themselves on opportunities for land-based care work; to conceptualize community outside of a human-centric lens; and to work to care for trees, gardens, animals, oceans, rivers, and all of our interconnected ecological communities. Here we share reflective questions to aid in this contemplation and examine further how our relationship with land might shape the field of human service.

### Questions for Reflection

1 How would you describe your relationship with land? How is it tied to concepts of home?
2 What natural resources are used in your daily life? How does the health of these resources shape your own?
3 What communities lived and worked the land before you? Where are their experiences recorded? What do these stories tell you about their health and well-being across time?
4 What are local care practices for the land? Who are your land-based care workers? Is there space for your skills in this work?
5 Sit quietly on this land and listen to your natural world. Write down all of the living beings you observe. What does life look like for them? How does their health, home, and liberation shape your own?

### References

Abbott, H. P. (2002). *The Cambridge introduction to narrative*. Cambridge University Press.
Atkinson, B. (2009). Teachers responding to narrative inquiry: An approach to narrative inquiry criticism. *The Journal of Educational Research, 103*(2), 91–102. DOI: 10.1080/00220670903323461
Baum, F., MacDougall, C., & Smith, D. (2006). Participatory action research. *Journal of Epidemiology and Community Health, 60*(10), 854–857. https://doi.org/10.1136/jech.2004.028662
Bradway, T. (2021). Queer narrative theory and the relationality of form. *PMLA, 136*, 711–727. https://doi.org/10/1632/S00030812921000407
Braun, V., & Clarke, V. (2006). Using thematic analysis in psychology. *Qualitative Research in Psychology, 3*(2), 77–101. https://doi.org/10.1191/1478088706qp063oa
Bretzlaff-Holstein, C. (2018). The case for humane education in social work education. *Social Work Education, 37*, 924–935. https://doi.org/10.1080/02615479.2018.1468428
Bronfenbrenner, U. (1994). Ecological models of human development. In *International Encyclopedia of Education, 3*. (2nd ed.). Oxford. Reprinted in: Gauvain, M., & Cole, M. (Eds.), *Readings on the development of children* (2nd ed.). (1993, pp. 37–43). Freeman.

Bronfenbrenner, U. (1979). *The ecology of human development: Experiments by nature and design.* Harvard University Press.

Bronfenbrenner, U. (1986). Ecology of the family as a context for human development: Research perspectives. *Developmental Psychology, 22,* 723–742.

Bronfenbrenner, U. (1994). Ecological models of human development. In *International Encyclopedia of Education, 3.* (2nd ed.). Oxford. Reprinted in: Gauvain, M., & Cole, M. (Eds.), *Readings on the development of children* (2nd ed.). (1993, pp. 37–43). Freeman.

Brown, A. M. (2017). *Emergent strategy: Shaping change, changing worlds.* AK Press.

Darling, N. (2007). Ecological systems theory: The person in the center of the circles. *Research in human development, 4*(3–4), 203–217. DOI: 10.1080/15427600701663023

Fine, M. D. (2018). *A caring society?: Care and the dilemmas of human services in the 21st century.* Bloomsbury Publishing.

Food and Agriculture Organization, United Nations Environment Programme, World Health Organization, & World Organisation for Animal Health. (2022). One Health Joint Plan of Action (2022–2026). https://www.who.int/publications/i/item/9789240059139

García-Carrión, R., Villarejo-Carballido, B., & Villardón-Gallego, L. (2019). Children and adolescents mental health: A systematic review of interaction-based interventions in schools and communities. *Frontiers in Psychology, 10,* 918. https://doi.org/10.3389/fpsyg.2019.00918

Glenn, E. N. (2015). Settler colonialism as structure: A framework for comparative studies of U.S. race and gender formation. *Sociology of Race and Ethnicity, 1*(1), 52–72.

hooks, b. (1984). *Feminist theory: From margin to center.* South End Press.

National Organization for Human Services. (2024). Ethical Standards for Human Services Professionals. Retrieved July 14, 2024, from https://www.nationalhumanservices.org/ethical-standards/

National Organization for Human Services. (n.d.). Our mission. Retrieved December 10, 2023, from https://www.nationalhumanservices.org/

Njoku, A. U. (2021). COVID-19 and environmental racism: Challenges and recommendations. *European Journal of Environment and Public Health, 5*(2), em0079. https://doi.org/10.21601/ejeph/10999

O'Connell, A. (2013). The deserving and non-deserving races: Colonial intersections of social welfare history in Ontario. *Intersectionalities: A Global Journal of Social Work Analysis, Research, Polity, and Practice, 2*(1), 1–18. https://journals.library.mun.ca/ojs/index.php/IJ/article/view/371/616

Patton, M. Q. (2014). Designing qualitative studies. In *Qualitative Research & Evaluation Methods* (4th ed.). Sage Publications.

Pearce, E. B. (2022). Understanding the historical context of human services in the United States. In *Introduction to human services: Second edition. Open Oregon Educational Resources.* https://openoregon.pressbooks.pub/introhumanservices2e/chapter/2-3-understanding-the-historical-context-of-human-services-in-the-united-states/

Piepzna-Samarasinha L. L. (2018). *Care work: Dreaming disability justice.* Vancouver: Arsenal Pulp.

Pollack, S., & Eldridge, T. (2015). Complicity and redemption: Beyond the insider/outsider research dichotomy. *Social Justice, 42,* 132–145. https://www.jstor.org/stable/24871287

Provan, K. G., & Milward, H. B. (2001). Do networks really work? A framework for evaluating public-sector organizational networks. *Public Administration Review, 61,* 414–423. https://doi.org/10.1111/0033-3352.00045

Riessman, C. K. (2008). *Narrative methods for the human sciences.* Sage.

Shahid, S., DiGiacomo, M., Lai, M., & Katona, L. (2021). Challenges and opportunities for cancer services in Aboriginal health in Australia: A systematic review. *Frontiers in Public Health, 9,* 637897. https://doi.org/10.3389/fpubh.2021.637897

Smith, L. T. (2012). *Decolonizing methodologies: Research and indigenous people* (2nd ed.). Zed Books.

Sosta, F. (2022). Decolonizing listening to decolonize memory. *From the European South, 11,* 10–23. https://www.fesjournal.eu/numeri/general-issue-4/decolonizing-listening-to-decolonize-memory/

Thompson, K. L., & Gullone, E. (2003). Promotion of empathy and prosocial behavior in children through humane education. *Australian Psychologist*, *38*(3), 175–182. https://doi.org/10.1080/000 50060310001707187

Ungunmerr, M. R. (2017). To be listened to in her teaching: Dadirri: Inner deep listening and quiet still awareness. *EarthSong Journal: Perspectives in Ecology, Spirituality and Education*, *3*(4), 14–15.

Ungunmerr-Baumann, M. R., Groom, R. A., Schuberg, E. L., Atkinson, J., Atkinson, C., Wallace, R., & Morris, G. (2022). Dadirri: An Indigenous place-based research methodology. *AlterNative: An International Journal of Indigenous Peoples*, *18*(1), 94–103. DOI: 10.2277/1177180122085353

Weaver, H. (2020). We are beauty and we walk in it: Native American women in leadership roles. In T. Kleibl, R. Lutz, N. Noyoo, B. Bunk, A. Dittman, & B. Seepamore (Eds.), *The Routledge handbook of postcolonial social work*. (pp. 174–184). Routledge. https://doi.org/10.4324/9780429468728

Wolfe, P. (2006). Settler colonialism and the elimination of the native. *Journal of Genocide Research*, *8*, 387–409. https://doi.org/10.1080/1462350601056240

World Health Organization. (2017, June 29). Protecting health from climate change: Country and regional profiles. Geneva: World Health Organization. ISBN: 9789241598880. Retrieved July 14, 2024, https://www.who.int/publications/i/item/protecting-health-from-climate-change

Yeo, R., & Dopson, S. (2018). Getting lost to be found: The insider–outsider paradoxes in relational ethnography. *Qualitative Research in Organizations and Management: An International Journal*, *13*, 333–355. https://doi.org/10.1108/QROM-06–2017-1533

# Appendix

## One Health Initiatives in the United States (publicly noted)

## Data Collected by Lincoln University Students Spring 2024

1 Appalachian State University
2 Auburn U—One Health Certificate Program
3 Berry College Center for One Health
4 Center for Animal and Human Health in Appalachia (CAHA), Lincoln Memorial U
5 Center for Emerging Infectious Diseases, University of Iowa
6 Center for Emerging, Zoonotic, and Arthropod-borne Pathogens (CeZAP), Virginia Tech University
7 Center for One Health Illinois, University of Illinois, Urbana
8 Center for One Health, Fontbonne University
9 Center for One Health Research, University of Alaska (COHR-University of Alaska)
10 Center for One Health Research, University of Washington (COHR-University of Washington)
11 Center for One Health Research, Virginia-Maryland CVM, and the Edward Via College of Osteopathic Medicine
12 Colorado State University One Health Institute
13 Colorado State University School of Public Health
14 Delaware Valley University One Health Working Group
15 Duke Comparative Oncology Group
16 Edward Via College of Osteopathic Medicine (VCOM)
17 Ferrum College One Health Undergraduate Minor
18 Fontbonne University One Health BSc
19 Georgetown University Medical Center
20 Georgetown University MSc in Global Infectious Disease
21 Global Health Institute, University Wisconsin-Madison
22 Global One Health Initiative, University of Minnesota College of Veterinary Medicine
23 Global One Health Initiative, Ohio State University (GOHI)
24 Health and Livelihoods Group (HEAL)
25 Horizon Solutions, Yale University
26 Initiative for One Health and the Environment, University of Maine
27 Institute for Global Health, Michigan State University
28 Iowa State University College of Veterinary Medicine
29 Massachusetts Institute of Technology
30 Michigan State University Canadian Studies Center One Health Initiative (CSC OHI)
31 Midwestern University One Health Center
32 Museums in One Health
33 Nebraska One Health and OH Lab Group, University of Nebraska-Lincoln

34  Nepal One Health, University of Michigan
35  One Health Center of Excellence, University of Florida
36  One Health Institute, University of California, Davi
37  One Health at Cornell University
38  One Health at Johns Hopkins University
39  One Health at Kansas State University
40  One Health at Purdue CVM
41  One Health at the University of Georgia
42  One Health Workforce Academies (OHWA)
43  One Health Workforce Next Generation, OHW-NG (University of Minnesota/USAID)
44  Pennsylvania State University Undergraduate One Health Mino
45  Princeton University
46  South Dakota One Health, University of South Dakota School of Medicine
47  Texas A&M University Global One Health
48  Texas A&M University Institute for Infectious Animal Diseases (IIAD)
49  Tufts University of Clinical and Translational Science, One Health Program, and MSC in Conservation Medicine/One Health
50  University of Arizona One Health Research Initiative, Mel & Enid Zuckerman School of Public Health
51  University of Idaho Institute for Interdisciplinary Data Sciences and Computational One Health
52  University of Maine
53  University of Maryland, U.S.-Middle East One Health Network
54  University of Missouri School of Medicine One Health BioRepository
55  University of Missouri College of Veterinary Medicine, Zalk Veterinary Medical Library
56  University of Pennsylvania School of Veterinary Medicine and School of Medicine, One Health Dual DVM/MPH
57  University of Tennessee One Health Initiative
58  University of Texas Medical Branch-Galveston (UTMB One Health)
59  U.S. Smithsonian Museum of Natural History
60  Utah State University, One Health
61  Veterinary One Health Association (VOHA), Cornell University College Vet Med
62  Virginia Tech University One Health/Public Health Program, Center for One Health and CZAP
63  Washington University School of Medicine
64  Westminster College Undergraduate One Health Major
65  Zoo New England One Health Program
66  Zoobiquity Research Initiative

**No HBCUs Listed**

# 10 Navigating Parental Challenges in Child Welfare

## Strategies for Enhancing Family Resilience

*Devin Senon-Garcia Wadley*

### Overview of Child Welfare

The child welfare system is a comprehensive network designed to ensure the safety, well-being, and stability of children. This system is multifaceted, involving various services and supports that work together to protect children from abuse and neglect and to promote their overall development.

The child welfare process typically begins with the reporting of suspected child abuse or neglect. Reports can be made by a wide range of individuals, including mandated reporters such as teachers, healthcare providers, and social workers, as well as by community members. Once a report is made, child protection services (CPS) investigates to determine the validity of the allegations and assess the risk to the child. This initial phase is critical, as it sets the stage for all subsequent actions. The investigation may involve home visits, interviews with the child and family members, and collaboration with other professionals.

If the investigation reveals that the child is at risk but can remain safely in the home, CPS may provide in-home services. These services are designed to address the underlying issues that put the child at risk, such as substance abuse, mental health problems, or domestic violence. In-home services can include family counseling, parenting classes, and case management. The goal is to strengthen the family unit and ensure a safe environment for the child. Social workers play a crucial role in this phase, working closely with the family to develop and implement a safety plan.

On the contrary, when it is determined that a child cannot safely remain at home, they may be placed in foster care. Foster care is a temporary arrangement where children live with foster families or in group homes while a long-term solution is sought. The primary objective during this phase is to provide a stable and nurturing environment for the child. Foster parents receive training and support to help them meet the needs of the child. Social workers are responsible for monitoring the child's well-being, facilitating visits with the biological family, and planning for the child's future.

Reunification with the biological family is the preferred outcome whenever it is safe and feasible. Reunification efforts involve working with the family to resolve the issues that led to the child's removal. This may include ongoing counseling, substance abuse treatment, and other supportive services. The decision to reunify is based on a thorough assessment of the family's progress and the child's safety. Social workers must balance the goal of reunification with the need to protect the child's well-being, often making complex and nuanced decisions.

If reunification is not possible, the system seeks to find a permanent home for the child through adoption or guardianship. Adoption provides a legal and permanent family for the

DOI: 10.4324/9781003531258-13

child, while guardianship grants long-term caregiving responsibilities without terminating parental rights. The process of adoption involves matching the child with prospective adoptive parents, conducting home studies, and finalizing the legal adoption. Social workers facilitate this process, ensuring that the child's needs are met and that the adoptive family is prepared for the responsibilities of parenting.

Lastly, the child welfare system also provides various support services to foster and adoptive families, as well as to older youth aging out of foster care. These services can include financial assistance, counseling, educational support, and life skills training. For older youth, transitioning out of foster care can be particularly challenging, and support services aim to help them achieve independence and stability.

Importance of family resilience

## Family Resilience

When looking at family resilience, this is a critical concept in social work, particularly within the child welfare system, where understanding and fostering resilience can significantly impact the well-being of families and children. Family resilience refers to the ability of a family unit to withstand and recover from significant stressors and challenges, such as economic hardships, health crises, or relational conflicts (Hawley, 2000). This capacity for resilience is not inherent but is developed through adaptive processes and supportive relationships within the family and the broader community (Becvar, 2007).

One of the primary reasons family resilience is important in the context of child welfare is that it promotes positive outcomes for children despite adversity. Resilient families are better equipped to manage stress and maintain functionality during difficult times (Walsh, 1996). This stability is crucial for the emotional and psychological well-being of children, who are more vulnerable to the negative impacts of family stress. When families can effectively navigate challenges, they provide a secure and nurturing environment that supports healthy development and reduces the risk of long-term psychological issues for children (Mullin & Arce, 2008).

Furthermore, family resilience is essential because it fosters a sense of empowerment and self-efficacy within families involved in the child welfare system. Families that develop resilience often feel more in control of their circumstances and more capable of influencing positive changes in their lives (Walsh, 1996). This empowerment can lead to increased problem-solving skills, improved communication, and stronger family bonds. These skills and attributes not only are beneficial in the immediate context but also contribute to the family's long-term ability to handle future challenges, which is particularly valuable in child welfare cases (Masten, 2001).

In addition, family resilience has a ripple effect that extends beyond the immediate family unit. Resilient families contribute to the strength and stability of their communities. They are more likely to engage in supportive social networks, participate in community activities, and provide mutual aid to other families in need. This collective resilience enhances the overall health and well-being of the community, creating a supportive environment where all families, especially those involved in the child welfare system, can thrive (Walsh, 1996).

## Understanding Parental Challenges in Child Welfare

Parental challenges within the child welfare system are multifaceted and complex, often exacerbated by systemic issues such as poverty, mental health problems, substance abuse, and lack of social support. These challenges not only impact the parents themselves but also have profound implications for the well-being and development of their children.

One of the most significant challenges faced by parents in the child welfare system is financial instability. Many families involved in child welfare are living in poverty, which can exacerbate other issues such as housing instability, food insecurity, and lack of access to healthcare (Kemp et al., 2009). Financial stress can lead to increased tension and conflict within the household, negatively affecting the parent–child relationship. Children in these situations are often exposed to environments that are not conducive to healthy development, potentially leading to issues such as poor academic performance and behavioral problems (Fong, 2017).

Mental health problems are another critical challenge for parents within the child welfare system. Conditions such as depression, anxiety, and post-traumatic stress disorder (PTSD) are prevalent among parents who have experienced trauma or ongoing stress. These mental health issues can impair a parent's ability to provide consistent and nurturing care, which is essential for a child's emotional and psychological development (Kemp et al., 2009). Children of parents with untreated mental health conditions are at a higher risk of developing mental health issues themselves, perpetuating a cycle of trauma and instability (Cao et al., 2019).

Substance abuse is a common issue among parents in the child welfare system. The misuse of drugs or alcohol can impair a parent's judgment and ability to care for their children, often leading to neglect or abuse. Substance abuse can also result in legal issues, further complicating the parent's ability to provide a stable environment (Kemp et al., 2009). For children, living with a parent who struggles with substance abuse can lead to emotional and behavioral issues, as well as an increased likelihood of substance abuse in their own lives (Taylor & Kroll, 2001).

Social support is crucial for parents navigating the child welfare system, yet many parents lack an extensive support network. This isolation can make it difficult for parents to access resources and assistance, exacerbating their challenges. Social support networks, including extended family, friends, and community organizations, can provide emotional support, practical help, and a sense of belonging (Kemp et al., 2009). A lack of social support can mean fewer positive role models for children. Furthermore, a family's limited access to extracurricular activities can stall a child's social development (Fong, 2017).

These challenges faced by parents in the child welfare system can have a profound impact on their well-being and ability to parent effectively. Financial instability, mental health issues, substance abuse, and lack of social support can all contribute to feelings of stress, anxiety, and hopelessness. These feelings can impair a parent's ability to provide consistent and nurturing care.

## Theoretical Frameworks for Family Resilience

### Resilience Theory

Resilience theory in the context of child welfare provides a framework for understanding how parents can thrive despite facing significant adversity. This theory emphasizes the dynamic process through which parents develop the capacity to adapt positively and recover from difficult circumstances, such as abuse, neglect, or exposure to domestic violence (Frankel et al., 1992).

One of the core elements of resilience theory is the identification of protective factors that can buffer parents against the negative impacts of adverse experiences. Protective factors include supportive relationships with children, teachers, or mentors; a positive self-concept; and effective coping strategies (Walsh, 1996). These factors can help parents build the emotional and psychological resources needed to navigate challenges.

Conversely, resilience theory also examines risk factors that can hinder a parent's well-being. Risk factors in the context of child welfare might include poverty, parental substance abuse, or a lack of stable housing (Hawley & De Haan, 1996, p. 285). Understanding these risk factors is crucial for developing targeted interventions that address the specific needs of at-risk parents.

Adaptive capacity is another key concept within resilience theory. It refers to a parent's ability to adjust to new circumstances and maintain functioning despite disruptions. This capacity is not static; it can be strengthened through supportive environments and targeted interventions (Carver, 1998). For example, programs that promote social and emotional learning can enhance a parent's adaptive capacity by teaching skills such as problem-solving, emotional regulation, and interpersonal communication. Building on the principles of resilience theory, which emphasizes the capacity of individuals and families to adapt and thrive despite adversity, we can further enhance our understanding by examining these dynamics through the lens of systems theory, which provides a comprehensive framework for analyzing the complex interactions within and between families.

## Systems Theory

Systems theory offers a comprehensive framework for understanding family dynamics by viewing the family as a complex, interrelated system. This approach, grounded in the principles of general systems theory, posits that individual family members cannot be understood in isolation but rather in the context of their relationships and interactions within the family unit (Cox & Paley, 1997).

At the core of systems theory is the concept of interdependence, which suggests that changes in one part of the family system will inevitably affect other parts (Weeland et al., 2021). For instance, a child's behavioral problems can influence parental stress levels, which in turn can affect marital satisfaction and sibling relationships. This interconnectedness highlights the importance of considering the family as a whole when addressing individual issues.

Another key concept is homeostasis, which refers to the family system's tendency to maintain stability and resist change. Families develop patterns and routines that help them function, but these patterns can sometimes become maladaptive (Cox & Paley, 1997). For example, a family might develop a pattern of avoiding conflict, which can lead to unresolved issues and increased tension over time. Understanding these patterns is crucial for identifying areas where intervention might be necessary.

Lastly, boundaries are also a significant aspect of systems theory. Boundaries define the limits of the family system and regulate the flow of information and influence between family members and external systems. Healthy boundaries are flexible and allow for appropriate levels of interaction and support, while rigid or diffuse boundaries can lead to dysfunction (Weeland et al., 2021).

In summary, systems theory and resilience theory both offer valuable perspectives for navigating resilience in the child welfare system. Systems theory provides a comprehensive view of the family's interactions with larger systems, while resilience theory focuses on the strengths and protective factors that help parents and families overcome adversity. Together, these theories help practitioners develop holistic and empowering interventions to support vulnerable children and their families. While systems theory offers a perspective on the interconnected elements influencing child welfare, incorporating cognitive-behavioral therapy (CBT) provides targeted interventions that can enhance family resilience by addressing and restructuring the cognitive and behavioral patterns of individuals within the system.

### CBT Techniques for Enhancing Family Resilience

CBT techniques can play a crucial role in enhancing family resilience. The first technique is cognitive restructuring. This technique helps individuals identify and challenge negative thought patterns and replace them with more positive and realistic ones (Clark, 2013). This can cause family members to develop healthier ways of thinking about conflicts and stressors, reducing misunderstandings and fostering a more supportive environment.

Consider a parent in the child welfare system who feels overwhelmed and believes they are a failure due to making a mistake. A social worker would first help the parent identify and articulate this negative automatic thought. Next, they would use techniques such as Socratic questioning to explore the validity of this belief (Clark, 2013). Questions could include, "What specific evidence supports the idea that you are a failure?" and "Are there instances where you have successfully managed similar situations?"

After identifying the cognitive distortion, the social worker would guide the parent in gathering evidence that contradicts the negative thought, such as recalling past successes or strengths. This process involves helping the parent reframe their thought to be more balanced and realistic (Clark, 2013). For instance, the social worker might assist them in developing a new thought like, "While I made a mistake, it does not define my overall abilities as a parent. I have the capacity to learn and improve."

The next technique is behavioral activation. This encourages individuals to engage in activities that they find rewarding and enjoyable. When family members participate in positive activities together, it strengthens their bonds and creates positive shared experiences, enhancing overall resilience (Boswell et al., 2017).

For example, consider a parent who feels overwhelmed and has withdrawn from daily activities due to stress. The social worker would first conduct a thorough assessment to identify the parent's values, interests, and the activities they find rewarding. Then they would collaboratively develop a plan to gradually reintroduce these activities into their routine. Next, they start with small, manageable goals that are aligned with the parent's values.

If a parent values spending quality time with their children but has been avoiding it due to feelings of inadequacy, the social worker could help them set a goal of having a 15-minute playtime with their child each day. They would also provide support and encouragement, helping them to overcome barriers and track their progress. By systematically increasing their engagement in positive activities, the parent can experience a sense of accomplishment and improved mood, which can, in turn, enhance their parenting skills and overall well-being.

CBT also teaches problem-solving and communication skills training to address specific issues effectively. This allows families to work together to identify problems, brainstorm solutions, and implement them, leading to more effective and collaborative resolution of conflicts (Egeci & Gencoz, 2011). Additionally, improved communication skills help family members express their needs and concerns more clearly and listen to each other more effectively, reducing conflicts and misunderstandings, further enhancing resilience.

Let's say a parent is having a hard time getting their child to complete homework. The social worker facilitates a session where the parent actively listens to the child's frustrations and acknowledges their feelings. Together, they discuss the importance of completing homework and collaboratively create a daily homework schedule. This plan includes a set time each day for homework and small rewards for task completion. The social worker supports the parent in consistently following the plan and regularly checking in. This approach helps the child develop better study habits, reduces homework-related stress, and strengthens the parent–child relationship.

CBT emphasizes the importance of reinforcing positive behaviors through rewards and positive feedback. Recognizing and reinforcing positive behaviors within the family can encourage more of these behaviors, creating a more positive and resilient family dynamic. While CBT effectively addresses individual cognitive and behavioral patterns to enhance resilience, dialectical behavioral therapy (DBT) builds on this by incorporating mindfulness and emotional regulation strategies, offering a comprehensive approach to fostering resilience within the entire family unit.

## DBT Techniques for Enhancing Family Resilience

DBT is a highly effective therapeutic approach that combines cognitive-behavioral techniques with principles of mindfulness. Originally developed for treating borderline personality disorder, DBT has been adapted for various populations and issues, including enhancing family resilience (Linehan, 2014).

The first technique is mindfulness. This is the cornerstone of DBT and involves being fully present and engaged in the current moment without judgment. For families, mindfulness practices can help members become more aware of their thoughts, feelings, and behaviors, which is essential for improving communication and reducing conflict. By practicing mindfulness, family members can learn to respond to each other with greater empathy and understanding (Linehan, 2014).

The next technique is emotional regulation. DBT teaches specific skills for managing and regulating intense emotions, which are crucial for maintaining family harmony and resilience. Emotion regulation skills include techniques for identifying and labeling emotions, increasing positive emotional experiences, and reducing vulnerability to negative emotions (Linehan, 2014).

Moving on, effective communication is vital for family resilience. DBT's interpersonal effectiveness skills focus on enhancing communication and relationship-building. These skills help family members assert their needs, set healthy boundaries, and navigate conflicts constructively. By fostering open and respectful communication, interpersonal effectiveness skills can help resolve conflicts and strengthen family bonds (Linehan, 2014).

DBT offers several valuable techniques that can enhance family resilience. Mindfulness practices help family members stay present and empathetic, emotion regulation skills promote emotional stability, and interpersonal effectiveness skills improve communication and conflict resolution. By incorporating these DBT techniques into their daily lives, families can build a stronger, more resilient foundation to navigate life's challenges together.

## Dignity-Centered Approach to Parental Support

Recognizing the intrinsic worth of parents is fundamental. Dignity-centered approaches affirm that every individual, including parents, possesses inherent value and deserves respect. This recognition can be transformative for parents who may feel marginalized or undervalued due to socioeconomic, cultural, or personal challenges (Grassi et al., 2024). By affirming their worth, social workers can help parents build self-esteem and confidence, which are crucial for effective parenting. When parents feel valued, they are more likely to engage positively with their children and make informed decisions that benefit the family unit.

Self-reflection is also a critical component of dignity-centered approaches. Social workers can facilitate opportunities for parents to reflect on their values, beliefs, and behaviors. This process of self-reflection can lead to increased self-awareness and personal growth (Wessels, 2017). For example, a parent who understands the impact of their actions on their children is better equipped to make positive changes. By promoting self-reflection, social workers empower parents to take ownership of their parenting journey and develop strategies that align with their values and goals.

Providing access to resources and support networks is another way dignity-centered approaches empower parents. Social workers play a crucial role in connecting parents with community resources, such as parenting classes, support groups, and financial assistance programs. These resources can provide practical assistance and emotional support, helping parents navigate the challenges of parenting (Jacobson, 2007). When parents have access to the resources they need, they are more likely to feel competent and capable in their parenting role.

Education about rights and the importance of dignity in family dynamics is also essential. Social workers can educate parents about their rights and the significance of upholding dignity within the family. This knowledge can empower parents to advocate for themselves and their children more effectively.

Positive reinforcement is a powerful tool in dignity-centered approaches. By acknowledging and celebrating the efforts and achievements of parents, social workers can boost their self-esteem and motivation. Positive reinforcement encourages parents to continue striving for positive family interactions, leading to healthier family dynamics.

Involving various stakeholders in supporting families is crucial for creating a comprehensive and effective child welfare system. The involvement of multiple stakeholders ensures a holistic approach that addresses the diverse needs of families and children. Stakeholders such as social workers, healthcare providers, educators, community organizations, and policymakkers each bring unique perspectives and resources that can significantly enhance the support provided to families (Jacobson, 2007).

Community organizations offer a wide range of services, from housing assistance to after-school programs, which can alleviate some of the pressures faced by families. These organizations often have strong ties within the community, making them effective in reaching and engaging families. Policymakers are crucial in creating and implementing policies that support families. Their decisions can lead to systemic changes that address the root causes of family instability, such as poverty, lack of access to healthcare, and inadequate housing (Wessels, 2017).

Collaboration among these stakeholders fosters a network of support that is more resilient and adaptive to the needs of families. It encourages the sharing of information and resources, leading to more coordinated and effective interventions. Furthermore, involving families themselves as stakeholders in the process ensures that their voices are heard and their specific needs are addressed, promoting empowerment and self-determination.

## Conclusion

Families often enter the child welfare system due to concerns such as child safety, abuse, neglect, or parental incapacity, which prompt investigations and interventions aimed at ensuring the child's well-being. Once in the system, families face a range of challenges, including navigating complex bureaucratic processes, dealing with social stigma, managing emotional stress, and accessing necessary resources and support services.

Understanding resilience is key in this context. Resilience refers to the ability to adapt positively in the face of adversity, trauma, or significant stress. It's important because it enables families to recover from difficulties and maintain functional and supportive relationships despite challenges. Resilience theory posits that resilience is not a static trait but a dynamic process that can be fostered through supportive relationships, adaptive skills, and positive experiences.

Incorporating systems theory provides further insight into how families interact with external systems, such as child welfare services. Systems theory highlights the importance of viewing families as interconnected units where changes in one part can affect the whole. By integrating resilience theory with systems theory, practitioners can better understand how to support families in building resilience within the context of their unique environments and relationships.

To enhance family resilience, CBT and DBT offer effective strategies. CBT helps parents and children identify and challenge negative thought patterns, fostering more adaptive and positive thinking. Behavioral activation, a component of CBT, encourages engagement in meaningful activities that can improve mood and reduce stress. DBT focuses on building emotional regulation, distress tolerance, and interpersonal effectiveness skills, which are essential for maintaining stable and supportive family relationships.

Finally, adopting a dignity-centered approach is crucial in supporting families within the child welfare system. This approach emphasizes respect, empathy, and empowerment, ensuring that families are treated with dignity and their voices are heard. It involves collaborating with families to identify their strengths and needs, providing culturally sensitive support, and advocating for their rights and well-being. By adopting a dignity-centered approach, practitioners can build trust and foster a more supportive and effective intervention process, ultimately enhancing family resilience and outcomes.

By understanding the complexities of how families enter the child welfare system, recognizing the challenges they face, and employing theories and techniques that promote resilience, we can better support families in overcoming adversity and thriving despite the difficulties they encounter.

## Questions for Reflection

1 How have the strategies discussed in this chapter helped you understand the complexities of parental challenges in the child welfare system?
2 Can you identify any personal biases you might have had before reading this chapter, and how they may have changed?
3 How can you apply the knowledge from this chapter to improve your practice as a social worker or human service?
4 In what ways can building stronger relationships with parents help address the challenges outlined in this chapter?
5 What role does cultural competence play in applying the interventions discussed in this chapter?

## Bibliography

Becvar, D. S. (2007). *Families that flourish: Facilitating resilience in clinical practice.* W. W. Norton.

Boswell, J. F., Iles, B. R., Gallagher, M. W., & Farchione, T. J. (2017). Behavioral activation strategies in cognitive-behavioral therapy for anxiety disorders. *Psychotherapy, 54*(3), 231.

Cao, Y., Hoffman, J. A., Bunger, A. C., Maguire-Jack, K., & Robertson, H. A. (2019). Identifying and addressing parental trauma and behavioral health need: The role of the child welfare system. *Journal of Public Child Welfare, 13*(3), 265–284. https://doi.org/10.1080/15548732.2019.1595259

Carver, C. S. (1998). Resilience and thriving: Issues, models, and linkages. *Journal of Social Issues, 54*(2), 245–266.

Clark, D. A. (2013). Cognitive restructuring. In S. G. Hofmann, D. J. A. Dozois, W. Rief, & J. A. J. Smits (Eds.), *The Wiley handbook of cognitive behavioral therapy* (pp. 1–22). Wiley Blackwell.

Cox, M. J., & Paley, B. (1997). Families as systems. *Annual Review of Psychology, 48*(1), 243–267. https://doi.org/10.1146/annurev.psych.48.1.243

Egeci, I. S., & Gencoz, T. (2011). The effects of attachment styles, problem-solving skills, and communication skills on relationship satisfaction. *Procedia-Social and Behavioral Sciences, 30*, 2324–2329.

Fong, K. (2017). Child welfare involvement and contexts of poverty: The role of parental adversities, social networks, and social services. *Children and Youth Services Review, 72*, 5–13.

Frankel, H., Snowden, L. R., & Nelson, L. S. (1992). Wives' adjustment to military deployment: An empirical evaluation of a family stress model. *International Journal of Sociology of the Family, 22*, 93–117.

Grassi, L., Nanni, M. G., Riba, M., & Folesani, F. (2024). Dignity in medicine: Definition, assessment and therapy. *Current Psychiatry Reports, 26*(6), 1–21.

Hawley, D. R. (2000). Clinical implications of family resilience. *American Journal of Family Therapy, 28*, 101–116.

Hawley, D. R., & De Haan, L. (1996). Toward a definition of family resilience: Integrating life-span and family perspectives. *Family Process, 35*(3), 283–298.

Helton, J. J., Cooper-Sadlo, S. C., House, N. G., Adler, H., & Norton, L. (2022). Resilience of families Involved in child welfare: A mixed-methods study. *Social Work Research, 46*(2), 153–161. https://doi.org/10.1093/swr/svac004

Kemp, S. P., Marcenko, M. O., Hoagwood, K., & Vesneski, W. (2009). Engaging parents in child welfare services: Bridging family needs and child welfare mandates. *Child Welfare, 88*(1), 101–126.

Jacobson, N. (2007). Dignity and health: A review. *Social Science & Medicine, 64*(2), 292–302.

Linehan, M. (2014). *DBT? Skills training manual*. Guilford Publications.

Masten, A. S. (2001). Ordinary magic: Resilience processes in development. *American Psychologist, 56*(3), 227.

Mullin, W. J., & Arce, M. (2008). Resilience of families living in poverty. *Journal of Family Social Work, 11*, 424–440.

Taylor, A., & Kroll, B. (2001). *Parental substance misuse and child welfare*. Jessica Kingsley Publishers.

Walsh, F. (1996). The concept of family resilience: Crisis and challenge. *Family Process, 35*(3), 261–281.

Weeland, J., Helmerhorst, K. O., & Lucassen, N. (2021). Understanding differential effectiveness of behavioral parent training from a family systems perspective: Families are greater than "some of their parts". *Journal of Family Theory & Review, 13*(1), 34–57.

Wessels, G. J. (2017). Promoting dignity and worth of people: Implications for social work practice. *Southern African Journal of Social Work and Social Development, 29*(3), 16–pages.

# 11 Nothing without Us! Working in Community with Disabled Persons

*Mia Ocean, Meagan Corrado, Melissa Hirschi, and Lashirah Warren Glenn*

The International Disability Alliance's call to action, "Nothing without us!" (National Democratic Institute, 2022), was our mantra as we wrote this chapter. If you are not familiar with this call, it may seem like common sense—it is! But if society was already integrating the voices of people with disabilities into programs, policies, and approaches, the Alliance would not have issued this call to action.

The Centers for Disease Control and Prevention (CDC, 2023) estimates that 27% of the U.S. population has a disability. Using common sense (i.e., including disabled individuals in all aspects of our society), individuals with disabilities should comprise approximately 27% of Congress. Yet it is estimated that less than 1% of Congress has a disability because we, as a nation, do not even inquire about the disability status of congressional members (National Council on Independent Living, 2022). We track race, ethnicity, gender, sexual orientation, age, immigration history, military service, education level, and religious demographics of congressional members but not disability status (Schaeffer, 2023). Think about that for a moment. What assumptions are embedded in the decision to refrain from collecting data on disability? What might that say about our expectations and values related to disabled people?

Within this chapter, we invite you to enact disability justice as a human services professional. As we document the tentacles of the past that continue to influence our conceptualization of disabilities and disabled communities, we also envision a new and different future. We begin by detailing institutionalization and disability conceptualizations in Western society (i.e., white, abled dominant, colonized countries) before moving into emancipatory ways to work alongside disabled people and communities. It is our hope, whether you have a disability or not, that you will learn, unlearn, and reflect on how you can actively make human services a safe, welcoming, and expansive space for people of all abilities.

The chapter includes direct quotes from writings on asylums and eugenics. Reading this ugly part of our ableist history can be traumatic. We included this painful information because we feel that moving forward requires us first to acknowledge our past. After sharing this difficult information, we provide you with an opportunity to pause and engage in reflection. We think it is important to be transparent so that you know what to expect before we begin. It is equally important to take moments to consider the many reasons to have hope, which are also included.

As we wrote this chapter, we were in conversation with each other. We have intentionally incorporated you into our discussion using first, second, and third person in our writing. Academic writing can depersonalize social problems and render them as static phenomena, but disability justice is a dynamic process that we, you, and they need to be a part of. Therefore, we purposefully violate the norms of conventional writing and APA format to make

DOI: 10.4324/9781003531258-14

our ideas accessible and bridge the divides between disabled communities, practitioners, and academics. We ask that you remain open rather than write us off because we do not present in *the typical* fashion.

We further use humor, including asides in parentheses (how dare we!), to connect with readers and infuse joy and humor into disability justice work (Ocean, 2024). While you may be reading this alone, you are welcome to be a part of a movement that is bigger than any one of us. Let's begin our exploratory journey together by first unearthing the past.

## Reckoning with the Atrocities Perpetrated by Our Professional Communities

Western society has a long history of treating individuals with disabilities in an exclusionary, inhumane way. As early as the 12th century, England opened its first psychiatric hospital; these hospitals, also referred to as asylums, were institutions where professionals abused, neglected, and confined disabled people without regard for fundamental human rights (Slater, n.d.). As the United States was colonized, our policies mirrored those of Europe, and Western countries fed off each other, passing more and more oppressive legislation ("The Education and Care," 1877). Abled people isolated and confined disabled people to prisons, almshouses, family attics and basements, and make-shift shacks or huts in the center of town out of an irrational fear that the disabled would contaminate the general population (Applebaum, 2018; Rothman, 1971). When a community no longer wanted to care for a disabled person, it was commonplace for the community to sneak the person away in the middle of the night and drop them off in another town's square so that the supervision and care of this person became another town's responsibility (Weihofen & Overholser, 1946). These were not isolated incidents. While oppression took many forms, stripping rights from disabled people and segregating them from society were socially acceptable practices (Applebaum, 2018).

In the 1800s, there were multiple asylums in the United States that incarcerated people with a wide range of disabilities and differences (Torrey, 1997). The first annual report (1852) published by the New York State Asylum for Idiots (yes, even the institution's name is offensive and problematic) provides insight into this era. They framed their work as "the management and education of young idiots," and their descriptions of the children in their care included "walked imperfectly … partial paralysis … excessive flow of saliva … very irritable … imperfect speech, the wandering gaze or fixed and vacant stare, imperfect hearing" and illiterate (The New York State Asylum for Idiots, 1852, p. 5). Descriptions like "defective or excessive sensation" and "excessive restlessness or inertia" meant that once a child was labeled, their fate was sealed for a lifetime (The New York State Asylum for Idiots, 1852, p. 5). The children were too much or not enough, but they could not escape the category of *idiot*.

In the report, the superintendent noted that the patients were commonly dehumanized:

> Even the witnessed or well authenticated results of efforts for their education are regarded as if they were the performances of trained animals…But it should be remembered that they have a human origin; that however they may differ in physical, mental or moral organization they are yet human beings.
>
> (The New York State Asylum for Idiots, 1852, p. 6)

Historians describe how asylum professionals sought to control or subdue disabled people by forcibly implementing protocols to indoctrinate people with disabilities with the dominant beliefs of the time and *cure* them of their disabilities (MacDonald, 1985). Scull (1989) believed no meaningful treatment was occurring, only abuse and ultimately death:

> Asylums were mere storage bins for human refuse, filled with chronic "patients" who seldom returned to the outside world ... the insane, if not the victims of violent assault by attendants or fellow inmates, passively rotted away, often spending their days restrained by camisoles and straitjackets and their nights locked into covered cribs.
>
> (p. 254)

The use of these facilities continued widely across the globe into the 1970s. At that time, populations decreased in psychiatric hospitals, and the populations in prison grew (Harcourt, 2011; Mechanic & Rochefort, 1990).

## Let's Pause

We just shared some deeply troubling information. It isn't easy to look back at the past, but it is necessary. We want to pause and take a breath. As we read and discussed this information, we, as co-authors, reached out to each other for support. We processed what we were learning and how emotionally overwhelmed we were by this information. We talked about how our loved ones were institutionalized and abused by helping professionals during these time periods.

As we reflect, it is equally important that we do not frame disabled communities as vulnerable populations who need human services professionals to save them (because—from who? The very same professionals?!). Therefore, during this pause, we also want to center leaders of the disability justice movement. Sins Invalid (2019) is a collective of disabled, Black Indigenous People of Color (BIPOC), and queer individuals who developed the disability justice principles evolving framework. One of the principles, interdependence, focuses on how disabled people cannot wait for government solutions and, to some extent, *should not* wait because of the accompanying exertion of control. Mutual aid is a viable alternative where people can care for and liberate each other. Whether we acknowledge it or not, as humans, we are all interconnected, share one planet, and impact each other. Let's be good to one another and treat each other with dignity, respect, and care.

When people read something like the disability justice principles, some may think, "*Why do we need that?*" But when we consider our professional history, it becomes obvious why we need them and how they can help us avoid repeating past mistakes. Speaking of past mistakes, let us take another breath and get back to it.

## The Introduction of *Normal*

It is important to consider how Western society's understanding of *normalcy* has also impacted our approach to disability and difference. The word "normal" was first introduced into the English language in 1840 (Davis, 2013, p. 1). According to Davis (2013), the idea of *normalcy* was based on the work of Adolphe Quetelet, a Belgian astronomer. Quetelet applied the *law of error* (used at the time to identify a star's location by averaging the sighting errors) to human features, like height and weight. This ultimately led to the development of the idea of the "average man" (Davis, 2013, p. 2). Anyone who fit within the normal distribution of the bell curve was in alignment with the expectations of the average person, and those who did not fit were considered *abnormal*.

Quetelet's work laid the foundation for the future marginalization of individuals who did not fit within the statistical expectations of *the average man.* By using statistics to determine if a person was *normal,* abled people then stigmatized and discriminated against those individuals who were different or who they determined had a disability (Davis, 2013; Watson, 2003). Watson (2003) explained that this conceptualization of disability allowed abled people "to grade individuals, providing us with hierarchies according to unspecified categories. Any violations of these situational norms [were] treated as signs of instability" (p. 36). Professionals (yes, professionals!) then developed formal classifications for mental and psychological functioning. These classifications impacted not only a disabled person's social standing but also their medical and psychological treatment (Applebaum, 2018; Mora, 1992). Yet the truth remained: "the 'problem' is not the person with disabilities; the problem is the way that normalcy is constructed to create the 'problem' of the disabled person" (Davis, 2013, p. 1).

With Western society's growing interest in the statistical *grading* of human bodies came eugenic ideologies because "almost all the early statisticians had one thing in common: they were eugenicists" (Davis, 2013, p. 3). As a result, the dominant group, in this case, abled people, stigmatized and forced individuals with disabilities and differences into a lower social stratum (Goffman, 1961). After abled people dehumanized disabled people, Western society felt justified to confine disabled people, subject them to inhumane treatment, silence their voices, take away their ability to reproduce, and deny their basic human rights.

## The Influence of Capitalism on Human Rights

Capitalism, an omnipresent force, cannot be ignored in any discussion on human rights in the United States. In the context of capitalist societies, disability and difference have historically been viewed as a threat to the established order because they have the potential to interfere with productivity standards (Stuckey, 2014; Snyder & Mitchell, 2006). Unfortunately, this line of reasoning fed eugenic dogmas. Bleecker Van Wagenen (1912) wrote the "Preliminary Report of the Committee of the Eugenic Section of the American Breeders' Association to Study and to Report on the Best Practical Means for Cutting Off the Defective Germ-Plasm in the Human Population" (where do we even begin with that title?!?). Within the report, he argued, on behalf of the committee, that people with disabilities, people who lived in poverty, and people convicted of crimes "must be considered as socially unfit, and their supply should, if possible, be eliminated from the human stock" (Van Wagenen, 1912, p. 462). Methods for accomplishing this included "segregation, sterilization, restrictive marriage laws and customs, eugenic education of the public ... (and) euthanasia" (Van Wagenen, 1912, p. 464).

## Let's Pause Again

We need to take another moment to pause and reflect. This is horrific to read. When we think about the people who lived through these atrocities, we cannot fathom the pain they endured. As we explored these original readings, we teared up and cried. It is important for us to sit with these intense emotions for a moment. If we gloss over them, we are setting ourselves up to repeat these mistakes in all their forms and harm people.

As we pause, it is again important to center disabled perspectives, this time through Mad Pride. Mad Pride is about rejecting the term *mental illness,* reclaiming the term *mad,* and refusing to feel shame for one's existence (Rashed, 2019). Teasing out all the nuances of Mad Pride is beyond this chapter's scope. However, we ask you to consider the idea of having pride in one's madness juxtaposed against our history presented here. Within its historical and environmental context, Mad Pride is a bold form of activism and resistance.

Ok. Hopefully by this point, you understand that our professional predecessors enacted monstrous atrocities. We do not want to continue digging up trauma for the sake of doing so. Instead, let's move forward, keeping in mind how our past can impact our present and simultaneously centering disability rights, progress, and hope.

## Disability Rights Activists

Disabled activists have aided and, at times, forced (wonder where they learned that) Western society to halt some of these oppressive practices and pass disability rights legislation. In the United States, with the pivotal help of the Black Panthers, disabled activists passed the Rehabilitation Act of 1973 and engaged in 504 sit-ins (Section 504 from the Act) to demand its implementation (Crowley, n.d.). This meaningful legislation requires accommodation at the federal level and is still being implemented to this day.

Disabled activists continued their activism for disability rights, using powerful public demonstrations that often led to their arrest. One such example was the Capitol Crawl, where people left their wheelchairs and crawled up the stairs of Capitol Hill. Their advocacy helped pass the Americans with Disabilities Act of 1990 (as amended) (Ervin, 2020). Moreover, disabled people, like Lois Curtis and Elaine Wilson, changed U.S. policy through the court system. They successfully sued the state of Georgia to be released from in-patient treatment and moved to community-based care (*Olmstead v. L.C.,* 1999). More recently, disabled activists were arrested as they helped save the Patient Protection and Affordable Care Act and the Medicaid expansion programs that the act enabled (Stein, 2017). Their efforts certainly helped disabled communities, but they also helped many abled people who rely on the Act to access healthcare.

## Present Conceptualizations of Disability

Definitions of disability are socially constructed but determine who has access to public and private financial assistance, to accommodations, to protection from discrimination, and, in some cases, to freedom. Language is powerful and has consequences for real people. Within this section, we explore the medical model, social model, and universal design (UD) conceptualizations of disability to understand where we have been. We will then imagine where we could be via an emerging philosophy of disability justice-informed practice.

### Medical Model

In the medical model, disabled individuals are framed as having a defect or impairment that should be medically corrected when possible. Examples that fit this model include someone who wants their back pain corrected or cancer to be removed from their body. However, this model is problematic because it situates abled people as *normal* and *healthy* and seeks to *cure* people who, in some cases, do not consent to, need, or desire such treatments. The Autistic Self-Advocacy Network (n.d.) is an example of a community organization run for and by people with autism who believe "autism cannot and should not be cured" ("Autism Research and Therapies" section). This network's message is important, and of course, the organization does not speak for every autistic person.

The medical model remains the dominant model in many realms. For instance, the current U.S. definitions of disability almost exclusively conform to the medical model and include remnants from the past that describe individuals as being deficient. A person with a disability is defined in the Americans with Disabilities Act (ADA, 1990) as someone who has "a physical or mental impairment that substantially limits one or more major life activities … a record of such an impairment; or being regarded as having such an impairment" (Section 12102). Here are a few examples of the diverse range of disabilities covered under the ADA and its impact on major life activities: asthma (breathing), attention-deficit/hyperactivity disorder (concentrating), bulimia (eating), insomnia (sleeping), leg paralysis (walking), and stuttering (speaking). Disability definitions, like the one presented in the ADA, situate the disabled individual as deviating from *the average man*. These definitions also place the onus on disabled people to prove that they meet the legal definition of disabled and request accommodations from people in power (which they may or may not grant).

### Social Model

The central premise of the social model of disability is that there is nothing wrong with disabled people; there is something wrong with society's ableist perceptions, attitudes, and norms. To be clear, by ableism, we mean the attitudes, beliefs, statements, behaviors, systems, policies, and laws that situate abled people as superior to disabled people (Purlang, 2020). Many Indigenous communities have embraced a socially inclusive perspective (before it was formally named in Western writings), living their core beliefs of connection, relationship, and interdependence and finding individual roles for all to contribute to society (Weaver, 2015). For people in Western societies, it took quite a bit of sorting through societal dysfunctions to progress beyond the medical model into the social model.

"(A) small, hardcore group of disabled people, inspired by Marxism," the Union of Physically Impaired Against Segregation (UPIAS), organized in Great Britain in the 1970s (Shakespeare, 2017, p. 196). The UPIAS (1976) wrote an interpretation of disability as they attempted to make sense of it in their own lives:

> In our view, it is society which disables physically impaired people. Disability is something imposed on top of our impairments by the way we are unnecessarily isolated and excluded from full participation in society. Disabled people are therefore an oppressed group in society.
>
> (p. 20)

In other words, the UPIAS viewed ableism as the disability.

Building on their conceptualization, Mike Oliver, a disabled sociologist, developed the formal social model of disability in the 1980s to help human service professionals engage in a more disability-just practice (Oliver, 2013). The social model proposes that disabilities are naturally occurring variances in human abilities and conditions in direct contrast to the medical model. According to the social model, the only barriers that disabled communities encounter are (1) society was built for abled people and (2) abled people or *the average man* are used as the reference point to judge other humans.

The foundational work of the UPIAS and the social model has been a powerful tool to reframe disability. Unfortunately, the model has also been misunderstood, criticized, and contorted into something that is more comfortable for abled people (Finkelstein, 2001; Oliver, 2013). However, we believe that the social model remains one (not the only) pivotal frame for human service professionals to conceptualize disability and engage in emancipatory practice with disabled communities.

### *Universal Design*

UD is a justice-oriented approach to accessible environments. UD is grounded in the idea that society can proactively plan for the naturally occurring variance in abilities so that disabled people can meet their needs seamlessly and autonomously without having to request special access. UD aligns with the World Health Organization's (WHO, 2023) perception of disability:

> Disability is part of being human. Almost everyone will temporarily or permanently experience disability at some point in their life. ... Disability results from the interaction between individuals with a health condition, such as cerebral palsy, Down syndrome and depression, with personal and environmental factors including, negative attitudes, inaccessible transportation and public buildings, and limited social support. A person's environment significantly affects the experience and extent of disability. Inaccessible environments create barriers that often hinder the full and effective participation of persons with disabilities in society on an equal basis with others.
>
> (para. 1–3)

While the focus of UD is on people with disabilities, the benefits are not limited to them. A common example is sidewalk cut-outs; they create access for people who use mobility aids while also helping people using strollers or dollies. Imagine if we designed our schools, organizations, businesses, and recreational environments planning for the natural variance that biologically occurs in human beings. If we did, ableism and its resulting barriers for persons with disabilities would cease to exist.

## How to Work in Community with Disabled Persons

Western society has had moments of both enlightenment and regression in its perspectives of disabled communities (Mora, 1992). However, Western society's long history of silencing, ignoring, and harming disabled people has resulted in a deep-seated mistrust of human service professionals within disability communities. We may not have directly caused this, but we have inherited it (Wilkerson, 2020). It is important to be mindful of our professional history and understand where our work begins. As we seek to honor the "Nothing without us!" call to action, we must respect disabled people as the foremost authorities in their own lives and begin to build trust. By sharing power, being transparent, and collaborating with individuals with disabilities, we can shift from *us versus them* to *we*.

Next, we share our emerging philosophy of disability justice-informed practice. These are practical ideas that can guide our work with clients, but they can also positively impact our encounters with colleagues, friends, and neighbors, helping us recognize and dismantle ableism within ourselves and our circles of influence. Our goal is to develop concrete and intentional ways to enact disability justice as human services professionals. We must challenge ourselves and our profession to consistently move equitably forward. As part of our ongoing reflective practice, it is crucial that we ask ourselves, "Are there ways that I can do this better? How can I work in community more completely than I already do?"

### Begin from a Place of Common Humanity

Treating people with respect and dignity, no matter who they are, where they come from, or the experiences they have had, is the essence of being a human services professional. When we understand our connectedness and how each of us plays a role in contributing to the greater good, it is easier to work as *we*. We must commit to co-creating spaces where we can learn from one another, draw strengths from one another, and collectively build a better community for all of us.

### Do Your Homework on Disabilities

Like all marginalized populations, disability communities are not homogeneous groups. There are differences across disabilities and within specific disabilities. Some people are born with disabilities, while others may acquire a disability as a child or an older adult. A person's disabilities may be dynamic (shifting throughout the day or month), or they may be stable. Because we live in an ableist society, it is easy for us to access information about abled culture. But it is essential that we intentionally seek out information about disabled culture. The information that is commonly shared often reinforces negative stereotypes and tropes.

One way to deprogram this inaccurate information is to replace it with more accurate information. Disabled people share their experiences and perceptions through scholarship, memoirs [even a fabulous complication of first-person narratives (Wong, 2020)], social media, blogs, *The Squeaky Wheel* (a disability focused satire publication), day-to-day interactions, and with us, as human services professionals, when we work together. We need to pay attention and seek out representative knowledge.

When you are working with someone who has a disability that you are unfamiliar with, seek out quality information from activists in the community and organizations that are led by people with that disability. Learn the basics so you can ask questions specific to your client's unique needs. Do your homework so that you are not putting your client in the position of an unpaid disability consultant.

### Know that People Are More Than Their Disability

Disability is just one aspect of a person's identity. A person's disability may or may not be one of their primary identities, and the intersection of a person's identities needs to be accounted for in our work (Crenshaw, 1991). Clients may be disabled, and they may also identify as pansexual, Muslim, a parent, male, and so on. The identity of a disabled person does not begin and end with their disability. It is just as important for us to also support clients in identifying their strengths, interests, relational connections, and aspirations.

### Say What You Mean

Language matters. Reflect on how the language that we use can either reinforce or dismantle ableist ideologies. Let's use this sentence as an example: *The person was blind to what was happening*. In this case, the word *blind* is used to mean *ignorant* and perpetuates ableist language. Consider the language used in your case notes and during treatment team meetings. Are you making an effort to eliminate ableism from your vocabulary by using direct and factual language? Similar to the campaign to end the use of the word *gay* in a derogatory manner, we have work to do regarding how disability-related words are used.

### If in Doubt, Ask

When working with a client, it is best to refrain from making assumptions. This means that you should not assume that a person has a disability based on how they present and should refrain from making assumptions about a person's identity related to their disability+ (i.e., race, gender, immigration status). Our first step should be to ask questions. After doing your homework, if you are still not sure how to interact with someone, ask. If you are wondering if someone wants your assistance, ask. If you learn that you will be working with an individual who might need some type of accommodation, ask. If you are unsure what language the person uses to describe their disability, ask. It is that simple. This may feel uncomfortable at first because we are conditioned to avoid talking about disability. But many people will appreciate your consideration and curiosity.

### Prioritize Your Client's Voice and Perspectives

Individuals with disabilities possess their own emotions, strengths, personalities, and aspirations (good ole' common sense again). The key to honoring a person's unique vantage point is engaging in meaningful dialogue with them. When an interpreter helps you communicate with a client, speak directly to the client, not the interpreter. Additionally, if a client brings a family member or support partner with them, make sure that you are prioritizing your client's perspective and needs. If the accompanying person speaks for the client, it is often appropriate to shift the conversation back to the client you are serving, but we must also consider the culture of the person and family. If the family makes decisions collectively, we want to honor that, making space for the complex, multifaceted nature of our work.

In exceptional circumstances where direct communication with the individual is not feasible, human service professionals may need to direct inquiries to a parent, guardian, or conservator to gain a better understanding of the individual. Nonetheless, it is crucial to acknowledge that this approach does not equate to direct communication with the individual, as family members might harbor differing perceptions of the individual or their disability.

### Respect Everyone's Right to Self-Determination

We must show respect for every person's autonomy. In our work, we may be tempted to make assumptions about what someone else may want. But it is rarely, if ever, our place to think *for* someone else. We must also work according to our client's pace and timeline. If additional information, time, or discussion is needed, it should be provided. We should avoid pressuring a client into a decision whenever possible. Additionally, we need to be transparent and provide quality, timely information so that disabled clients, disabled colleagues, disabled supervisors, disabled supervisees, and disabled community partners (and those without disabilities) can make informed decisions and determine how they want to proceed.

### Learn about Legislation Related to Your Work

Become familiar with oversight agencies, including the Department of Justice (primarily for public access), the Equal Employment Opportunity Commission (primarily for potential, current, and former employees), and the Office for Civil Rights (primarily for students). Learn about disability legislation to ensure that you are meeting or exceeding legal accessibility requirements. Familiarity with legislation can also help you inform disabled clients about their rights and support them in filing a complaint if they believe they have been discriminated against. Attend professional development workshops and review publicly available resources like the Job Accommodation Network and the U.S. Access Board to learn about new guidance as it becomes available and to engage in our commitment to lifelong learning.

### Meet or Exceed Ethical Standards

Human service professionals should always adhere to their ethical standards of practice. Certain standards are especially important when working with persons with disabilities. According to the National Organization for Human Services' (NOHS, 2024) ethical standards, professionals should ensure that they do not impose their personal values or biases on their clients (Standard 7). This means that helping professionals should be aware of their biases and take the necessary steps to ensure that these biases do not negatively impact their work with clients.

Additionally, NOHS (2024) Standard 34 states that professionals should maintain awareness of their culture, values, and biases. This means we need to recognize how these factors may impact clients and our relationships with clients. Further, we need to commit to delivering culturally informed services. Consider asking yourself, "What preconceived thoughts or feelings do I have about this client or their disability? Are there any biases that I need to check prior to meeting with my client?"

### Think Critically and Act Creatively

Sometimes people do things in a particular manner because it's the way things have always been done. When reviewing our professional history, we believe that is a scary way to approach human services work. We contend that it is ok and even necessary to be creative, to be innovative, and to expand how we do things. If we regularly took the time to slow down and observe the social environments in which we work, interact, play, and live, we would be amazed! Think about these places and spaces from a different perspective, not our traditional world as seen through an ableist lens. Ask questions and critically observe how our world is designed. How might we change our spaces to be more universally accessible? How can we introduce creative ideas into our workplaces and communities? Not all changes need to be built into legislation or policy. We can go beyond what is required by law and design human services centering equity. Think critically about our world and work to increase accessibility and minimize (or eliminate!) oppression.

We also need to develop new interventions to truly partner with communities. The Storiez Trauma Narrative intervention, developed by Dr. Meagan Corrado (2016), was created for urban youth who have experienced trauma. Corrado (2023) developed the intervention in collaboration with the youth she supported as a clinician. The intervention guides youth as they look back at their past experiences, process those experiences creatively, and develop a vision for the future (Corrado, 2015a, 2015b). Through Storiez, youth have created narratives in various formats—from written stories to videos, paintings, and collages. Youth are encouraged to actively use their own voices throughout the storytelling process and are given control and autonomy over their own narratives (Corrado et al., 2022). Storiez is a great example of how to creatively work in community and how we must continually develop innovative ways to work effectively as human services professionals.

### Be an Imperfect Human. Take Responsibility. Learn. Repeat.

We are going to make mistakes, and there is no singular way to do disability justice work. Lizzo, American singer, rapper, and flautist, provided a model for how to handle a situation when a person uses language that a disabled person or community finds offensive. She included what can be considered an ableist slur, *spaz*, in a song. When there was public outcry, she acknowledged what happened, educated herself, and released a new version of the song without the word. She was then able to move forward in a positive way, making our world a more beautiful and musical place.

When you find yourself in a similar situation, apologize, take responsibility, and do not do it again. Language and our conceptualization of disability, equity, and power sharing are constantly in flux. We have the opportunity to respect the needs of those who have been marginalized, actively build alliances, and enact the disability justice principles in our work.

## Conclusion

It is our sincere hope that, after reading this chapter, you understand that there is not one way to be in this world. There are infinite ways to express ourselves, and none are necessarily better or worse, but some are closer to the definition of *normal*. Our writing models one way to overcome ableist standards without sacrificing rigorous content. We chose to make this topic personal rather than continue to dehumanize. But this required support from active allies, like our book editor. You are also in a gatekeeping role as a human services professional. Please question traditional human services practices and use creativity to invite, nudge, and sometimes shove progress forward.

Because there are many wondrous ways to live, engage, and achieve, it can complicate things. It means that sometimes we need to do our homework and ask questions. It means that there are no clear-cut answers for what to do and when to do it. It means that being disabled in an ableist world takes more work, but to be disabled is also to be filled with joy, community, strength, and innovation. Let's face it. If we wanted neat and tidy answers, we would have chosen a different discipline.

We also realize that our chapter touches on very basic information. Unfortunately, based on our professional and personal experiences, our documented history, and current research, there is a need for fundamental education on how to work in community with persons with disabilities (even if it should be common sense). If we invest in implementing a disability justice-informed practice, we can quickly render our work a gruesome relic of the past (that we can make fun of) and move into a more emancipatory phase of our profession's development.

To close, we want to revisit the International Disability Alliance's call to action, "Nothing without us!" As hard as it was to dig up and rummage through our professional history, we did it for the generations before us, and we did it for the generations to come. We seek to honor the truth that is too frequently buried, justified, and overlooked. Disability justice work is a lifelong journey, not a destination, and it will take all of us working as a community to eradicate ableism. We commit to doing better as professionals and people, and we hope you will join us as an active member of the disability justice movement.

## Questions for Reflection

- What are the implications of how we frame disability?
- Beyond the examples shared in this chapter, how does our ableist, professional history still influence human services?
- What will you do when you encounter ableism as a human services professional?
- What are you willing to do over the next month, six months, and year to be an active member of the disability justice movement?

## References

Americans with Disabilities Act of 1990, 42 U.S.C. § 12101 et seq. (1990). https://www.ada.gov/pubs/adastatute08.htm

Applebaum, L. I. (2018). Deviancy, dependency, and disability. *Duke Law Journal, 68*(3), 417–468. https://www.jstor.org/stable/48563657

Autistic Self-Advocacy Network. (n.d.). *What we believe.* https://autisticadvocacy.org/about-asan/what-we-believe/

Centers for Disease Control and Prevention. (2023, May 15). *Disability impacts all of us.* https://www.cdc.gov/disability-and-health/articles-documents/disability-impacts-all-of-us-infographic.html

Corrado, M. (2015a). *Storiez: A guide for children and teenagers.* Ingram Spark.

Corrado, M. (2015b). *Storiez: A guide for therapists.* Ingram Spark.

Corrado, M. (2016). *Trauma narratives with inner city youth: The Storiez intervention* [Doctoral dissertation, University of Pennsylvania]. https://repository.upenn.edu/handle/20.500.14332/32953

Corrado, M. (2023). Storiez with urban youth: The evolution of a trauma narrative intervention. *Clinical Social Work Journal, 52*, 37–47. https://doi.org/10.1007/s10615-023-00906-x

Corrado, M., Murray, G., & Ghose, T. (2022). It gives them a voice the way they want the voice: A qualitative exploration of clinicians' use of Storiez with urban youth. *Journal of Poetry Therapy, 36*(2), 144–159. https://doi.org/10.1080/08893675.2022.2117999

Crenshaw, K. (1991). Mapping the margins: Intersectionality, identity politics, and violence against women of color. *Stanford Law Review, 43*(6), 1241–1299. https://doi.org/10.2307/1229039

Crowley, M. (n.d.). *Disability history: The 1977 504 sit-in.* https://disabilityrightsflorida.org/blog/entry/504-sit-in-history

Davis, L. J. (2013). Introduction: Disability, normality, and power. In L. J. Davis (Ed.), *The disability studies reader* (4th ed., pp. 1–16). Routledge.

"The education and care of idiots, imbeciles, and harmless lunatics." (1877, July 28). *The British Medical Journal, 2*(865), 108–110. https://www.jstor.org/stable/25245188

Ervin, M. (2020, July 1). An oral history of the capitol crawl. *New Mobility.* https://newmobility.com/the-capitol-crawl/

Finkelstein, V. (2001). *The social model of disability repossessed.* https://disability-studies.leeds.ac.uk/wp-content/uploads/sites/40/library/finkelstein-soc-mod-repossessed.pdf

Goffman, E. (1961). *Asylums: Essays on the social situation of mental patients and other inmates.* Anchor Books.

Harcourt, B. E. (2011). Reducing mass incarceration: Lessons from the deinstitutionalization of mental hospitals in the 1960s. *Ohio State Journal of Criminal Law, 9*(1), 53–88. https://hdl.handle.net/1811/73369

MacDonald, M. (1985). Review: Madness and healing in the nineteenth-century America. *Reviews in American History, 13*(2), 211–216. https://www.jstor.org/stable/2702412

Mechanic, D., & Rochefort, D. A. (1990). Deinstitutionalization: An appraisal of reform. *Annual Review of Sociology, 16*, 301–327. https://doi.org/10.1146/annurev.so.16.080190.001505

Mora, G. (1992). The history of psychiatry in the United States: Historiographic and theoretical considerations. *History of Psychiatry, 3*(10), 187–201. https://doi.org/10.1177/0957154X9200301003

National Council on Independent Living. (2022). *Current elected officials with disabilities in 2022.* https://web.archive.org/web/20241013112607/https://ncil.org/elected-officials/

National Democratic Institute. (2022, March 28). *From "Nothing about us without us" to "Nothing without us."* https://www.ndi.org/our-stories/nothing-about-us-without-us-nothing-without-us

National Organization for Human Services. (2024). *Ethical standards.* https://www.nationalhumanservices.org/ethical-standards/

The New York State Asylum for Idiots. (1852). *First Annual Report.* https://www.disabilitymuseum.org/dhm/lib/detail.html?id=758&page=all

Ocean, M. (2024). The potential of humor to joyously dismantle ableism+: Considerations for social workers. *The Journal of Sociology & Social Welfare, 51*(1), Article 6. https://doi.org/10.15453/0191-5096.4720

Oliver, M. (2013). The social model of disability: Thirty years on. *Disability & Society, 28*(7), 1024–1026. https://doi.org/10.1080/09687599.2013.818773

Olmstead v. L. C., 527 U.S. 581 (1999). https://supreme.justia.com/cases/federal/us/527/581/

Purlang, A. (2020, October 25). Words matter, and it's time to explore the meaning of "ableism." *Forbes.* https://www.forbes.com/sites/andrewpulrang/2020/10/25/words-matter-and-its-time-to-explore-the-meaning-of-ableism/

Rashed, M. A. (2019). In defense of madness: The problem of disability. *The Journal of Medicine & Philosophy, 44*(2), 150–174. https://doi.org/10.1093/jmp/jhy016

Rehabilitation Act of 1973, 29 U.S. Code § 701 et seq. (1973). https://www.govinfo.gov/content/pkg/COMPS-799/pdf/COMPS-799.pdf

Rothman, D. J. (1971). *The discovery of the asylum: Social order and disorder in the New Republic.* Little, Brown and Company.

Schaeffer, K. (2023, February 7). *The changing face of Congress in 8 charts.* Pew Research Center. https://www.pewresearch.org/short-reads/2023/02/07/the-changing-face-of-congress/

Scull, A. (1989). *Social order/mental disorder: Anglo-American psychiatry in historical perspective.* Routledge.

Shakespeare, T. (2017). The social model of disability. In L. J. Davis (Ed.), *The disability studies reader* (pp. 195–203). Routledge.

Sins Invalid. (2019). *Skin, tooth, and bone: The basis of movement is our people* (2nd ed.). https://www.sinsinvalid.org/disability-justice-primer

Slater, C. (n.d.). *Idiots, imbeciles, and intellectual impairment.* http://caslater.freeservers.com/ancient.htm

Snyder, S., & Mitchell, D. T. (2006). *Cultural locations of disability.* University of Chicago Press.

Stein, J. (2017, June 22). "No cuts to Medicaid!": Protesters in wheelchairs arrested after release of health care bill. *Vox.* https://www.vox.com/policy-and-politics/2017/6/22/15855424/disability-protest-medicaid-mcconnell

Stuckey, Z. (2014). *A rhetoric of remnants: Idiots, half-wits, and other state-sponsored interventions.* State University of New York Press.

Torrey, E. F. (1997). *Out of the shadows: Confronting America's mental health crisis.* Wiley.

The Union of Physically Impaired Against Segregation. (1976). *Aims and policy statement.* https://disability-studies.leeds.ac.uk/wp-content/uploads/sites/40/library/UPIAS-UPIAS.pdf

Van Wagenen, B. (1912). *Preliminary report of the Committee of the Eugenic Section of the American Breeders' Association to study and to report on the best practical means for cutting off the defective germ-plasm in the human population.* https://readingroom.law.gsu.edu/cgi/viewcontent.cgi?article=1073&context=buckvbell

Watson, N. (2003). Daily denials: The routinization of oppression and resistance. In S. Riddell, & N. Watson (Eds.), *Disability, culture, and identity* (pp. 34–52). Taylor & Francis.

Weaver, H. N. (2015). Disability through a Native American Lens: Examining influences of culture and colonization. *Journal of Social Work in Disability & Rehabilitation, 14*(3–4), 148–162. https://doi.org/10.1080/1536710X.2015.1068256

Weihofen, H., & Overholser, W. (1946). Commitment of the mentally ill. *Texas Law Review, 24*(3), 307–348.

Wilkerson, I. (2020). *Caste: The origins of our discontents.* Random House.

Wong, A. (Ed.). (2020). *Disability visibility: First-person stories form the twenty-first century.* Vintage.

World Health Organization. (2023, March 7). *Disability.* https://www.who.int/health-topics/disability#tab=tab_1

# 12 Supporting Graduate Students' Mental Health

## Addressing Challenges for Underrepresented Communities

*Adrian Rodriguez*

Graduate school requires students to balance rigorous academic demands with family, work, and financial concerns. This challenge can elevate graduate students' stress and anxiety, increasing their risk for depression and suicide and negatively impacting their academic performance (Satinsky et al., 2021). Mental health concerns worsened for this population during the COVID-19 pandemic and persist today (Herrell & Foster, 2024; Zhai & Du, 2020). Underrepresented Graduate Students (UGS), including Black, Indigenous, and People of Color (BIPOC), Lesbian, Gay, Bisexual, Transgender, Queer, and additional identities (LGBTQ+) and non-binary individuals, first-generation graduate students (i.e., first in the family to attend graduate school), international students, and those from low-income backgrounds, as well as other groups face additional systemic barriers such as discrimination and marginalization. These challenges can lead to impostor syndrome (IS), or the intense feeling of not belonging, such as to a graduate program and fear of exposure as unqualified (Levine, 2020; Murguía Burton & Cao, 2022; Schwartz, 2019). Addressing barriers for UGS can improve the effectiveness of graduate programs and enhance student outcomes (Powell et al., 2019).

This chapter examines graduate student mental health, including how faculty can identify distress and engage in supportive conversations. It highlights the unique challenges faced by underrepresented groups, such as discrimination, microaggressions, marginalization, and IS, and the use of an intersectional framework to provide support. The chapter also offers practical strategies to respond to these issues at the individual, classroom, and department levels, along with suggestions to integrate graduate students' cultural identities into the curriculum to build resilience and well-being to improve their academic success.

## The Mental Health Landscape for Graduate Students

A quarter of U.S. graduate students experience severe mental health issues due to the high academic demands and hectic schedules of their programs (Herrell & Foster, 2024). These challenges are compounded by the ongoing impact of the COVID-19 pandemic and additionally by systemic discrimination for underrepresented groups (Lipson et al., 2022; Quan et al., 2023; Wildey et al., 2022). A Spring 2024 survey by the American College Health Association found that 30% of graduate students were stressed, 24.4% were anxious, and 16.1% were depressed (ACHA, 2024). Some students cope with these pressures by turning to substances. In Allen et al.'s (2022) study, 85% of graduate students disclosed drinking alcohol during a 12-month period, while 20% used marijuana, and 7% took prescription drugs non-medically. While one-third of graduate students utilize mental health services, non-white and first-year students are least likely to seek help (Wildey et al., 2022).

DOI: 10.4324/9781003531258-15

Universities must work to destigmatize mental health discussions and make resources more relatable and accessible (Hopley, 2019).

## Signs of Mental Illness

In ACHA's (2024) assessment, 44.1% of graduate students felt lonely. These feelings are shaped by personality, the academic environment, and perceived support from faculty and peers and can lead to psychological distress and lowered academic performance (Kalubi et al., 2020). Key signs of psychological distress include prolonged sadness or withdrawal indicative of major depression; sudden overwhelming fear with accompanying physiological symptoms such as a racing heart, characteristic of panic attacks; and severe changes in mood representative of bipolar disorder (SAMHSA, 2023). These emotional fluctuations often lead to negative behavioral changes and a sense of instability and result in the loss of interest in studies, struggles with coursework, and contemplation over whether to drop out (Murguía Burton & Cao, 2022).

## Faculty as Gatekeepers of Mental Health

Students often turn to faculty first when in distress, and many faculty members view being gatekeepers of mental health as part of their role. While faculty are not counselors, they can still engage in meaningful conversations with students about their well-being (Speicher Sarraf, 2021). In a recent survey by TimelyCare, 76% of faculty believed it is one of their job duties, while 45% of students in a 2023 StudentVoice survey shared this sentiment (Mowreader, 2024). However, many faculty request more training on identifying signs of distress and referring students to appropriate resources (Kalkbrenner & Sink, 2018; Mowreader, 2024). Training programs should cover suicide prevention, integrate well-being in learning environments, and offer role-play strategies to assist distressed students.

### Talking about Mental Health

Graduate students, when contemplating whether to disclose mental health issues, consider the stigma and emotional risks, as well as how faculty might respond (LaBelle et al., 2024). Those who share often do so to seek help with their academic performance, to maintain transparency, and to build relationships. Positive faculty responses help graduate students trust the process and expand on their concerns, while dismissive reactions can deter further help-seeking. As faculty members determine how to respond to students' mental health concerns, attending mental health trainings can help them better recognize the signs of distress, such as excessive anxiety and agitation, and guide students toward proper care (Hopley, 2019; Kalkbrenner & Sink, 2018).

Faculty can initiate well-being check-ins with observational comments such as, "I noticed you haven't been in class as much lately. I know that's not like you, and I wanted to check in to see how you're holding up (Franko, 2022)." When students respond, faculty can practice active listening by attending to both spoken words and non-verbal cues, such as tone, body language, and facial expressions, to better assess their emotional state. For example, a student may claim, "Everything is great," yet their body language (e.g., folded arms and glossy eyes) reveals otherwise (Corey, 2017). Faculty can express care by responding, "It sounds like you're carrying a lot right now," "I'm here to support you," and "If or when you're ready, I'd be glad to talk about what that might look like" (Franko, 2022). Such statements, along with active listening, can help students feel seen and heard, which normalizes their experiences, shows appreciation for their trust, and encourages openness. Faculty might also encourage resilience by asking about past coping strategies, "What has helped you during past difficulties?" and inviting them to apply those strategies now, "How might you build upon what you did then?" (Rodriguez & Mallinckrodt, 2021). Comments such as "That sounds really creative," "That took a lot of courage," or "That's a resourceful approach" can help validate their efforts.

Following up regularly demonstrates a commitment to students' well-being (Franko, 2022; Speicher Sarraf, 2021). When doing so, it is important to remain nonjudgmental. Students may not have used the resources provided or followed through on next steps. Faculty should check in discreetly, either in private or via email, using phrases like, "I wanted to see how things have been going since we last spoke," or "If there's anything else I can do, such as offering you additional resources or support, please let me know" (Franko, 2022). Some faculty may feel engaging with students about mental health issues is outside of their comfort zone and skillset. A licensed psychologist in a university counseling center with expertise in graduate student support suggests validating this viewpoint and ensuring faculty have the tools they need to connect students with appropriate resources (A. Petrossian, personal communication, September 19, 2024). Counseling centers, for instance, can present workshops to academic departments on available services and provide strategies for connecting with and referring students in ways that align with each faculty member's perspective. Beneficial campus student resources include Counseling and Psychological Services, the Student Health Center, Title IX, and Diversity Initiatives. Faculty can also include a Student Resources section in their syllabi with names and links for mental health services and reference this during the first class. It is essential to refer students for additional support when their issues: (1) go beyond the scope of faculty's competence or comfort zone, (2) involve self-harm or harm to others, and (3) include elevated anxiety or unusual behavior (Speicher Sarraf, 2021; When to refer, 2023). When considering a referral, faculty can avoid mislabeling culturally appropriate behaviors by becoming proficient in the mental health needs of the populations they assist (Corey, 2017).

### Unique Challenges for Underrepresented Graduate Students

Graduate students often work beyond the standard workweek, juggling coursework, research, teaching, and sometimes outside employment with smaller support networks, especially if they moved away for school (Hopley, 2019). This can lead to stress, loneliness, and isolation, resulting in mental health concerns that can hinder academic performance through burnout, decreased productivity, and diminished capacity to manage academic responsibilities. Success in graduate school requires **social capital** or the essential skills and resources for adapting to the elite academic spaces and social norms of graduate life (Mishra, 2020; Okpych & Gray, 2021).

Two forms of social capital are critical in this process. **Bonding capital** affords students the emotional and practical support from family, peers, and home communities to "get by" as they begin their programs. **Bridging capital**, on the contrary, involves the skills students develop to "get ahead" by forming connections with faculty, staff, and peers that offer them access to necessary research, teaching, and internship placements (Mishra, 2020; Okpych & Gray, 2021). These networks enhance graduate students' academic development and professional advancement. Successful students can combine the personal support from family and friends with their newfound academic networks to access a wider range of resources.

For BIPOC and LGBTQ+ students, the lack of faculty and peers who share their identities limits their ability to build necessary social capital. This sociocultural power imbalance often upholds white privilege and heteronormativity, which inherently perpetuates discrimination toward and the marginalization of people in these groups (Gunaratne & Lumb, 2023; Misawa, 2015). Those UGS lacking sufficient social capital must **code-switch** or adjust how they speak, present themselves, and communicate with faculty and peers to fit in, which can lead to stress, psychological fatigue, and feelings of isolation, and negatively affect their academic performance (Allen & Stewart, 2022; McCluney et al., 2021).

### Barriers to Inclusivity

Discrimination and microaggressions are common barriers for UGS that can impact their well-being and retention in graduate school. **Discrimination** involves the unfair or prejudicial treatment of people based on their race, gender identity, age, sexual orientation and identity, or other characteristics (APA, 2023). Examples include questioning the credibility or intelligence of students based on their race or gender identity. Day-to-day discrimination takes the form of **microaggressions** or subtle, often unintentional, but offensive comments or actions directed at members of a non-dominant group that make them feel invalid or that they do not belong.

UGS experience more frequent discrimination and racial microaggressions at predominately white institutions (PWIs), such as questions by white peers over their intelligence and cultural stereotyping that leads to feelings of invisibility; at Historically Black Colleges and Universities, these acts, while less frequent, may involve exclusion or stereotyping of non-Black minority students (e.g., Asian American and Latina/o) by their Black/African American peers (Berger et al., 2020). An example of a microaggression that undermines a BIPOC individual's competence is: "I wouldn't have guessed you were the TA for the class"—spoken by a white graduate student to a graduate student of Mexican heritage, who is the class's teaching assistant.

Daily microaggressions contribute to chronic stress, which diminishes individuals' mental health (APA, 2023). Additionally, these experiences can trigger UGS's self-censorship of thoughts, lowering their self-esteem and self-efficacy, or belief in their ability to be successful in graduate school, causing them to question their belonging in their programs (Conway-Klaassen & Maness, 2017; Perez-Lopez et al., 2022). These students may lose respect for their offending peers and mentors and may ultimately drop out of their majors and/or fields of study.

UGS often experience a sense of otherness compared to their peers. **Marginalization** is a form of social exclusion that can make underrepresented individuals feel like they are outsiders culturally and intellectually, leading to isolation (Gay, 2004). Examples include attending a graduate program that fails to offer culturally relevant curricula and being surrounded by faculty and peers who show indifference or hostility toward UGS's struggles, both of which make them feel invisible. Consistent marginalization, like microaggressions, erodes UGS's self-worth and elevates their mental health concerns. Through repeated exposure to discrimination, microaggressions, and marginalization, UGS feel alienated, powerless, and meaningless in their academic environments. These concerns manifest in strong doubts about their capabilities and worthiness to remain in their programs.

IS often arises from discrimination and marginalization (Levine, 2020; Schwartz, 2019). A lack of role models and mentors who share one's racial and/or gender identity can also lead to IS, which intensifies UGS's worries and doubts over their right to belong in their graduate programs. Schwartz's (2019) study of IS among Indigenous law students showed that they found course curricula irrelevant to their future needs, felt socially isolated, and believed they were less intelligent than their peers. Racial and ethnic minorities and women in graduate STEM programs are more likely to experience IS, which can lead to disengagement and reduced motivation (Collier & Blanchard, 2023; Levine, 2020; Schwartz, 2019). To combat IS, the students in Schwartz's (2019) study found support through the Nura Gili program, an Indigenous campus unit that provided belonging, solidarity, and a space where they could share their struggles and anxieties. The law students also sought encouragement from family and advocated for events to connect the school with their families and the Indigenous community.

## Dismantling Barriers: Addressing Exclusionary Practices in Graduate Education

Eliminating barriers to inclusivity is critical for UGS's success. Drawing from APA (2023) and Gunaratne and Lumb (2023), the following are three key faculty strategies to promoting inclusivity: (1) **Establish Academic Support Networks**: Inclusive mentorship programs and UGS groups help students reframe their negative experiences, enhance self-worth, and provide guidance and practical advice on handling discrimination and microaggressions. (2) **Offer Workshops on Coping Strategies and Building Resilience**: These workshops, in partnership with college counselors and other healthcare professionals, can teach students to respond to stress and anxiety using relaxation techniques (e.g., deep breathing and mindfulness). Through role-playing exercises, students can practice articulating and combating instances of discrimination. (3) **Strengthen and Publicize Reporting Mechanisms**: Campus departments and affiliated networks can encourage students to report discrimination through straightforward and simple processes, anonymously if they so choose. To build students' trust in the system, departments should promptly address their concerns and remedy the offending behaviors.

To help students diminish the impact of IS often associated with the preceding barriers to inclusivity, faculty can employ the following strategies based on work by Levine (2020): (1) **Encourage Students to Acknowledge Their Feelings**: Remind students it is normal and acceptable to feel inadequate at times during their academic and professional journey. (2) **Help Students to Redirect Their Anger**: Show them how to channel their frustration away from themselves and toward confronting IS through reflective exercises that highlight their achievements and reaffirm their professional worth. Lastly, (3) **Nurture Their Self-Compassion**: Motivate students to move forward compassionately by reminding themselves that their doubts do not define their overall capabilities.

### Utilizing an Intersectional Approach

An intersectional approach deepens understanding of UGS's varied experiences. Dr. Kimberlé Crenshaw asserts that to fully understand how Black women are subordinated in society, we must consider their intersectional experience, which is greater than the sum of the sexism and racism they face (Crenshaw, 1989). Expanding this to additional groups, **intersectionality** encompasses the various ways individuals' social identities, including their race, ethnicity, gender identity, sexual orientation and identity, socioeconomic status, and ability, act and interact within larger systems of privilege and oppression (Bowleg, 2012). This approach illuminates how systemic issues contribute to UGS's unique experiences of discrimination, microaggressions, and marginalization, with detriment to their mental health and challenges within their graduate departments and institutions (Rodriguez et al., 2024).

By adopting an intersectional lens, faculty can implement tailored support structures, creating a more inclusive and supportive environment. Take, for example, international graduate students at a PWI in the United States. They face the typical academic pressures but also unique hurdles such as visa restrictions, potential language difficulties, and cultural unfamiliarity, which can hinder their acculturation process and leave them feeling isolated and hesitant to seek mental health support (Rodriguez et al., 2024). International and first-generation college students also carry added pressures to succeed, such as bringing success to their families. They may hide their struggles to avoid disappointing their families and burdening others (Murguía Burton & Cao, 2022; Soria & Horgos, 2021). These students' intersecting identities shape their unique acculturation, academic, and wellness challenges.

Consider the following two MBA students: Sara, a 22-year-old Korean American, cisgender lesbian woman, and single parent, and Aicha, a 54-year-old cisgender straight Algerian woman, devout Muslim, and an international student. Both have become noticeably withdrawn in class. During office hours, they each express feelings of sadness, loneliness, instances of belittlement by several peers and faculty, and growing doubts about their fit in the program. Through an intersectional analysis, faculty can explore how each student's experiences are influenced by their age, cultural background, relationship status, parenting status, religion, sexual orientation and identity, and resident status, which distinctly affect their experiences of depression, isolation, and disconnection. To effectively connect with students using Crenshaw's (1989) framework, faculty can (1) recognize that discrimination and microaggressions differ by culture and individual experience, (2) embrace the complexity of intersecting identities, and avoid reducing students' experiences to one issue, and (3) approach each interaction with flexibility, practicing empathy as they adjust to each student's unique needs.

Sara and Aicha likely have a mix of similar and differing experiences and needs. Both students may benefit from broader inclusion initiatives like support groups or mentorship programs that offer connections to faculty and classmates who share similar backgrounds and/or face relatable challenges (Crenshaw, 1989). Sara, individually, may also benefit from resources for single parents, including flexible scheduling and childcare services (Goldrick-Rab & Sorensen, 2010), whereas programs that support language proficiency and facilitate religious accommodations may be helpful to Aicha (Rajendram et al., 2019; Stubbs & Sallee, 2013). By recognizing Sara and Aicha's unique circumstances and multiple identities, faculty can help mitigate their feelings of isolation and empower them to engage more fully and successfully within their academic and social environments (Sims-Schouten & Gilbert, 2022).

### Fostering Resilience

Faculty can enhance graduate students' well-being by promoting **resilience**, a process that enables individuals to access their positive emotions, successful traits, and coping mechanisms to adapt to and move forward from hardships (Luthar et al., 2000). It should also encompass mental, physical, and spiritual development and acknowledge the experiences and support structures that enable underrepresented communities to thrive despite systemic challenges (Sims-Schouten & Gilbert, 2022). For instance, Muslim women immigrants to the United States post-9/11 found resilience through their Islamic faith and collective supportive relationships in and outside of their families, while young Black men in the UK overcame exclusion from the school system by utilizing cultural community wealth (i.e., family and community support; Aziz, 2012; Wright et al., 2016). Faculty can promote graduate students' resilience by encouraging goal setting, self-reflection, and engagement in altruistic practices such as affirming their cultural ties through community volunteering and service-learning projects.

### Creating Culturally Responsive Academic Spaces

Using culturally responsive teaching methods, faculty can further enhance the resilience of UGS. **Culturally relevant pedagogy** (CRP) is a student-centered approach that recognizes and develops each student's distinct cultural assets to improve their well-being and academic performance, while creating community within the classroom (Brown, 2020). Through CRP, faculty can guide the integration of students' cultural knowledge, prior experiences, and unique performance styles into the curriculum, making learning more relevant and effective. Faculty can refine their teaching to best meet their students' needs by seeking ongoing feedback on their delivery of course content and engagement style, using questions like, "How am I doing?" and "How well am I reflecting who you are in the classroom?" Through clear communication of academic expectations and attention to the "hidden curriculum" or unwritten rules and social norms for success in graduate school (Perez-Lopez et al., 2022), faculty can help students gain the social capital and academic competence necessary for success.

Additionally, through open discussions about mental health in the classroom and departmental settings, faculty can create spaces that encourage students to share their struggles and seek help (Mowreader, 2024; Perez-Lopez et al., 2022). By advocating for a cultural shift within academic departments to prioritize mental health, faculty can promote an inclusive graduate community and enhance the recruitment and success of minoritized candidates. By engaging in university mental health trainings, inviting teaching and research assistants to departmental planning discussions on wellness, and implementing regular well-being check-ins during faculty meetings, classroom sessions, research lab meetings, and student organization gatherings, faculty can establish a more resilient support system (Gunaratne & Lumb, 2023).

## Applying Your Learning: A Case Study

As you read the following case of Manny, adapted from McGill University and the California Senate (Case Studies, n.d.), consider how you might help him access effective strategies and support systems as he navigates the complexities of graduate school.

Manny is a 28-year-old, cisgender, bisexual Puerto Rican male, and the first in his family to attend graduate school. As the only Latino in a Data Analytics program, he often feels misunderstood and frustrated, especially when peers repeatedly ask him about Mexican culture. He faces financial strain but does not want to take on more student loans. After coming out as bisexual, Manny's parents are increasingly pressuring him to marry his girlfriend, Terri, despite his ongoing feelings for his best friend, Daniel. To cope with stress, Manny has turned to alcohol. Long lab hours, self-criticism, and isolation have worsened his anxiety, impacting his academic performance. His recent negative thesis review led to a stipend reduction, prompting thoughts of dropping out. He sought his father for advice, who said only that "Winners never quit, and quitters never win!" Those words invoked in Manny the value of perseverance and expectation to push through despite challenges. They also heightened his fear of failure and feelings of isolation in his struggles. Hesitant to approach his preoccupied thesis chair, Manny confided in a classmate, Dalton, who suggested counseling. Manny is open to the idea but worries about how it might affect his reputation in the program and with his family.

You, as Manny's professor, notice his distressed appearance and fidgety behavior. After class, you invite him to talk to you.

1  **How do discrimination, microaggressions, marginalization, IS, intersectionality, and resilience collectively shape Manny's concerns?**

Manny grapples with a lack of representation in his program and familial and financial pressures that impact his exploration of his sexual identity and ability to focus on coursework. Microaggressions by his peers and a lack of support from his faculty advisor fuel his IS, anxiety, and isolation. These stresses lead Manny to use alcohol to manage his increasing anxiety. Despite cultural norms against help-seeking, Manny confides in a friend, valuing his own well-being enough to break his silence and consider counseling.

2  **How would you check in with Manny?**

Consider establishing a confidential space, like your office, to express your concern for Manny's well-being. You might say:

> Manny, thank you for meeting with me. I've noticed you've seemed distracted in our recent classes. How is everything going for you? You can share as much or as little as you feel comfortable. I'm here to support you.

3  **How would you support Manny after he shares more of his situation?**

Consider validating Manny's feelings by normalizing his struggles and highlighting the strength in help-seeking. Offer referrals to campus mental health services and diversity resources, including the Latine/x Resource Center and LGBTQ+ Resource Center. Discuss ways to alleviate stress, like flexible assignment due dates or a reduced workload. You might say:

> I appreciate your sharing. It sounds quite overwhelming for you, and I'm glad we're discussing this. Last semester, when I found it difficult to balance my research deadlines with family concerns, talking with my therapist helped me regain focus. Let's explore some options to assist you, like adjusting your assignments, and connecting with campus resources for further strategies. What would help you most right now?

## Conclusion

Supporting graduate students' mental health is fundamental to a successful, thriving academic environment. Recognizing the signs of mental health issues and offering initial support make a significant difference. Challenges for UGS are compounded by discrimination, microaggressions, marginalization, and IS. Through open conversations, an intersectional framework, culturally responsive teaching, and structural changes to academic departments, faculty can perpetuate an inclusive and equitable academic culture that promotes well-being, normalizes help-seeking, and builds resilience.

## Reflective Questions for Consideration

1  How can you balance the need to support students' mental health with the academic pressures and expectations inherent in graduate programs?

2  What strategies can you utilize, beginning with the admissions process and throughout the graduate program, to establish and maintain a supportive and inclusive academic environment for students facing mental health challenges and/or IS?
3  How can you integrate culturally responsive approaches in your teaching and mentorship to cultivate resilience for students of diverse backgrounds and appropriately address discrimination, microaggressions, and marginalization?

## References

Allen, H. K., Lilly, F., Green, K. M., Zanjani, F., Vincent, K. B., & Arria, A. M. (2022). Substance use and mental health problems among graduate students: Individual and program-level correlates. *Journal of American College Health*, 70(1), 65–73. https://doi.org/10.1080/07448481.2020.1725020

Allen, A. M., & Stewart, J. T. (Eds.). (2022). *We're not ok: Black faculty experiences and higher education strategies*. Cambridge University Press.

American College Health Association [ACHA]. (2024). *NCHA-III Spring 2024 Reference Group Data Report*. https://www.acha.org/wp-content/uploads/NCHA-IIIb_SPRING_2024_GRADUATE_PROFESSIONAL_REFERENCE_GROUP_DATA_REPORT.pdf

American Psychological Association. [APA]. (2023). *Discrimination: What it is and how to cope*. APA.org. https://www.apa.org/topics/racism-bias-discrimination/types-stress

Aziz, S. F. (2012). From the oppressed to the terrorist: Muslim-American Women in the crosshairs of intersectionality. *Hastings Race and Poverty Law Journal, 9*, 191. https://scholarship.law.tamu.edu/facscholar/100

Berger, M., Luster-Teasley, S., Poleacovschi, C., Smith, K. C., Feinstein, S. G., & Jones-Johnson, G. (2020). A tale of two universities: An intersectional approach to examining microaggressions among undergraduate engineering students at an HBCU and a PWI. In *Proceedings of the American Society for Engineering Education (ASEE) Annual Conference*, Montreal, Canada. https://www.asee.org/public/conferences/172/papers/30929/view

Bowleg, L. (2012). The problem with the phrase Women and Minorities: Intersectionality—An important theoretical framework for public health. *American Journal of Public Health (1971), 102*(7), 1267–1273. https://doi.org/10.2105/AJPH.2012.300750

Brown, E. (2020). *Using culturally relevant pedagogy to promote student achievement* [Webinar]. Brandman University School of Extended Education. https://files.constantcontact.com/652e7816401/8516a2a2-370e-4f75-b2e5-b083d09ec45f.pdf

*Case studies for roundtable discussions*. (n.d.). McGill, California Senate. https://www.mcgill.ca/senate/files/senate/case_studies.pdf

Collier, K., & Blanchard, M. (2023). Investigating graduate students' experiences through structural equation modeling (SEM). *Trends in Higher Education, 2*(4), 718–746. https://doi.org/10.3390/higheredu2040042

Conway-Klaassen, J., & Maness, L. (2017). Developing cultural competency in laboratory practice. *American Society for Clinical Laboratory Science, 30*(1), 43–50. https://doi.org/10.29074/ascls.30.1.43

Corey, G. (2017). *Theory and practice of counseling and psychotherapy* (10th ed.). Cengage Learning.

Crenshaw, K. (1989). Demarginalizing the intersection of race and sex: A Black feminist critique of antidiscrimination doctrine, feminist theory and antiracist politics, *University of Chicago Legal Forum, 1989*(1), 139–161. https://chicagounbound.uchicago.edu/uclf/vol1989/iss1/8

Franko, D. L. (2022). *Faculty guide: Supporting student mental health*. Northeastern University, Office of the Senior Vice Provost for Academic Affairs; University Health and Counseling Services; Office of Prevention and Education at Northeastern. https://bpb-us-e1.wpmucdn.com/sites.northeastern.edu/dist/7/7597/files/2024/08/faculty-mental-health-guide-2.8.22.pdf

Gay, G. (2004). Navigating marginality en route to the professoriate: Graduate students of color learning and living in academia. *International Journal of Qualitative Studies in Education, 17*(2), 265–288. https://doi.org/10.1080/09518390310001653907

Goldrick-Rab, S., & Sorensen, K. (2010). Unmarried parents in college. *The Future of Children, 20*(2), 179–203. https://doi.org/10.1353/foc.2010.0008

Gunaratne, D., & Lumb, P. (2023, February 5). Ensuring underrepresented grad students' well-being. *Inside Higher Ed.* https://www.insidehighered.com/opinion/career-advice/carpe-careers/2023/02/05/ensuring-underrepresented-grad-students-well-being

Herrell, C., & Foster, S. (2024). Can't stop won't stop: Problematic phone use, sleep quality, and mental health in U.S. graduate students. *Journal of American College Health, 28*, 1–7. https://doi.org/10.1080/07448481.2024.2334068

Hopley, S. (2019, November 13). Grad students left out of mental health conversation FRESH TALK. *Hartford Courant.* https://www.proquest.com/newspapers/grad-students-left-out-mental-health-conversation/docview/2313883034/se-2

Kalkbrenner, M. T., & Sink, C. A. (2018). Development and validation of the College Mental Health perceived competency scale. *The Professional Counselor, 8*(2), 175–189. https://doi.org/10.15241/mtk.8.2.175

Kalubi, J., Bertrand, Y., Dagenais, B., Houde, R., Marcoux, S., & Bujold, M. (2020). Graduate students' mental health: Exploring experiences of isolation and loneliness. *European Journal of Public Health, 30*(5), v126. https://doi.org/10.1093/eurpub/ckaa165.340

LaBelle, S., White, A., & Forman, E. R. (2024). Graduate students' privacy boundaries in communicating about mental health with their advisors. *Communication Education, 73*(2), 143–167. https://doi.org/10.1080/03634523.2023.2281325

Levine, A. (2020, July 1). How to banish imposter syndrome. *Science.* https://www.science.org/content/article/how-banish-impostor-syndrome

Lipson, S. K., Lattie, E. G., & Eisenberg, D. (2022). Trends in college student mental health and help-seeking by race/ethnicity: Findings from the national healthy minds study, 2013–2021. *Journal of Affective Disorders, 306*, 138–147. https://doi.org/10.1016/j.jad.2022.03.038

Luthar, S. S., Cicchetti, D., & Becker, B. (2000). The construct of resilience: A critical evaluation and guidelines for future work, *Child Development, 71*(3), 543–562. https://doi.org/10.1111/1467-8624.00164

McCluney, C. L., Durkee, M. I., Smith, R. E., Robotham, K. J., & Lee, S. S.-L. (2021). To be, or not to be...Black: The effects of racial codeswitching on perceived professionalism in the workplace. *Journal of Experimental Social Psychology*, 97, 104199–. https://doi.org/10.1016/j.jesp.2021.10419

Misawa, M. (2015). Cuts and bruises caused by arrows, sticks, and stones in academia: Theorizing three types of racist and homophobic bullying in adult and higher education. *Adult Learning, 26*(1), 6–13. https://doi.org/10.1177/1045159514558412

Mishra, S. (2020). Social networks, social capital, social support and academic success in higher education: A systematic review with a special focus on 'underrepresented' students. *Educational Research Review*, 29, 100307. https://doi.org/10.1016/j.edurev.2019.100307

Mowreader, A. (2024, January 30). Student wellness tip: Helping faculty help students. *Inside Higher Ed.* https://www.insidehighered.com/news/student-success/health-wellness/2024/01/30/strategies-professors-support-student-mental-health

Murguía Burton, Z. F., & Cao, X. E. (2022). Navigating mental health challenges in graduate school. *Nat Rev Mater, 7*, 421–423. https://doi.org/10.1038/s41578-022-00444-x

Okpych, N. J., & Gray, L. A. (2021). Ties that bond and bridge: Exploring social capital among college students with foster care histories using a novel social network instrument (FC-Connects). *Innovative Higher Education, 46*(6), 683–705. https://doi.org/10.1007/s10755-021-09553-x

Perez-Lopez, E., Gavrilova, L., Disla, J., Goodlad, M., Ngo, D., Seshappan, A., Sharmin, F., Cisneros, J., Kello, C. T., & Berhe, A. A. (2022). Ten simple rules for creating and sustaining antiracist graduate programs. *PLoS Computational Biology, 18*(10), e1010516. https://doi.org/10.1371/journal.pcbi.1010516

Powell, J. A., Menendian, S., & Ake, W. (2019). Targeted universalism: Policy & practice. *Othering & Belonging Institute*. https://escholarship.org/uc/item/9sm8b0q8

Quan, L., Lu, W., Zhen, R., & Zhou, X. (2023). Post-traumatic stress disorders, anxiety, and depression in college students during the COVID-19 pandemic: A cross-sectional study. *BMC Psychiatry, 23*(1), 228–228. https://doi.org/10.1186/s12888-023-04660-9

Rajendram, S., Sinclair, J., & Larson, E. (2019). International graduate students' perspectives on high-stakes english tests and the language demands of higher education. *Language & Literacy (Kingston, Ont.), 21*(4), 68–92. https://doi.org/10.20360/langandlit29428

Rodriguez, A. A., & Mallinckrodt, B. (2021). Native American-Identified students' transition to college: A theoretical model of coping challenges and resources. *Journal of College Student Retention: Research, Theory & Practice, 23*(1), 96–117. https://doi.org/10.1177/1521025118799747

Rodriguez, M., Zammarrippa Roman, B., Mohamed, M., & Barthelemy, R. (2024). Social and cultural barriers reported by STEM international graduate students of color. *Journal of International Students, 14*(3), 276–302. https://doi.org/10.32674/jis.v14i3.6694

SAMHSA. (2023, April 24). *For educators. Substance abuse and mental health services administration*. SAMHSA. https://www.samhsa.gov/mental-health/what-is-mental-health/how-to-talk/educators

Satinsky, E. N., Kimura, T., Kiang, M. V., Abebe, R., Cunningham, S., Lee, H., Lin, X., Liu, C. H., Rudan, I., Sen, S., Tomlinson, M., Yaver, M., & Tsai, A. C. (2021). Systematic review and meta-analysis of depression, anxiety, and suicidal ideation among Ph.D. students. *Scientific Reports, 11*(1), 14370–14370. https://doi.org/10.1038/s41598-021-93687-7

Schwartz, M. (2019). Retaining our best: Imposter syndrome, cultural safety, complex lives and Indigenous student experiences of Law School. *Legal Education Review, 28*(2), 1–23. https://doi.org/10.53300/001c.7455

Sims-Schouten, W., & Gilbert, P. (2022). Revisiting "resilience" in light of racism, "othering" and resistance. *Race & Class, 64*(1), 84–94. https://doi.org/10.1177/03063968221093882

Soria, K. M., & Horgos, B. (2021). Factors associated with college students' mental health during the COVID-19 pandemic. *Journal of College Student Development, 62*(2), 236–242. https://doi.org/10.1353/csd.2021.0024

Speicher Sarraf, K. (2021, October 24). Beyond gatekeepers. *Inside Higher Ed*. https://www.insidehighered.com/views/2021/10/25/how-professors-can-support-students-mental-health-opinion#:~:text=Invite%20students%20to%20discuss%20their,services%20(the%20gatekeeper%20model

Stubbs, B. B., & Sallee, M. W. (2013). Muslim, too: Navigating multiple identities at an American university. *Equity & Excellence in Education, 46*(4), 451–467. https://doi.org/10.1080/10665684.2013.838129

When to refer a student. (2023). SUNY Broome Counseling Services. https://www2.sunybroome.edu/counseling/when-to-refer-a-student/#:~:text=Anytime%20a%20student%20shares%20a,a%20referral%20to%20Counseling%20Services

Wildey, M. N., Fox, M. E., Machnik, K. A., & Ronk, D. (2022). Exploring graduate student mental health and service utilization by gender, race, and year in school. *Journal of American College Health, 72*(8), 2982–2990. https://doi.org/10.1080/07448481.2022.2145898

Wright, C., Maylor, U., & Becker, S. (2016). Young Black males: Resilience and the use of capital to transform school 'failure.' *Critical Studies in Education, 57*(1), 21–34. https://doi.org/10.1080/17508487.2016.1117005

Zhai, Y., & Du, X. (2020). Addressing collegiate mental health amid COVID-19 pandemic. *Psychiatry Research, 288*, 113003. https://doi.org/10.1016/j.psychres.2020.113003

# 13  Shifting the Narrative in Healthcare

## From "Limited English Proficiency" to "Limited Linguistic and Cultural Competence"

*Neda Moinolmolki*

As the United States continues to grow and diversify, the number of Limited English Proficiency (LEP) individuals is continually rising. LEP status is defined by the U.S. Department of Justice as "Individuals who do not speak English as their primary language and who have a limited ability to read, speak, write, or understand English" (U.S. Department of Justice, n.d.). According to the 2023 U.S. Census Bureau, approximately 29.6 million U.S. residents have been identified as LEP, compared to 25.9 million in 2015. Paralleling this, scholars and practitioners are seeing an increase in the diversity of languages spoken by LEP households. Between 2021 and 2022, there was a drastic increase in the total number of households speaking the following languages: Spanish, Chinese, French, German, Vietnamese, Arabic, and Korean. Nationwide, these household-level rate increases ranged from 11,280 households (for Arabic-speaking households) to 569,943 (for Spanish-speaking households; U.S. Census Bureau, 2023).

With the rising levels of LEP residents in the United States, it is essential to recognize the systemic inequities they face, particularly when it comes to healthcare. Individuals with LEP status often encounter systemic barriers to receiving high-quality healthcare services, including inefficient patient–physician communication, poor healthcare service quality, subpar healthcare insurance coverage, and limited access to stable healthcare providers as well as preventive care services (Berdahl & Kirby, 2019; Kilbourne, 2005; Ramirez et al., 2023)—all of which have significant implications on their general health. Given these barriers, it is not surprising that LEP patients are more likely to have inconsistent sources of healthcare and unmet healthcare needs and often overdue for preventive care services, even when they have health insurance coverage (Graves et al., 2020; Jang & Kim, 2019).

LEP status today is recognized as a social determinant of health and is considered a risk factor for achieving optimal healthcare (Coren et al., 2009). The root causes of healthcare disparities among LEP populations are often theorized to be centered on language and literacy barriers. These barriers, along with cultural obstacles, restrict their access to medical/health services, healthcare resources, and informational capital (Fischer et al., 2021). In addition, LEP populations are often faced with other Social Determinants of Health risk factors, such as living in poverty and having low levels of education. Despite their increased vulnerability, the responsibility for addressing these healthcare-related disparities often falls on the LEP patients themselves rather than the broader healthcare system. Addressing healthcare inequities necessitates a shift away from a focus on terms such as "LEP status," which place the blame on patients, to terms such as "Limited Linguistic and Cultural Competence," which illuminate the accountability of healthcare systems in meeting the needs of their diversifying multilingual populations. Systemic efforts are warranted if we truly want to dismantle the healthcare inequities faced by LEP patients.

DOI: 10.4324/9781003531258-16

LEP individuals are legally entitled to access healthcare services and information in their preferred language. These rights have long been protected since the establishment of Title VI of the Civil Rights Act of 1964, which prohibits discrimination based on national origin, including language discrimination, and requires healthcare organizations receiving federal funding to provide meaningful access to their services (Civil Rights Act of 1964). This mandate was further expanded through subsequent legislation, including the Patient Protection and Affordable Care Act (ACA), which now also requires health insurers and providers to offer language assistance services to improve access for LEP patients (Patient Protection and Affordable Care Act, 2010). More recently, the ACA's nondiscrimination provisions have mandated that hospitals post accessible "patients' rights" taglines on their websites in the top 15 languages spoken in their state. Despite these federal mandates, many hospital systems still lag behind in providing such assurances, particularly within web-based domains. These lapses are of grave concern as Americans across all socioeconomic and language proficiencies are increasingly relying on the Internet for healthcare-related information, resources, and services (Graves et al., 2020; Rodriguez & Singh, 2018).

The internet has proven to be a valuable and widely available tool for LEP patients in seeking information about cultural and healthcare resources (Kim et al., 2020). Hospital websites often serve as crucial sources of healthcare information and accessible services, including language assistance (Graves et al., 2020; Rodriguez & Singh, 2018). Expanding cultural and linguistic materials on hospital websites can significantly enhance healthcare accessibility and quality for LEP populations.

Despite the known benefits and federal mandates in place, many hospital websites remain insufficiently accessible, both linguistically and culturally, for LEP patients. A study in 2021 found that only 22.5% of the top 40 hospitals nationwide (according to U.S. News & World Report and Newsweek) had Spanish translation capabilities on their websites (Honeycutt et al., 2021). Even more concerning was that children's hospitals, hospitals affiliated with public medical schools, and those in communities with higher proportions of Latinx populations were not more likely to offer Spanish-translated websites. Often, the costs and administrative burdens associated with revamping hospital websites to make them more accessible are cited as reasons many hospitals choose not to translate their websites (U.S. Department of Health and Human Services, 2020). Another study conducted in the state of Washington found that only about 10.8% of the 93 acute care hospitals in that state had translatable websites (Graves et al., 2020). Of that 10.8%, the top four translated languages were Spanish, Japanese, Korean, and Russian.

With the increasing number of Afghan and Middle Eastern refugees resettling in the United States since the official withdrawal from Afghanistan, an empirical study was conducted in 2023 by the author of this chapter, assessing the accessibility of hospital websites for Middle Eastern LEP patient populations. Regarding positionality, the author of this chapter is a second-generation Iranian American Higher Education professional who identifies as a woman. She is passionate about serving her community and is actively engaged in volunteering as an English tutor for recently resettled Afghan refugees, whose experiences have significantly contributed to her pursuit of this particular study. The study had targeted three major Afghan refugee resettlement hubs—Houston, TX; San Diego, CA; Sacramento, CA; and Connecticut (the state where the author resides). In the spring of 2023, 61 hospital websites were systematically reviewed using a Structured Assessment Checklist to assess the availability of translated content and information about language assistance services on hospital websites. The checklist evaluated the presence of information on hospitals' language services, the types of language assistance available, the translated website content, and the availability of translated health literacy materials. The checklist demonstrated strong inter-rater reliability among the three reviewers: two trained student research assistants and the study's principal investigator.

The results of the study revealed significant variations between cities and states in the percentage of hospital websites with accessible translation features, translated health literacy resources, and information regarding accessible language assistance services. San Diego had the highest percentage of hospitals with translated websites (60%), followed by Sacramento (33%), Connecticut (29%), and Houston (18%). Sacramento had the highest percentage of hospitals with accessible translated health literacy resources (89%), followed by San Diego (60%), Houston (35%), and Connecticut (14%). Connecticut had the highest percentage of hospitals including information on interpretation/language assistance services (100%), followed by Sacramento (89%), San Diego (80%), and Houston (53%). On average, hospitals with translated websites offered 1.7 languages (SD = 2.0), with Spanish, Chinese, and Arabic being the most frequent. Besides Arabic, no other commonly spoken Middle Eastern languages by Afghan refugees, such as Dari, Farsi, and Pashto, were found to be accessible on any of the investigated hospital websites.

These findings, along with the previous literature, highlight that, despite federal regulations regarding healthcare equity related to language and literacy accessibility, digital media platforms of hospital systems still fall short. Expanding the accessibility of hospital websites through translated resources is crucial for reducing healthcare barriers, improving healthcare outcomes, and addressing disparities in our communities. Although federal regulations are currently in place and the evidence is clear regarding the benefits of language and literacy accessibility in healthcare, the ambiguity in how federal policies are conceptualized and defined often absolves healthcare systems from being held accountable.

## The Problematic Conceptualization of "LEP" and Its Implications on Healthcare Policy and Practice

The term LEP has long posed challenges in healthcare policies and the healthcare industry due to three key assumptions: its ethnocentric perspective, its deficit orientation, and its ambiguity. The first major assumption focuses on the ethnocentric view of "primary language," which suggests that individuals learn languages sequentially—first acquiring one language before moving on to another. This idea, known as Successive Language Acquisition, is rooted in a Western understanding of language learning. This is in contrast to Simultaneous Language Acquisition, which is the most prominent form of language acquisition worldwide. This form of language acquisition occurs when an individual, often a child, learns two languages at the same time, challenging the Westernized notion of bilingualism.

The second major assumption underpinning the conceptualization of LEP is its ambiguity in the notion of "Limited Ability," which is often complex, multifaceted, and fluid. Individuals with LEP are frequently conceptualized as having intrinsically linked abilities in speaking, reading, writing, and understanding English; however, proficiency in these areas can vary considerably from one context to another. Furthermore, speaking, reading, writing, or understanding English are not inextricably linked skills, with some skills being more proficient than others. The third major assumption underpinning the concept of LEP is its deficit orientation. The notion of "Limited Proficiency" in itself presupposes a deficit that must be remedied, addressed, or assisted. The identification of LEP individuals as in need of "language assistance" easily absolves healthcare systems from shedding light on their own deficits (Ortega et al., 2022).

The above problematic assumptions of LEP have contributed to the ambiguity in the interpretation of healthcare policies by hospital systems, often absolving healthcare systems from accountability. Addressing healthcare inequities necessitates a shift away from focusing on the term "LEP status," which emphasizes patients' deficits, to one that illuminates the accountability of healthcare systems in meeting the needs of their diversifying multilingual populations, such as "Limited Linguistic and Cultural Competence."

"Limited Ability" is often used to describe patients' deficits but is seldom applied to doctors, nurses, and/or clinicians. Although many hospitals report that they regularly provide language assistance to those who prefer to communicate in languages besides English, very few hospitals genuinely assess the language proficiency of their healthcare staff (Diamond et al., 2019; Ortega et al., 2022). Even when language proficiency is assessed, it is often done superficially with a simple binary question, disincentivizing the value of physicians' language and literacy skills (e.g., "Do you speak another language? Yes/No") (Ortega, 2018). Not surprisingly, many clinicians report using limited language skills to "get by" during encounters with linguistic minority patients (Andres et al., 2013; Ortega et al., 2022). Even more concerning is that such language-discordant health encounters are known to lead to negative patient outcomes, higher healthcare costs, decreased patient satisfaction, and increased rates of medical errors (Diamond et al., 2019; Schulson & Anderson, 2022)—all of which can be mitigated by providing language-concordant (Diamond et al., 2019) or interpreter-mediated care (Schulson & Anderson, 2022). Despite the critical role of language-concordant healthcare encounters in fostering optimal healthcare outcomes and cost efficiency, ad hoc interpreters (family members, untrained medical staff, etc.) remain in widespread use in the medical field. Data analyzed from the 2020 CLAS Physician Survey found that only 30% of physicians reported regular use of professional interpreters (Schulson & Anderson, 2022). It is clear that there is a tremendous amount of work that needs to be done to help combat the stark language-related healthcare inequities prevalent within the United States.

## Theoretical and Political Recommendations

When it comes to improving language-appropriate healthcare accessibility, equity, and outcomes, the first and most crucial recommendation is to systematically move away from terms such as "LEP" in favor of more strength-based ones, such as the term "Non-English Language Preference (NELP)" coined by Ortega et al. (2022). Such reframing should be not only strength-based but also patient-centered and accurately reflect the diversity and fluidity of the languages spoken within the United States. Shifting the focus away from deficit-oriented terms will help not only in embracing a more strength-based perspective but also in illuminating the accountability of healthcare agencies and systems for accommodating the linguistic preferences of their target populations.

The words and terms we use when describing populations matter tremendously in shaping how we as a society perceive them and the quality of care they receive. It is crucial for federal guidelines and policies to be explicitly reframed by discarding the term "LEP" and replacing it with one that is more strength-based in nature and that better reflects the increasingly diverse populations within the United States. One wonderful example would be the utilization of the term "Non-English Language Preference (NELP)" proposed by Ortega and colleagues, which instills a sense of patient agency, empowerment, and choice in its conceptualization.

These federal guidelines and policy changes must be made alongside the illumination of detailed narratives describing the rationale behind such reframing, with clearly established, objective, and operationally defined criteria in place to hold hospitals and healthcare systems accountable and prevent any ambiguity in the interpretation of such mandates.

## Conclusions

Improving the quality of communication and information exchange in healthcare systems through various pathways is crucial for enhancing the optimal health of NELP patients. Despite federal mandates on language equity and accessibility within healthcare, many hospital systems still lag behind in providing such assurances, particularly in web/digital media domains and platforms. As Americans across all socioeconomic and linguistic proficiency levels increasingly rely on the internet for information regarding health conditions, resources, and services (Graves et al., 2020; Rodriguez & Singh, 2018), these lapses by hospital systems are gravely concerning. Expanding the accessibility of hospital websites through translation resources is essential for reducing healthcare barriers, improving health outcomes, and addressing disparities in our communities. Although federal regulations are in place and there is evidence clearly supporting the benefits of enforcing language-related healthcare accessibility, the ambiguity of how federal policies conceptualize and define the term LEP often absolves healthcare systems from being held accountable. Addressing healthcare inequities necessitates a systemic shift away from focusing on terms such as "LEP status" to ones that illuminate the accountability of healthcare systems in meeting the needs of their diversifying multilingual populations. These efforts must be multifaceted and targeted at all systemic levels of our healthcare industry to holistically help shift this narrative.

## Questions for Reflection

1 How does the shift from the term "LEP," focused on patient status, to "Limited Linguistic Accessibility" or "Limited Linguistic and Cultural Competence," related to hospital systems, alter the framing of healthcare disparities? What implications might this have for the accountability of healthcare systems?

*Reflect on how changing terminology might influence perceptions and responsibilities within healthcare systems and whether this shift can lead to more effective policy and practice changes.*

2 In what ways can hospital websites be optimized to better serve non-English Language Proficient (NELP) populations, and what are the potential barriers to achieving this optimization?

*Consider the practical steps hospitals can take to improve website accessibility and identify any systemic or resource-related obstacles they might face.*

3 How can healthcare systems address the underlying causes of language and cultural barriers in patient care, beyond just translating written materials?

*Explore strategies for improving healthcare delivery for NELP patients that go beyond language translation, such as cultural competency training and more inclusive communication practices.*

4 What are the potential consequences of continuing to use deficit-oriented terms like "LEP" in healthcare policy and practice, and how might these consequences affect patient outcomes and system accountability?

*Reflect on how terminology can shape policies and practices and how using deficit-oriented language might perpetuate existing inequities and hinder effective solutions.*

5 How can federal guidelines and policies be restructured to ensure clearer and more actionable definitions of terms related to language accessibility, and what role should stakeholders play in this process?

*Consider the role of different stakeholders—such as policymakers, healthcare providers, and community organizations—in refining and enforcing guidelines to improve language accessibility and accountability.*

## References

Affordable Care Act, 42 U.S.C. § 18116. (2010). https://www.congress.gov/bill/111th-congress/house-bill/3590/text

Andres, E., Wynia, M., Regenstein, M., & Maul, L. (2013). Should I call an interpreter?—How do physicians with second language skills decide?. *Journal of Health Care for the Poor and Underserved, 24*(2), 525–539. https://doi.org/10.1353/hpu.2013.0060

Berdahl, T. A., & Kirby, J. B. (2019). Patient-provider communication disparities by limited English proficiency (LEP): Trends from the US Medical Expenditure Panel Survey, 2006–2015. *Journal of General Internal Medicine, 34*(8), 1435–1440. https://doi.org/1434-1440.10.1007/s11606-018-4757-3

Coren, J. S., Filipetto, F. A., & Weiss, L. B. (2009). Eliminating barriers for patients with limited English proficiency. *Journal of Osteopathic Medicine, 109*(12), 634–640. https://doi.org/10.7556/jaoa.2009.109.12.634

Diamond, L., Izquierdo, K., Canfield, D., Matsoukas, K., & Gany, F. (2019). A systematic review of the impact of patient–physician non-English language concordance on quality of care and outcomes. *Journal of General Internal Medicine, 34,* 1591–1606. https://doi.org/10.1007/s11606-019-04847-5

Fischer, A., Conigliaro, J., Allicock, S., & Kim, E. J. (2021). Examination of social determinants of health among patients with limited English proficiency. *BMC Research Notes, 14,* 1–6. https://doi.org/10.1186/s13104-021-05720-7

Graves, J. M., Moore, M., Gonzalez, C., Ramos, J., Nguyen, L., & Vavilala, M. S. (2020). Too little information: Accessibility of information about language services on hospital websites. *Journal of Immigrant and Minority Health, 22*(3), 433–438. https://doi.org/10.1007/s10903-020-00978-8

Honeycutt, C. C., Bueno, K. M., Tran, T., Gao, M., Balu, S., & Sendak, M. (2021). Assessment of Spanish translation of websites at top-ranked US hospitals. *JAMA Network Open, 4*(2), e2037196. https://doi.org/e2037196-e2037196.

Jang, Y., & Kim, M. T. (2019). Limited English proficiency and health service use in Asian Americans. *Journal of Immigrant and Minority Health, 21,* 264–270. https://doi.org/10.1007/s10903-018-0763-0

Kilbourne, A. M. (2005). Care without coverage: Too little, too late. *Journal of the National Medical Association, 97*(11), 1578. https://doi.org/10.17226/10367

Kim, W., Kim, I., Baltimore, K., Imtiaz, A. S., Bhattacharya, B. S., & Lin, L. (2020). Simple contents and good readability: Improving health literacy for LEP populations. *International Journal of Medical Informatics, 141,* 104–230. https://doi.org/10.1016/j.ijmedinf.2020.104230

Ortega, P. (2018). Spanish language concordance in US medical care: A multifaceted challenge and call to action. *Academic Medicine, 93*(9), 1276–1280. https://doi.org/10.1097/ACM.0000000000002307

Ortega, P., Shin, T. M., & Martínez, G. A. (2022). Rethinking the term "limited English proficiency" to improve language-appropriate healthcare for all. *Journal of Immigrant and Minority Health, 24*(3), 799–805. https://doi.org/10.1007/s10903-021-01257-w

Patient Protection and Affordable Care Act, 42 U.S.C. § 18116. (2010).

Ramirez, N., Shi, K., Yabroff, K. R., Han, X., Fedewa, S. A., & Nogueira, L. M. (2023). Access to care among adults with limited English proficiency. *Journal of General Internal Medicine*, *38*(3), 592–599. https://doi.org/10.1007/s11606-022-07690-3

Rodriguez, J. A., & Singh, K. (2018). The Spanish availability and readability of diabetes apps. *Journal of Diabetes Science and Technology*, *12*(3), 719–724. https://doi.org/10.1177/19322968177496

Schulson, L. B., & Anderson, T. S. (2022). National estimates of professional interpreter use in the ambulatory setting. *Journal of General Internal Medicine*, *37*, 472–474. https://doi.org/10.1007/s11606-020-06336-6

Title IV of the Civil Rights Act of 1964, 42 U.S.C. § 2000d. (1964).

U.S. Census Bureau. (2023). Press kit: 2018–2022 American community survey 5-year estimates. https://www.census.gov/newsroom/press-kits/2023/acs-5-year.html

U.S. Department of Health and Human Services. (2020). *Nondiscrimination in health and health education programs or activities; delegation of authority* (42 U.S.C. § 18116). 85 Fed. Reg. 37160–37248. https://www.govinfo.gov/content/pkg/FR-2020-06-19/pdf/2020-11758.pdf

U.S. Department of Justice. (n.d.). *Commonly asked questions and answers regarding Limited English Proficient (LEP) individuals.* https://www.lep.gov/node/3456

# 14 Reframing Adolescent Development through the Lens of Cascading Collective Trauma

*Daya Patton*

## Understanding Cascading Collective Trauma

Cascading collective trauma describes a phenomenon where traumatic events occur consecutively or overlap (Silver et al., 2021). These events can include natural disasters, acts of terrorism, social injustice, mass shootings, civil unrest, community violence, refugee displacement, and global pandemics. Such traumas affect large population segments either directly or indirectly through media exposure. The chronic nature and uncertain outcomes of cascading collective traumas create worry and anxiety. Each new traumatic event exacerbates the impact of previous ones, potentially overwhelming adolescents' coping capacities. Rather than leading to diminished psychological and emotional responses, this pattern may trigger increasingly intense emotional reactions with each successive exposure (Silver et al., 2021).

Cascading collective trauma can spread rapidly via social networks, social media, or other institutional structures, adversely affecting adolescents and communities who did not directly experience the traumatic event. The interconnectedness of social systems and real-time broadcasting across multiple media platforms amplify the emotional and psychological impact of these events. The effects of a traumatic event can ripple outward, influencing many aspects of people's social lives and potentially leading to further traumatic events (Alexander et al., 2004). Addressing the effects of cascading collective trauma requires a comprehensive approach that considers the interconnectedness of our social systems and the complex ways trauma impacts communities. Exposure to trauma affects both individuals and society pervasively, constituting a public health crisis (Magruder et al., 2017).

## Historical Context and Theoretical Foundations

The concept of "cascading collective trauma" evolves from theories in trauma studies, sociology, and psychology. It builds on ideas of community and collective trauma, rooted in the broader framework of cultural trauma (Alexander et al., 2004). Cultural trauma occurs when a community experiences a traumatic event that profoundly impacts its collective consciousness. This experience leaves a lasting mark on the group's collective memory, significantly shaping its future identity. Understanding collective identity and cultural trauma is crucial for comprehending how trauma and its potential cascading effects impact communities and society.

Sztompka (2000) argues that cultural trauma represents a crucial aspect of social change, causing dramatic disruption to cultural patterns and collective identity. Traumatic events can destabilize community structures and social norms, triggering further traumatic experiences

DOI: 10.4324/9781003531258-17

as communities adapt to new realities. Significant social disruptions lead to cultural trauma by disturbing established norms and values, resulting in an identity crisis. Groups struggle to adapt to new realities while longing for their previous sense of self and community. This adaptation process elicits intense emotional responses, including fear, grief, and anger, influencing individual and collective behavior. Collective trauma involves a complex relationship between initial trauma and successive traumatic experiences. Cultural trauma constitutes an ongoing intergenerational process, requiring continuous renegotiation and reinterpretation to manage social change and encourage societal resilience.

Traumatic events create vulnerabilities to further trauma. For instance, communities affected by natural disasters may experience additional traumas such as displacement, social fragmentation, and economic hardship (Erikson, 1994). The social construction of meaning from collective trauma influences the likelihood of cascading collective trauma (Hirschberger, 2018). If a group perceives an event as an existential threat, it intensifies feelings of insecurity, anxiety, and vulnerability, leading to additional traumatic experiences. Historical traumas like colonization and genocide have long-lasting effects that cascade through generations, impacting the descendants of those who initially experienced the trauma firsthand (Kirmayer et al., 2014). Severely traumatic events like the Holocaust and the genocides in Rwanda and Iraq have been linked to long-term genocide memories and post-traumatic stress among impacted individuals (Ahmed, 2024; Blumenthal et al., 2024). Additionally, genocide is linked to cross-generational trauma, negatively impacting the mental health of both survivors and younger generations impacted by the cultural and familial aftermath (Ahmed, 2024). Studies have shown that the colonization of Indigenous populations has contributed to intergenerational trauma, negatively impacting Indigenous youth's mental and emotional health (Smallwood et al., 2021). Colonization across Canada, Australia, New Zealand, and the United States disrupted access to education, proper healthcare, and cultural continuity among indigenous populations, contributing to negative intergenerational impact (Smallwood et al., 2021).

## Adolescent Development and Cascading Collective Trauma

Cascading collective trauma profoundly affects adolescent development, impacting emotional, psychological, social, and academic growth. The interconnected nature of trauma exacerbates its impact on adolescent populations, resulting in long-term developmental challenges. Adolescents exposed to cascading collective traumas often exhibit increased levels of worry, anxiety, depression, and post-traumatic stress disorder symptoms (Nader, 2008). Ongoing stress, anxiety, and fear associated with trauma disrupt adolescent emotional regulation, causing difficulties in managing emotions and creating heightened susceptibility to mental health challenges.

Cascading collective trauma can impair adolescent cognitive functions, including attention, memory, and executive functioning. Affected adolescents may struggle with focus, problem-solving, and academic performance, hindering their academic progress and intellectual development (Beers & De Bellis, 2002). Furthermore, cascading collective trauma adversely impacts social development by affecting peer relationships and social interactions. Traumatized adolescents may experience difficulties trusting others, face challenges in forming and maintaining friendships, and exhibit social isolation or withdrawal (La Greca et al., 1996).

Adolescents at a critical stage of identity formation may experience disruptions in this process due to trauma. Exposure to cascading collective trauma can lead to behavioral issues, with adolescents responding through aggression, substance abuse, and risk-taking behaviors as unhealthy coping mechanisms. These behaviors exacerbate developmental challenges and lead to long-term adverse outcomes (Kilpatrick et al., 2000). The stress and instability caused by cascading collective trauma induce confusion, negative self-perceptions, and difficulties in developing a coherent and positive sense of identity among adolescent populations. Additionally, cascading collective trauma significantly impacts family dynamics, increasing family stress and parental trauma and causing changes in family roles that create an unstable home environment. This disruption in family dynamics challenges adolescents' coping mechanisms and impedes healthy development (Walsh, 2007).

## COVID-19 Pandemic and Cascading Collective Trauma

The COVID-19 pandemic has exposed the cascading trauma facing adolescents in society, revealing how compounding stressors significantly impact their mental and physical health (Robinson et al., 2021; Silver et al., 2021). This pandemic created unprecedented social isolation and cultural trauma, affecting all population segments and exacerbating existing disparities (Sztompka, 2000). For adolescents, the sudden disruption of school routines and social structures interrupted crucial developmental experiences (Erikson, 1994). The pandemic further amplified digital inequalities, widening the gap between the educational experiences of urban and affluent adolescents and those from lower socioeconomic backgrounds or remote areas (Robinson et al., 2021). Marginalized adolescent populations affected by disparities in access to technology include racial and ethnic minorities, those from low-income families or who live in rural areas, adolescents with disabilities, and LGBTQ+ adolescents (Anderson & Perrin, 2018). These disparities in technology access compounded social and educational isolation, especially for marginalized adolescent populations (Hirschberger, 2018).

The COVID-19 pandemic significantly escalated stress among American adolescents already experiencing other societal crises (Silver et al., 2021). These crises, characterized by their chronic nature, ambiguous endpoints, and intensified media coverage, amplified their psychological impact on adolescents (Sztompka, 2000). The murders of unarmed Black Americans, including Ahmaud Arbery, Breonna Taylor, and George Floyd, contributed to racialized trauma among many adolescent populations and their communities (Hirschberger, 2018). The United States also faced extreme weather events such as tornadoes, hurricanes, wildfires, and record-breaking heatwaves, further compounding stress levels (Robinson et al., 2021). Economic instability, marked by looming financial crises, inflation, and pandemic-related job losses, added to the collective trauma exposure for adolescents. While any single crisis could potentially cause lasting traumatic impacts, the concurrent nature of these events contributed to compounding exposure to cascading collective trauma (Silver et al., 2021).

Adolescents are particularly susceptible to cascading collective trauma due to several developmental factors. The ongoing development of the prefrontal cortex, responsible for executive functioning and decision-making, renders adolescents vulnerable to impaired emotional regulation and risk assessment when exposed to trauma (Steinberg, 2005). Furthermore, traumatic events can significantly influence identity formation, potentially leading to long-lasting negative effects on an adolescent's worldview and self-concept (Erikson, 1968).

Heightened emotional reactivity and limited coping skills characteristic of adolescence exacerbate vulnerability to trauma's emotional impacts (Compas et al., 2001; Casey et al.,

2008). Collective cascading trauma can interfere with crucial developmental processes, disrupting education and social skills development (Masten & Narayan, 2012). Exposure to trauma during this period can impair the development of healthy social relationships, causing difficulties with attachment and interpersonal skills (Cook et al., 2005).

Moreover, trauma exposure increases the risk of mental health disorders and substance use problems in adolescents (McLaughlin et al., 2010). Neurobiological changes resulting from trauma can lead to alterations in stress response systems, affecting long-term stress regulation (De Bellis & Zisk, 2014).

## School Shootings and Cascading Collective Trauma

Mass school shootings represent a severe form of violence with profound and lasting effects on adolescents, resulting in widespread collective trauma. These events impact direct victims and reverberate through communities, affecting students, families, educators, and society at large. Survivors and witnesses of mass school shootings experience immediate psychological distress, including acute stress disorder, anxiety, depression, and post-traumatic stress disorder (PTSD). This trauma can persist, leading to long-term mental health challenges (Nader, 2008).

Such traumatic events disrupt the fundamental sense of safety and security that schools provide, leading to heightened vigilance, fear, and anxiety about attending school, extending beyond the directly affected community (Newman et al., 2004). School shooting trauma adversely affects students' academic performance and social relationships. It can disrupt cognitive functions, resulting in difficulties with concentration, memory, and learning. Additionally, social relationships may deteriorate as students struggle with trust and feelings of safety in social settings (Cornell & Mayer, 2010).

Witnessing or hearing about mass school shootings can re-traumatize individuals with prior traumatic experiences. Extensive media coverage can lead to secondary trauma among adolescents not directly involved but exposed to the event through news reports and social media (Pfefferbaum et al., 2014). Mass school shootings can generate a collective sense of grief and loss within the affected community, potentially extending to other communities as cultural trauma. This collective trauma can impact community cohesion, trust in institutions, and cultural narratives surrounding safety and violence (Erikson, 1994). The trauma experienced by adolescents during school shootings can have intergenerational effects, as parents, educators, and community members may also experience trauma, affecting their interactions with and support for adolescents, thus perpetuating a cycle of trauma across generations (Yehuda & Bierer, 2009).

## Direct and Media-Based Exposure and Cascading Collective Trauma

The proliferation of 24-hour news cycles, smartphones, and social media platforms provides unprecedented access to real-time coverage of traumatic events. Many students now have direct access to social media and personal devices, leading to frequent indirect exposure to such events through media. Research links repeated media-based exposure to traumatic events with both mental and physical health issues (Silver et al., 2021), suggesting that ongoing media exposure to collective trauma can perpetuate a cycle of exposure and PTSD symptoms over time.

Both direct and media-based exposure to traumatic events, such as mass school shootings, significantly contributes to cascading collective trauma among adolescents. These exposures exacerbate psychological distress, foster pervasive fear and insecurity, and amplify trauma's impact across communities, thereby perpetuating a cycle of collective trauma. Adolescents directly exposed to traumatic events, such as being present during a school shooting, face a high risk of developing acute stress reactions and long-term mental health issues. Such direct exposure can trigger a cascade of trauma effects within the immediate community as individuals process their experiences and interact with others who have shared similar traumas (Nader, 2008).

Media coverage of traumatic events profoundly affects adolescents, even if they are not directly involved. Continuous exposure to graphic images, distressing narratives, and repeated broadcasts can result in secondary trauma, causing individuals to experience symptoms akin to those directly involved in the event (Pfefferbaum et al., 2014). Both direct and media-based exposure amplify fear and anxiety among adolescents. This heightened state of fear can spread through social networks, influencing peers and contributing to a pervasive sense of insecurity (Comer & Kendall, 2007).

Trauma exposure disrupts normal developmental processes in adolescents, including emotional regulation, social relationships, and academic performance. These disruptions can lead to cascading effects, as affected adolescents may struggle to manage additional stressors, resulting in further trauma (Layne et al., 2011). Secondary trauma, which occurs when individuals experience trauma symptoms through exposure to others' trauma, can arise from media coverage, leading to vicarious trauma where viewers identify with victims and experience trauma responses themselves (Torres & Bergner, 2010). Extensive exposure to graphic news coverage of traumatic events or social media content related to traumatic events can produce secondary trauma among adolescent populations (Holman et al., 2014). For example, repeated exposure to graphic news content about school shootings and exposure to social media cyberbullying can contribute to the development of secondary trauma among adolescent populations. Trauma can also be transmitted socially and culturally as stories, symbols, and meanings related to the traumatic event spread within and across communities. Media plays a crucial role in this transmission, often perpetuating narratives that reinforce collective trauma (Alexander et al., 2004).

## The Role of School-Based Human Services Professionals in Addressing Cascading Collective Trauma

School-based human services professionals offer crucial support to students within the educational setting, enhancing their academic, emotional, social, and psychological well-being. School counselors and social workers occupy a unique position to support students who have experienced cascading collective trauma. They play a key role in fostering supportive school environments that contribute to students' success and well-being. Their specialized training equips them to address the complex nature of cascading collective trauma and enables them to understand and mitigate its impacts on students' lives and learning through collaboration within the school system.

School counselors and social workers receive ongoing training in trauma-informed care, crisis intervention, counseling techniques, and emotional and psychological support (American School Counselor Association, 2019). They develop and implement comprehensive counseling programs designed to address the needs of all students, including those affected by cascading collective trauma. School social workers specifically focus on understanding family dynamics, leveraging community resources, and addressing systemic issues that adversely impact students. They also take specialized coursework in trauma, crisis intervention, and child welfare (School Social Work Association of America, 2020).

Additional support for students experiencing cascading collective trauma comes from school psychologists, nurses, behavioral specialists, and special education educators. School psychologists receive training in psychological assessment, mental health interventions, and behavior management, with a specific focus on the effects of trauma on student learning and behavior (National Association of School Psychologists, 2020). School nurses, trained in physical and mental health management, can identify physical and psychological symptoms of trauma (National Association of School Nurses, 2016). Behavioral support specialists provide intervention strategies for students with behavioral issues ("Bacb—about behavior analysis," 2023). Special education educators understand how trauma affects student behavior and learning and develop positive behavioral supports and interventions (Council for Exceptional Children, 2018).

## Identifying Adolescents at Risk of Cascading Collective Trauma

School-based human services professionals must prepare to provide interventions and support for adolescents experiencing cascading collective trauma. This process begins with identifying at-risk adolescents or those who have already experienced such trauma. Professionals can utilize standardized screening and assessment tools to identify signs of trauma and related mental health issues. Given the complex, layered effects of cascading collective trauma on entire communities, societies, or nations, often across generations, screening and assessment tools must thoroughly consider individual and group experiences. Some trauma screening and assessment tools for individuals include the Primary Care PTSD Screen for DSM-5 (PC-PTSD-5) and the Trauma Screening Questionnaire (TSQ) (Brewin et al., 2002; Prins et al., 2016). Trauma screening and assessment tools for groups include the Trauma and Life Events Checklist (TALE) and the Harvard Trauma Questionnaire (HTQ) (Carr et al., 2018; Mollica et al., 1992).

The National Child Traumatic Stress Network (2018b) recommends that trauma screening evaluate two critical elements: (1) exposure to potentially traumatic events/experiences, including traumatic loss, and (2) traumatic stress symptoms/reactions. The screening and assessment process should involve both children and their families. Professionals can employ child-completed tools (Self-Report), caregiver-completed tools, or provider-completed screening tools. Examples include the Child PTSD Symptom Scale, Trauma Symptom Screening for Children and Adolescents, Pediatric Emotional Distress Scale, and the Child Trauma Screen.

Initial trauma screening results determine the necessity for formal assessment. Qualified school-based human services professionals may complete the evaluation or refer the child to a qualified professional for assessment. Formal assessments for cascading collective trauma include the UCLA PTSD Reaction Index for DSM-5 (Child Version), Trauma Assessment for Adults and Children (TAA/TAAC), Traumatic Events Screening Inventory-Parent Report Revised (TESI-PRR), and the Behavior Assessment System for Children (BASC-3). The National Child Traumatic Stress Network webpage offers additional screenings and measures for specific populations and trauma exposures.

## Supporting Students Experiencing Cascading Collective Trauma

School counselors and social workers play a vital role in supporting students experiencing cascading collective trauma. They help mitigate its impact on student academic performance, mental health, social relationships, and physical well-being. This support requires a comprehensive, multifaceted approach. These professionals establish clear policies promoting trauma-informed care and create calm, safe physical environments for de-escalation. They foster inclusive, respectful school cultures that validate students' experiences. Regular staff development on trauma impacts and practices, along with ongoing support for implementing trauma-informed practices, is crucial. They also offer training and educational workshops for parents on recognizing, understanding, and supporting children affected by trauma.

School counselors and social workers regularly observe student behavior, social interactions, and academic performance to detect changes indicating trauma exposure. They review dispensary records, attendance logs, and grades to identify patterns suggesting trauma impact. Noticeable drops in grades, increased absenteeism, and failure to complete assignments following traumatic events may indicate a need for additional support. These professionals administer surveys to students, teachers, and parents to gather information about overall student well-being following traumatic events. They collaborate with teachers and parents to collect data on changes in student behavior post-trauma.

Engaging families and caregivers in the support process following student exposure to collective trauma is key to providing continuous care and a consistently supportive environment at school and home (Alvord & Grados, 2005). School counselors and social workers educate parents about trauma effects and offer parenting support. They facilitate referrals and access to mental health services for students needing more intensive support and connect parents with community mental health providers (Atkins et al., 2010). Partnerships with community agencies and organizations help coordinate resources for students and families. These partnerships provide support services such as healthcare, food security, housing, and socioeconomic assistance to alleviate additional stressors associated with cascading collective trauma (Weist et al., 2014).

Ongoing professional development keeps school-based human services professionals up-to-date on the latest research and best practices in trauma-informed care. This ensures they remain prepared and equipped to identify and respond to students' trauma-related needs (Paccione-Dyszlewski, 2016). Creating a safe, supportive, and inclusive school environment encourages students to seek help. Implementing school-based crisis intervention teams enables quick responses to traumatic events and immediate triage and support. This sense of safety and security within schools reduces anxiety and promotes normalcy (Hobfoll et al., 2007). Social-emotional learning programs help students develop skills to cope with traumatic events, manage emotions, establish positive relationships, and make responsible decisions. These programs benefit students who have experienced trauma, providing tools for stress coping and resilience-building (Durlak et al., 2011).

While limited empirical research exists on cascading the effects of collective traumatic experiences on adolescents' mental and physical health, substantial evidence demonstrates the impact of cumulative lifetime adversity. Studies show that lifetime adversity exposure is associated with difficulties coping with additional stressors, higher distress rates, overall functional impairment, and lower life satisfaction (McLaughlin et al., 2012; Seery et al., 2010). Contrary to the idea that adolescents might adjust to cascading collective trauma, research suggests these experiences may produce stronger emotional responses with each new exposure (Garfin et al., 2020).

Teaching coping skills effectively prepares adolescents to manage repeated or cascading collective traumas (Seery et al., 2010). Personal and environmental factors influence adolescents' physical and mental responses to cascading collective trauma (Norris et al., 2002). Adverse childhood experiences, pre-existing mental health conditions, lower family socioeconomic status, and lack of social support can increase vulnerability to negative outcomes from cascading collective traumatic events (Forbes & Krueger, 2019). Conversely, strong family and social support, access to personal resources, and higher socioeconomic status can promote resilience, enabling adolescents to thrive despite exposure to such events (Gelkopf et al., 2012).

### Evidence-Based Direct Interventions for Cascading Collective Trauma

School-based human services professionals can utilize evidence-based strategies to directly intervene with students affected by cascading collective trauma. Given the complexity of cascading collective trauma, employing evidence-based curricula and interventions is essential to achieving successful outcomes. Evidence-based interventions are strategies, programs, or practices evaluated through scientific research and proven effective. These interventions are designed to achieve specific outcomes based on empirical evidence, systematic reviews, and randomized controlled trials. Some evidence-based interventions or curricula may incur costs for materials, training, or monitoring.

Trauma-focused cognitive-behavioral therapy (TF-CBT) effectively addresses cascading collective trauma (Cohen, 2018). TF-CBT integrates cognitive-behavioral and humanistic theories and includes interventions such as psychoeducation about trauma, coping skills building, stress management techniques, and cognitive processing of traumatic experiences. School-based human services professionals can implement TF-CBT in individual or group settings for students affected by cascading collective trauma.

Cognitive Behavioral Interventions for Schools (CBITS) is another evidence-based curriculum supporting students who have experienced cascading collective trauma. CBITS is suitable for students in grades 5 through 12 who have experienced or witnessed traumatic events, including community violence, school violence, natural disasters, physical abuse, and domestic violence (National Child Traumatic Stress Network, 2018a).

Multimodality trauma treatment, also known as trauma-focused coping, is a cognitive-behavioral approach for children exposed to single-incident trauma and experiencing residual symptoms such as depression, anxiety, anger, or external locus of control. This skills-oriented curriculum is appropriate for individuals aged 6–18 and can be used in both individual and group settings (National Child Traumatic Stress Network, 2018a).

Psychological first aid (PFA) is an evidence-informed intervention suitable for immediate application after traumatic events. PFA has been used worldwide following natural disasters, acts of terrorism, and other traumatic events. The intervention comprises eight helping actions: contact and engagement, safety and comfort, stabilization, information gathering, practical assistance, connection with social supports, information on coping support, and linkage with collaborative services. PFA applies to any age group, in individual settings, and for emergency triage (Brymer et al., 2006).

Integrative Treatment of Complex Trauma for Children (ITCT-C) is a multimodal, evidence-based, assessment-driven treatment model. It involves interviews and standardized trauma-specific measures administered at two to three-month intervals to identify symptoms and issues requiring clinical attention. ITCT-C is culturally adapted, developmentally appropriate, and suitable for use in clinics, schools, hospitals, and in-patient and residential treatment settings. It is designed for children aged 5–12, particularly those who are economically disadvantaged and culturally diverse (National Child Traumatic Stress Network, 2018a).

Bounce Back is a cognitive-behavioral, group skills-based intervention for elementary school students exposed to traumatic or stressful events (Langley et al., 2015). The curriculum helps children develop coping skills to recover from traumatic experiences. It is especially useful for children who have experienced community and school violence, natural disasters, traumatic separation through the death of a loved one, incarceration or deportation, or child welfare placement. The curriculum, deliverable in group or individual sessions, aids children aged 5–11 in problem-solving, conflict resolution, and building positive social support (National Child Traumatic Stress Network, 2018a).

### Addressing Cultural and Socioeconomic Factors

Research indicates that Black, Indigenous, and People of Color (BIPOC) communities in the United States disproportionately experience negative effects from cascading collective trauma (Curtice & Choo, 2020). This disparity arises from the compounding effects of historical collective trauma, systemic racism, and poverty (Bryant-Davis & Ocampo, 2005). Students from BIPOC populations may require additional support after traumatic events; thus, school-based human services professionals must provide culturally sensitive and competent care. Professionals should avoid making assumptions based on students' backgrounds and recognize that individual trauma experiences are unique. Potential interventions to mitigate these effects include increased mental health support, training in positive coping strategies and resilience-building activities, and life skills programs (Holmes et al., 2020).

Awareness of the unique traditions, social norms, and values of BIPOC students is crucial for school-based human services professionals. Strong community support, commitment, and emotional support act as protective factors against the impacts of cascading collective traumas (Gelkopf et al., 2012). Professionals should collaborate with community organizations trusted by students and their families for additional support. Given the disproportionate impact of cascading collective trauma on BIPOC communities, targeted outreach efforts are necessary to address their specific needs and vulnerabilities (Silver et al., 2021).

Professionals working with students from marginalized communities who have experienced cascading traumatic events should engage in targeted professional development to support these communities. Additionally, they should routinely practice reflective techniques to acknowledge and address any personal biases they may hold.

### Questions for Reflection

1 How might the increasing prevalence of real-time media exposure to traumatic events influence future approaches to supporting adolescents exposed to cascading collective trauma? What role should digital literacy play in these interventions?
2 What ethical considerations regarding privacy and stigmatization should school-based human services professionals keep in mind when identifying and supporting students who have been impacted by cascading collective trauma?
3 How might the implementation of schoolwide trauma-informed practices influence the overall school culture and climate beyond supporting individual students impacted by cascading collective trauma? What comprehensive strategies can be implemented to mitigate cascading collective trauma?
4 How can school-based human services professionals identify and address the complex impact of cascade and collective trauma on student cognitive, social, and emotional development?

# References

Ahmed, D. R. (2024). From Holocaust to Anfal: The impact of genocide and cross-generational trauma on the mental health of Kurds. *International Journal of Social Psychiatry, 70*(3), 621–625.

Alexander, J. C., Eyerman, R., Giesen, B., Smelser, N. J., & Sztompka, P. (2004). *Cultural trauma and collective identity.* University of California Press.

Alvord, M. K., & Grados, J. J. (2005). Enhancing resilience in children: A proactive approach. *Professional Psychology: Research and Practice, 36*(3), 238–245.

American School Counselor Association. (2019). The school counselor and student mental health. https://www.schoolcounselor.org/Standards-Positions/Position-Statements/ASCA-Position-Statements/The-School-Counselor-and-Student-Mental-Health

Anderson, M., & Perrin, A. (2018). *Nearly one-in-five teens can't always finish their homework because of the digital divide.* Pew Research Center, 26.

Atkins, M. S., Hoagwood, K. E., Kutash, K., & Seidman, E. (2010). Toward the integration of education and mental health in schools. *Administration and Policy in Mental Health and Mental Health Services Research, 37*(1–2), 40–47.

*Bacb—about behavior analysis.* (2023, June 22). Behavior Analyst Certification Board. https://www.bacb.com/about-behavior-analysis/

Beers, S. R., & De Bellis, M. D. (2002). Neuropsychological function in children with maltreatment-related posttraumatic stress disorder. *American Journal of Psychiatry, 159*(3), 483–486.

Blumenthal, A., Caparos, S., & Blanchette, I. (2024). Understanding the structure of autobiographical memories: A study of trauma memories from the 1994 Rwandan genocide. *Memory and Cognition, 52*(7), 1597–1608.

Brewin, C. R., Rose, S., Andrews, B., Green, J., Tata, P., McEvedy, C., Turner, S., & Foa, E. B. (2002). Brief screening instrument for post-traumatic stress disorder. *British Journal of Psychiatry, 181*(2), 158–162.

Bryant-Davis, T., & Ocampo, C. (2005). Racist incident-based trauma. *The Counseling Psychologist, 33*(4), 479–500.

Brymer, M. J., Jacobs, A., Layne, C. M., Pynoos, R. S., Ruzek, J. I., Steinberg, A. M., Vernberg, E. M., & Watson, P. J. (2006). *Psychological first aid: Field operations guide* (2nd ed.). National Child Traumatic Stress Network and National Center for PTSD.

Carr, S., Hardy, A., & Fornells-Ambrojo, M. (2018). The Trauma and Life Events (TALE) checklist: Development of a tool for improving routine screening in people with psychosis. *European Journal of Psychotraumatology, 9*(1), 1512265.

Casey, B. J., Jones, R. M., & Hare, T. A. (2008). The adolescent brain. *Annals of the New York Academy of Sciences, 1124*(1), 111–126.

Cohen, J. A., Deblinger, E., & Mannarino, A. P. (2018). Trauma-focused cognitive behavioral therapy for children and families. *Psychotherapy Research, 28*(1), 47–57.

Comer, J. S., & Kendall, P. C. (2007). Terrorism: The psychological impact on youth. *Clinical Psychology: Science and Practice, 14*(3), 179–212.

Compas, B. E., Connor-Smith, J. K., Saltzman, H., Thomsen, A. H., & Wadsworth, M. E. (2001). Coping with stress during childhood and adolescence: Problems, progress, and potential in theory and research. *Psychological Bulletin, 127*(1), 87.

Cook, A., Spinazzola, J., Ford, J., Lanktree, C., Blaustein, M., Cloitre, M., DeRosa, R., Hubbard, R., Kagan, R., Liautaud, J., Mallah, K., Olafson, E., & Van der Kolk, B. (2005). Complex trauma in children and adolescents. *Psychiatric Annals, 35*(5), 390–398.

Cornell, D. G., & Mayer, M. J. (2010). Why do school order and safety matter? *Educational Researcher, 39*(1), 7–15.

Council for Exceptional Children. (2018). *Special education professional standards.* https://exceptionalchildren.org/professional-preparation-standards

Curtice, K., & Choo, E. (2020). Indigenous populations: Left behind in the COVID-19 response. *The Lancet, 395*(10239), 1753.

De Bellis, M. D., & Zisk, A. (2014). The biological effects of childhood trauma. *Child and Adolescent Psychiatric Clinics, 23*(2), 185–222.

Durlak, J. A., Weissberg, R. P., Dymnicki, A. B., Taylor, R. D., & Schellinger, K. B. (2011). The impact of enhancing students' social and emotional learning: A meta-analysis of school-based universal interventions. *Child Development, 82*(1), 405–432.

Erikson, E. H. (1968). *Identity: Youth and crisis.* W. W. Norton & Company.

Erikson, K. (1994). A new species of trouble: The human experience of modern disasters. W.W. Norton & Company. Erikson explores the long-term psychological and social effects of disasters, offering insights into how trauma can cascade through communities.

Forbes, M. K., & Krueger, R. F. (2019). The great recession and mental health in the United States. *Clinical Psychological Science, 7*(5), 900–913.

Garfin, D. R., Silver, R. C., & Holman, E. A. (2020). The novel coronavirus (COVID-2019) outbreak: Amplification of public health consequences by media exposure. *Health Psychology, 39*(5), 355–357.

Gelkopf, M., Berger, R., Bleich, A., & Silver, R. C. (2012). Protective factors and predictors of vulnerability to chronic stress: A comparative study of 4 communities after 7 years of continuous rocket fire. *Social Science & Medicine, 74*(5), 757–766.

Hirschberger, G. (2018). Collective trauma and the social construction of meaning. *Frontiers in Psychology, 9*, 1441.

Hobfoll, S. E., Watson, P., Bell, C. C., Bryant, R. A., Brymer, M. J., Friedman, M. J., ... & Ursano, R. J. (2007). Five essential elements of immediate and mid-term mass trauma intervention: Empirical evidence. *Psychiatry: Interpersonal and Biological Processes, 70*(4), 283–315.

Holman, E. A., Garfin, D. R., & Silver, R. C. (2014). Media's role in broadcasting acute stress following the Boston Marathon bombings. *Proceedings of the National Academy of Sciences, 111*(1), 93–98.

Holmes, E. A., O'Connor, R. C., Perry, V. H., Tracey, I., Wessely, S., Arseneault, L., Ballard, C., Christensen, H., Cohen Silver, R., Everall, I., Ford, T., John, A., Kabir, T., King, K., Madan, I., Michie, S., Przybylski, A. K., Shafran, R., Sweeney, A., Worhtman, C,. Yardley, L., Cowan, K., Cope, C., Hoyopf, M., & Bullmore, E. (2020). Multidisciplinary research priorities for the COVID-19 pandemic: A call for action for mental health science. *The Lancet Psychiatry, 7*(6), 547–560.

Kilpatrick, D. G., Acierno, R., Saunders, B., Resnick, H. S., Best, C. L., & Schnurr, P. P. (2000). Risk factors for adolescent substance abuse and dependence: Data from a national sample. *Journal of Consulting and Clinical Psychology, 68*(1), 19–30.

Kirmayer, L. J., Gone, J. P., & Moses, J. (2014). Rethinking historical trauma. *Transcultural Psychiatry, 51*(3), 299–319.

La Greca, A. M., Silverman, W. K., Vernberg, E. M., & Prinstein, M. J. (1996). Symptoms of posttraumatic stress in children after Hurricane Andrew: A prospective study. *Journal of Consulting and Clinical Psychology, 64*(4), 712.

Langley, A. K., González, A., Sugar, C. A., Solis, D., & Jaycox, L. H. (2015). Bounce back: Effectiveness of an elementary school-based intervention for multicultural children exposed to traumatic events. *Journal of Consulting and Clinical Psychology. 83*(5), 853–865.

Layne, C. M., Ippen, C. G., Strand, V., Stuber, M., Abramson, D., Reyes, G., ... & Pynoos, R. S. (2011). The core curriculum on childhood trauma: A tool for training a trauma-informed workforce. *Psychological Trauma: Theory, Research, Practice, and Policy, 3*(3), 243–252.

Magruder, K. M., McLaughlin, K. A., & Elmore Borbon, D. L. (2017). Trauma is a public health issue. *European Journal of Psychotraumatology, 8*(1), 1375338.

Masten, A. S., & Narayan, A. J. (2012). Child development in the context of disaster, war, and terrorism: Pathways of risk and resilience. *Annual Review of Psychology, 63*(1), 227–257.

McLaughlin, K. A., Conron, K. J., Koenen, K. C., & Gilman, S. E. (2010). Childhood adversity, adult stressful life events, and risk of past-year psychiatric disorder: A test of the stress sensitization hypothesis in a population-based sample of adults. *Psychological Medicine, 40*(10), 1647–1658.

McLaughlin, K. A., Green, J. G., Gruber, M. J., Sampson, N. A., Zaslavsky, A. M., & Kessler, R. C. (2012). Childhood adversities and first onset of psychiatric disorders in a national sample of US adolescents. *Archives of General Psychiatry, 69*(11), 1151–1160.

Mollica, R. F., Caspi-Yavin, Y., Bollini, P., Truong, T., Tor, S., & Lavelle, J. (1992). The Harvard Trauma Questionnaire: Validating a cross-cultural instrument for measuring torture, trauma, and posttraumatic stress disorder in Indochinese refugees. *The Journal of Nervous and Mental Disease, 180*(2), 111–116.

Nader, K. O. (2008). *Understanding and assessing trauma in children and adolescents: Measures, methods, and youth in context*. Routledge.

National Association of School Nurses. (2016). Framework for 21st century school nursing practice. https://www.nasn.org/nasn/nasn-resources/professional-topics/framework

National Association of School Psychologists. (2020). *The provision of school psychological services: A comprehensive model*.

National Child Traumatic Stress Network. (2018a, August 14). *Interventions*. https://www.nctsn.org/treatments-and-practices/trauma-treatments/interventions

National Child Traumatic Stress Network. (2018b, March 27). Trauma screening. https://www.nctsn.org/treatments-and-practices/screening-and-assessments/trauma-screening

Newman, K. S., Fox, C., Harding, D. J., Mehta, J., & Roth, W. (2004). *Rampage: The social roots of school shootings*. Basic Books.

Norris, F. H., Friedman, M. J., Watson, P. J., Byrne, C. M., Diaz, E., & Kaniasty, K. (2002). 60,000 disaster victims speak: Part I. An empirical review of the empirical literature, 1981–2001. *Psychiatry: Interpersonal and Biological Processes, 65*(3), 207–239.

Paccione-Dyszlewski, M. R. (2016). Trauma-informed schools: A must. *The Brown University Child and Adolescent Behavior Letter, 32*(7), 8–8.

Pfefferbaum, B., Newman, E., & Nelson, S. D. (2014). Mental health interventions for children exposed to disasters and terrorism. *Journal of Child and Adolescent Psychopharmacology, 24*(1), 24–31.

Prins, A., Bovin, M. J., Smolenski, D. J., Marx, B. P., Kimerling, R., Jenkins-Guarnieri, M. A., Kaloupek, D. G., Schnurr, P. P., Kaiser, A. P., Leyva, Y. E., & Tiet, Q. Q. (2016). The Primary Care PTSD Screen for DSM-5 (PC-PTSD-5): Development and evaluation within a veteran primary care sample. *Journal of General Internal Medicine, 31*(10), 1206–1211.

Robinson, L., Schulz, J., Ball, C., Chiaraluce, C., Dodel, M., Francis, J., Huang, K.T., Johnston, E., Khilnai, A., Kleinmann, O., Kwon, K.H., McClain, N., Ng, Y.M.M., Pait, H., Ragnedda, M., Reisdorf, B.C., Ruiu, M., Silva, C., Trammel, J., Wiborg, Ø., & Williams, A. A. (2021). Cascading crises: Society in the age of COVID-19. *American Behavioral Scientist, 65*(12), 1608–1622.

School Social Work Association of America. (2020). *School social work services*. https://www.sswaa.org/school-social-work

Seery, M. D., Holman, E. A., & Silver, R. C. (2010). Whatever does not kill us: Cumulative lifetime adversity, vulnerability, and resilience. *Journal of Personality and Social Psychology, 99*(6), 1025–1041.

Silver, R. C., Holman, E. A., & Garfin, D. R. (2021). Coping with cascading collective traumas in the United States. *Nature Human Behaviour, 5*(1), 4–6.

Smallwood, R., Woods, C., Power, T., & Usher, K. (2021). Understanding the impact of historical trauma due to colonization on the health and well-being of indigenous young peoples: A systematic scoping review. *Journal of Transcultural Nursing, 32*(1), 59–68.

Steinberg, L. (2005). Cognitive and affective development in adolescence. *Trends in Cognitive Sciences, 9*(2), 69–74.

Sztompka, P. (2000). Cultural trauma: The other face of social change. *European Journal of Social Theory, 3*(4), 449–466.

Torres, A. C., & Bergner, R. M. (2010). Vicarious trauma in mental health professionals: Toward a deeper understanding. *Journal of Loss and Trauma, 15*(1), 78–96.

Walsh, F. (2007). Traumatic loss and major disasters: Strengthening family and community resilience. *Family Process, 46*(2), 207–227.

Weist, M. D., Lever, N. A., Bradshaw, C. P., & Owens, J. S. (2014). Further advancing the field of school mental health. *School Mental Health, 6*(2), 95–97.

Yehuda, R., & Bierer, L. M. (2009). The relevance of epigenetics to PTSD: Implications for the DSM-V. *Journal of Traumatic Stress, 22*(5), 427–434.

*Claude large language model was used for language improvement in this document.*

# 15  Treating Adults Living with Perinatally Acquired HIV

*Angela M. Wilbon*

## The Global and National Landscape of HIV

The human immunodeficiency virus (HIV) is a significant global public health challenge, affecting 38 million people worldwide as of 2020 (UNAIDS, 2020). This figure includes approximately 36.2 million adults and 1.8 million children under the age of 15. HIV is a virus that compromises the immune system, making those infected more vulnerable to other infections and diseases. The primary modes of HIV transmission include the exchange of bodily fluids such as blood, semen, pre-seminal fluid, rectal fluids, vaginal fluids, and breast milk. Despite advances in treatment and prevention, HIV continues to be a pervasive issue, particularly in certain demographics and regions. The widespread availability of antiretroviral therapy (ART) has significantly improved the quality of life and life expectancy of those living with HIV, turning what was once a fatal disease into a manageable chronic condition.

## HIV in the United States

In the United States, an estimated 1.2 million people were living with HIV at the end of 2018 (Centers for Disease, 2020). Of these, a significant proportion were adults and adolescents aged 13 years and older, accounting for 1,040,352 of the total number. The distribution of HIV cases within the U.S. population highlights significant disparities based on race, ethnicity, and age. In 2018, there were approximately 36,400 new HIV infections reported in the country.

## Demographic Disparities

The prevalence and incidence of HIV vary considerably across different racial and ethnic groups in the United States. African Americans are disproportionately affected, representing 42% of all new HIV diagnoses despite comprising only 13% of the U.S. population. This discrepancy underscores the significant racial and ethnic health disparities present in the country. In 2018, approximately 482,900 African Americans were living with HIV (CDC, 2020).

In contrast, white Americans, who make up 60% of the U.S. population, accounted for 29% (340,700) of the total number of people living with HIV. The Hispanic/Latinx community, comprising 19% of the U.S. population, represented 23% (274,100) of those living with HIV. Other racial and ethnic groups, including people who identify as multiracial, Asians, American Indians, Alaska Natives, Native Hawaiians, and Pacific Islanders, have lower prevalence rates but still face significant challenges related to HIV prevention, treatment, and care.

DOI: 10.4324/9781003531258-18

### Trends in HIV Diagnoses

The number of new HIV diagnoses provides a critical measure of the ongoing spread of the virus. In 2018, there were approximately 37,968 new HIV diagnoses in the United States (CDC, 2020). The distribution of these new diagnoses mirrors the patterns seen in the overall prevalence data. African Americans accounted for 42% (16,002) of new diagnoses, while the Hispanic/Latinx community made up 27% (10,300), and white Americans constituted 25% (9,000). Smaller percentages were seen in other racial and ethnic groups, reflecting both the size of these populations and the success of targeted prevention and treatment programs.

### Gender and HIV

Gender also plays a significant role in the epidemiology of HIV in the United States. Of the estimated 1.2 million people living with HIV, 245,154 were women (CDC, 2020). African American women are particularly affected, representing 58% of all women diagnosed with HIV in the United States, despite making up a smaller proportion of the population. Hispanic/Latinx women accounted for 20% of HIV diagnoses among women, while white women made up 16%. Women identifying as multiracial, Asian, Native Hawaiian/Other Pacific Islanders, and American Indian/Alaska Natives accounted for smaller percentages.

In 2018, women constituted 19% of the 37,968 new HIV diagnoses in the United States. The primary mode of transmission for women was heterosexual contact, accounting for 85% of new cases. Injection drug use was responsible for 15% of new diagnoses, with a negligible percentage attributed to other transmission routes. African American women bore the brunt of new diagnoses, representing 57% of the total, highlighting the intersection of race, gender, and socioeconomic factors in HIV transmission and prevention.

### Perinatal HIV Transmission

Perinatal HIV transmission, also known as vertical transmission, occurs when HIV is transmitted from a mother to her child during pregnancy, childbirth, or breastfeeding. The transmission modes from mother to child are (1) in utero or during pregnancy, (2) intrapartum or during delivery, or (3) postpartum or after birth through breastfeeding (Kamya, 2012). At the start of the disease in the United States, mothers were unwittingly transmitting HIV to their children due to their lack of knowledge regarding their own HIV status and modes of transmission to their infants. This mode of transmission accounts for a low percentage but a significant number of HIV cases. In 2020, there were 12,588 people in the United States living with HIV who had been perinatally infected, including children, youth, and adults. This includes approximately 1,447 children under the age of 13 diagnosed with perinatal HIV (CDC, 2020).

### Historical Data and Trends

An estimated 21,732 infants were born HIV-positive from 1978 to 2018 (Taylor et al., 2017). Approximately 16,000 infants were infected with HIV between 1978 and 1995 (Faucher, 2002; Krist & Crawford- Nesheim et al., 2017). The CDC reports that 70 infants were born HIV-positive in 1978, with an incidence rate of 2.1 per 100,000 live births (CDC, 2008). The estimated incidence of vertical HIV transmission peaked in 1992 with

43.1 infants per 100,000 live births, totaling 1,750 new perinatally HIV infections in that year alone (Nesheim et al., 2017). African Americans accounted for 63% of perinatal HIV infections from 2002 through 2013 (Taylor et al., 2017). These rates of infection were attributed to low rates of prenatal care, late or nonmaternal HIV diagnoses, lack of mothers and infants on Highly Active Antiretroviral Therapy (HAART) treatments and prophylaxis, and a non-existent universal HIV testing policy for expectant mothers.

### Interventions to Decline Transmission Rates

The rate of HIV transmission from mother to child has seen a steady decline in the last two decades. In 1994, governmental public health agencies, including the CDC, healthcare institutions, and providers, instituted a plethora of intervention programs to stop the transmission of HIV from mother to child (CDC, 2008). The HIV screening standard established in the United States for maternal health HIV testing includes two approaches. The first approach was an HIV screening opt-in service, where expectant mothers are provided HIV pretest counseling and the opportunity to consent to be tested. The other approach, opt-out, informs pregnant women that an HIV test is part of their prenatal tests. If women do not decline the specific HIV test, they are tested for HIV. Medical facilities utilizing the opt-out approach observed higher rates of HIV testing of expectant mothers than sites utilizing the opt-in method (CDC, 2017).

### Effective Prevention of Vertical HIV Transmission

The intervention services, such as testing, counseling, and provision of antiretroviral medications, were shown to be effective in reducing mother-to-child HIV transmission. Between 2002 and 2005, 37.5% of expectant mothers who were HIV-positive were diagnosed before their pregnancy. Between 2010 and 2013, 51.5% of HIV-positive mothers were diagnosed before becoming pregnant (Taylor et al., 2017). According to Brandon et al., the retrospective study indicated an increase in preconception HIV diagnosis from 73% to 90% between the period of 2008–2013 and 2014–2019 (Brandon, Chakravarti & Hemelaar, 2022). Due to these advancements in medical treatments and screening of HIV-positive women, vertical HIV transmission rates decreased from 216 infants diagnosed with HIV in 2002 to 69 infants in 2013 (Taylor et al., 2017). By 2013, HIV vertical transmission in the United States was 1.75 per 100,000 live births, which is an approximate 96% decline since the 1992 transmission peak (CDC, 2017). Lastly, between 2014 and 2018, the number of infants born with HIV in the United States declined from 141 to 65 (CDC, 2020).

### Medication and Treatment Adherence in Perinatal HIV Transmission

The remarkable 96% reduction in vertical HIV transmission in the United States showcases the effectiveness of medical protocols and HIV screening programs. However, before these measures were established, many infants contracted HIV. By 1995, AIDS had become the leading cause of death among children in the United States (Krist & Crawford-Faucher, 2002). The following factors contributed to the alarming AIDS death rates in children: lack of universal HIV testing in pregnant women, lack of widespread antiretroviral therapies, lack of early HIV testing and prophylaxis treatment of infants, opportunistic infections in children, delayed public health responses to the HIV/AIDS epidemic, and healthcare disparities in impoverished and marginalized communities (Brandon et al., 2022; Lampe et al., 2023; Selph et al., 2019). According to UNICEF (2018), without treatment, 30% of children infected with HIV perinatally die before their first birthday, and half die before turning two.

Healthcare providers specializing in infectious diseases and immunology strongly recommend immediate treatment for newborns exposed to or infected with HIV. This treatment involves administering antiretroviral medications (HAART) at birth to reduce viral replication and prevent further transmission. These medications, combined with regular monitoring of HIV viral loads and CD4 T-cell counts, are crucial for managing HIV-positive individuals' health. These healthcare strategies support and enable optimal health despite a compromised immune system. These medical advancements have also extended children's lives into adulthood. As children and adolescents live into adulthood, it poses unique challenges for these individuals.

### Quality of Life and Challenges for People Living with HIV

Advances in HIV treatment, particularly HAART medications, have enabled HIV-positive individuals to achieve life expectancies comparable to those of the general population (Pozniak, 2014). Despite this progress, living with HIV presents unique challenges due to the disease's stigmatized nature. Factors such as HIV symptoms, family dynamics, societal stigmas, and psychological issues associated with chronic illness profoundly impact the health and quality of life for people living with perinatally acquired HIV (PHIV). Understanding these specific needs and challenges is crucial for developing effective practices to enhance their quality of life.

Quality of life for individuals with chronic illnesses involves assessing their lives in relation to culture, values, goals, expectations, standards, and interests (Bishop et al., 2009). It also considers their level of functioning and disease symptoms. The stigma associated with HIV adds another layer of complexity as individuals navigate their lives and manage their condition. Clinicians who understand these complexities can collaborate effectively with patients to implement interventions that improve overall quality of life and self-perception. Research by Miners et al. (2014) indicated that the health-related quality of life of HIV-positive individuals with controlled HIV was significantly lower than that of the general population, highlighting the need for targeted strategies to address this disparity.

### Mental and Behavioral Health Challenges in Perinatally HIV Infected Adults

Research indicates that PHIV youth and young adults face significant behavioral health challenges. Studies conducted across various countries, including the United States, South Africa, and Kenya, show that PHIV youth exhibit higher rates of psychiatric disorders and behavioral issues compared to their uninfected peers. For instance, Kamau et al. (2012) found that nearly half of the youth in their study met the criteria for a psychiatric disorder, with anxiety and major depression being prevalent, especially among those with low CD4 counts. Similarly, Santamaria and Dolezal (2011) observed that while HIV status disclosure did not correlate with increased anxiety, it did not reduce depression or internalizing behavior problems. These findings highlight the complexities of managing mental health in PHIV youth, where factors like knowledge of HIV status and immune suppression play significant roles.

Additional studies underscore the prevalence of behavioral health issues among PHIV youth. Malee et al. (2011) reported that behavioral impairments such as conduct disorder, learning problems, and hyperactivity were two to three times more common in PHIV youth compared to the general population. This higher prevalence was linked to suboptimal viral suppression and potential neurocognitive impairments from inadequate HAART regimens. Wood and Shah (2009) also identified psychiatric illnesses like mood and psychotic disorders in nearly half of their study participants, associating these conditions with neurological impairments caused by HIV-related illnesses. Tadesse et al. (2012) further identified socioeconomic status and parental loss as significant factors contributing to behavioral and emotional problems in PHIV youth. These studies collectively suggest that a deeper understanding of the multifaceted challenges faced by PHIV youth is essential for developing targeted interventions and support systems.

### Locus of Control in HIV Disease

The impact of HIV as a chronic illness extends beyond individual health to societal contributions. The level of health management influences how HIV+ individuals participate in daily activities, work, and social settings. Poorly managed HIV can limit their ability for autonomy, self-care, and contribution to their communities, affecting broader societal dynamics. Understanding patients' perspectives on their disease control through the lens of locus of control (LOC) is essential for developing effective interventions. LOC helps determine whether patients attribute their health outcomes to personal efforts (internal LOC) or external factors (external LOC), guiding tailored support strategies to improve health behaviors and outcomes.

Research highlights the significance of internal and external LOC in managing HIV. Studies like those by Ubbiali et al. (2008) and Jenkins and Patterson (1998) show that HIV+ patients with a higher internal LOC often exhibit better health behaviors and outcomes. However, internal LOC can sometimes lead to increased anxiety and self-blame. Conversely, an external LOC, particularly belief in powerful others, can reduce depression and enhance mental health, especially in collectivist cultures. Studies also show that interventions designed to shift patients' LOC toward a more beneficial orientation can improve overall well-being and quality of life. Understanding these dynamics enables healthcare providers to offer more effective, culturally sensitive care to people living with HIV.

### HIV Stigma

Living with a stigmatized chronic illness such as HIV presents unique challenges that providers must understand to deliver effective support. While Goffman (1963) described stigma as a discrediting quality that reduces an individual to a "tainted" status. Recent research continues to emphasize the pervasive impact of stigma on the psychosocial well-being of people living with HIV (PLWH). Stigma persists globally, with individuals experiencing societal misconceptions and fear that lead to exclusion and discrimination. A study by Turan et al. (2019) highlights how HIV stigma remains a barrier to care, particularly in healthcare settings, where PLWH face discrimination from medical providers, which exacerbates both physical and mental health challenges (Selph et al., 2019). These stigmas can lead individuals to avoid physical contact with HIV+ people or exhibit other fear-based behaviors. Such stigma can severely impact the social and emotional well-being of those infected, causing them to hide their diagnosis, refrain from discussing their medical treatment, or avoid romantic relationships to prevent rejection or harm. By understanding these nuanced issues, providers can develop interventions to combat stigma and empower HIV+ individuals.

Moreover, the forms of stigma categorized by Earnshaw and Chaudoir (2009) into enacted, anticipated, and internalized stigma continue to shape the experiences of PLWH. Studies have found that internalized stigma, in particular, is associated with higher levels of depression, anxiety, and social isolation. A study by Nachega et al. (2020) underscores how internalized stigma correlates with poor adherence to ART and reduced engagement in care. As previously observed, these stigmas can prevent individuals from seeking support, disclosing their status, or engaging in relationships.

Stigmatizing behaviors toward HIV-positive individuals can still range from subtle avoidance to overt acts of violence, as noted by recent studies. Hegazi et al. (2020) emphasize that stigma can manifest as microaggressions or social exclusion, both of which have profound impacts on the mental health and social engagement of PLWH. Additionally, research by Pantelic et al. (2022) draws attention to how stigma can lead to a reluctance to access healthcare, which delays diagnosis, treatment, and overall health outcomes, thereby perpetuating a cycle of poor health and further stigmatization.

### Social Support Needs for PHIV+ Youth and Adults

As PHIV+ youth transition into adulthood, their need for social support increases significantly (Toth et al., 2018). Living with HIV presents various psychosocial, emotional, physical, financial, and vocational challenges. These challenges include frequent hospitalizations, medication toxicity, and opportunistic infections, which create daily stressors. The stigma associated with an HIV diagnosis can lead to distress and social isolation. Multiple forms of social support are crucial in mitigating these challenges, helping individuals navigate the complexities of living with HIV.

HIV+ patients face numerous health-related responsibilities, such as adhering to daily HAART regimens, managing immune system vulnerabilities, coping with symptom distress, and attending frequent medical appointments. These responsibilities often result in missed school or work, medication resistance, and an ongoing struggle with their mortality. Consequently, disclosing their status and participating in routine activities become secondary to managing their health. These circumstances hinder their ability to build and maintain social connections. Social support, encompassing family, friends, peers, medical professionals, and community organizations, plays a vital role in helping HIV+ individuals cope with their condition.

Studies highlight the importance of social support in enhancing health outcomes and reducing stress for those with chronic illnesses, including HIV. Social support is defined as interpersonal transactions involving aid, affirmation, and affection or being part of a network of giving and receiving support (Kimmel, 2000; Williams et al., 2004). Effective social support includes tangible, emotional, informational, and appraisal components. Research shows that strong social support networks improve survival rates and mitigate the psychological impact of chronic illnesses (Cohen, 2004; Thoits, 1985). For HIV+ individuals, identifying and fostering appropriate social supports can significantly enhance their ability to manage their diagnosis and related stressors, ultimately improving their overall quality of life.

### Demographic Overview of Study Participants

This study explored various factors, including health LOC, HIV-related stigma, social support, quality of life, anxiety, and depression, among 128 adults who acquired HIV

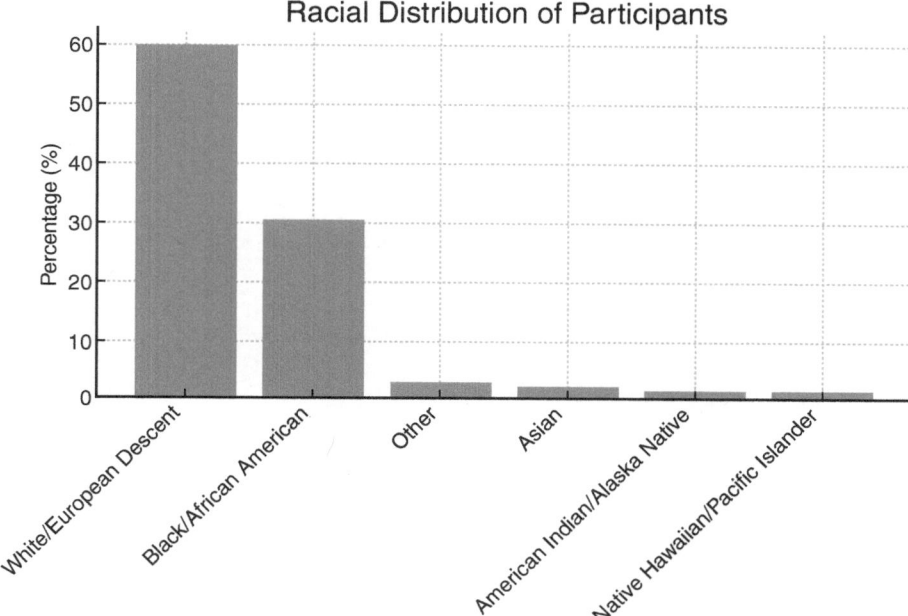

*Figure 15.1* Bar graph showing racial distribution of participants.

perinatally. The sample consisted of 68 males (53.1%) and 60 females (46.9%), with one non-binary participant whose responses were excluded due to insufficient representation. The participants' ages ranged from 18 to 50, with a mean age of 31.41 years. The age distribution included 35.9% aged 18–29, 50.8% aged 30–39, 12.5% aged 40–49, and one participant aged 50. Racially, over 60% were white or of European descent, 30.5% were Black or African American, 3.1% identified as Other, 2.3% were Asian, and both American Indian/Alaska Native and Native Hawaiian/Other Pacific Islander, each comprising 1.6% of the participants. Additionally, 17% identified as Hispanic or Latino.

The participants in our study exhibited a wide range of educational attainment, employment status, and income levels. In terms of educational attainment, less than 1% had not completed high school, 22.7% had a high school diploma, 17.2% had a trade school certification or an associate's degree, 32% had a bachelor's degree, 21.1% had a master's degree, and 6.2% had terminal degrees. The employment status varied, with the majority (80.5%) employed full-time, 12.5% part-time, 1.6% unemployed, 2.3% self-employed, 2.3% unable to work, and 0.8% retired. Income levels also showed diversity, with 2.3% reporting no income, 25.8% earning less than $49,999, 24.1% earning between $50,000 and $74,999, 27.3% earning between $75,000 and $99,999, and 20.3% earning over $100,000.

## Gender Differences in Locus of Control, HIV Stigma, and Quality of Life

The study examined gender differences among adults with perinatally acquired HIV in terms of LOC, HIV stigma, and quality of life. It found that males reported higher levels of LOC compared to females, indicating a greater perception that their personal traits and

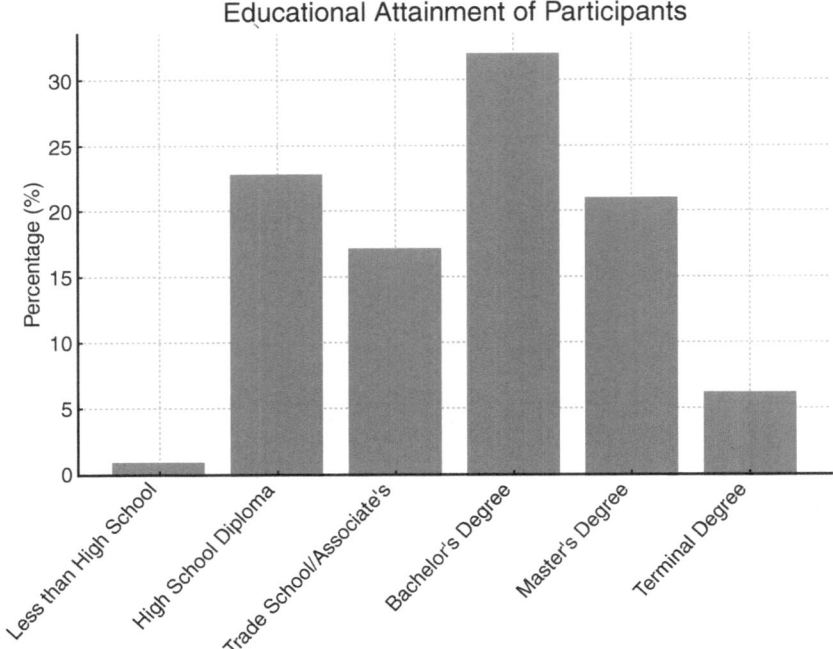

*Figure 15.2* Bar graph showing the educational attainment of participants.

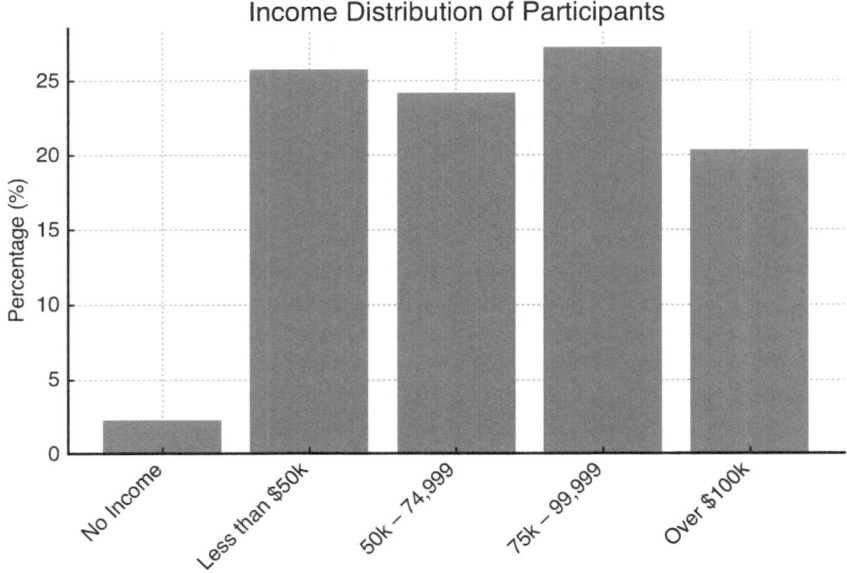

*Figure 15.3* Bar graph showing the income distribution of participants.

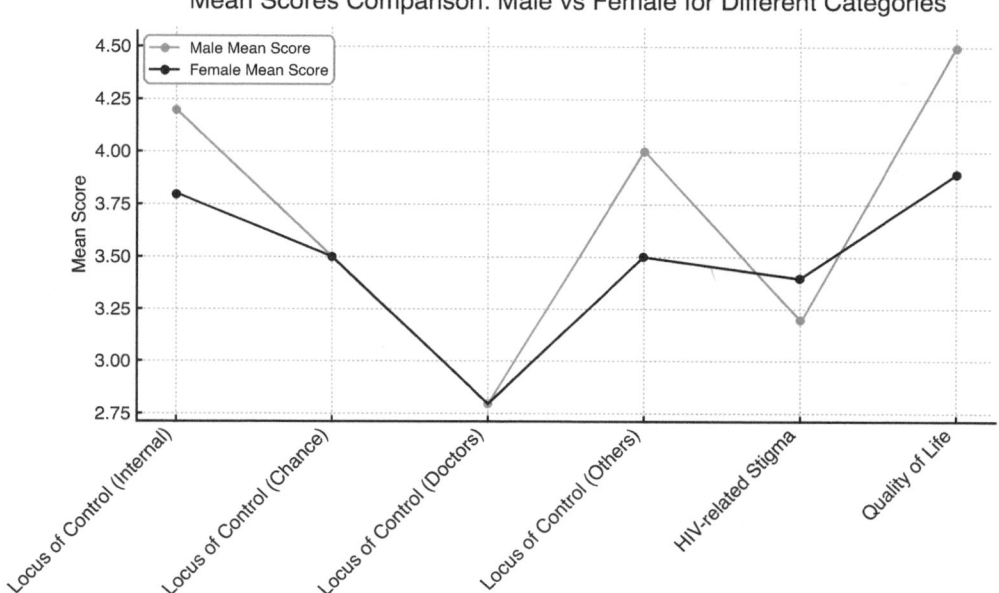

*Figure 15.4* Line graph showing mean scores comparison (male vs female) among different categories.

efforts influence their HIV management. Additionally, males showed higher reliance on significant others to manage their condition. Males endorsed a higher quality of life than females, reflecting better appraisal of their lives in the context of their HIV status. However, no significant differences were found between genders in terms of attributing their health status to luck, fate, or medical providers. HIV-stigma levels were similar between genders, with females showing a marginally higher mean score.

### Socioeconomic Status and Its Impact

The analysis of socioeconomic status, defined by education and income levels, revealed no statistically significant differences in LOC, HIV stigma, or quality of life among the participants. However, clinically significant trends were noted. Participants with higher education levels tended to believe more in their personal attributes for managing HIV and those with higher incomes reported similar trends. Specifically, participants earning $100k or more showed higher internal LOC and belief in their own skills. Those earning between $50k and $99,999 indicated higher reliance on healthcare providers. Despite the lack of statistical significance, these trends suggest that education and income may influence perceptions of control and quality of life among HIV+ individuals.

### Age and Racial Differences in LOC, HIV Stigma, and Quality of Life

Age was found to have a significant positive correlation with internal and chance loci of control, with older participants showing higher beliefs in their abilities and attributing health status to fate. Conversely, younger participants reported lower quality of life. No

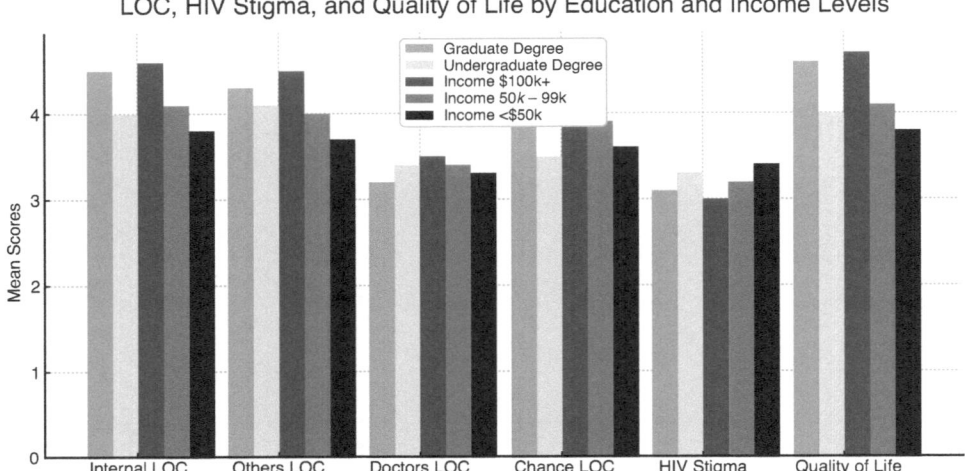

*Figure 15.5* Grouped bar graph showing LOC, quality of life, and HIV stigma by education and income levels.

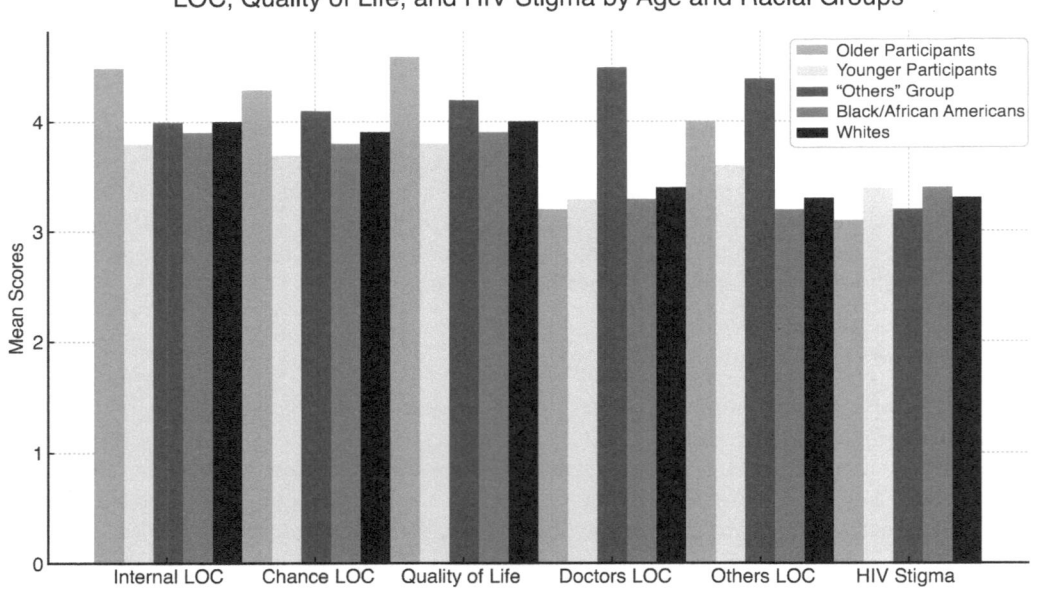

*Figure 15.6* Grouped bar graph showing LOC, quality of life, and HIV stigma by age and racial groups.

significant relationship was found between age and HIV stigma. Racial analysis revealed that the "Others" group attributed their health status more to medical providers and significant others compared to Black/African Americans and whites. No additional significant differences were found for internal LOC, chance LOC, HIV stigma, or quality of life across racial groups.

## Mediating Role of HIV Stigma

HIV stigma was found to mediate the relationship between LOC and quality of life. Higher internal LOC was associated with better quality of life, while higher HIV stigma correlated with lower quality of life. Participants attributing their health status to their medical providers also reported higher quality of life. These findings highlight the importance of addressing HIV stigma to improve the overall well-being of individuals with perinatally acquired HIV.

The study identified significant relationships between demographics, self-perception variables, and overall well-being. Higher internal LOC, lower HIV stigma, and greater social support were associated with better quality of life. Higher HIV stigma and lower social support influenced anxiety, while depression was linked to higher HIV stigma and reliance on medical providers. These results emphasize the complex interplay between this population's psychological factors, social support, and health outcomes.

## Discussion

The global HIV landscape highlights the persistent challenge the virus poses, with millions affected worldwide, including vulnerable populations, including adults living with perinatally acquired HIV. In the United States, HIV disproportionately impacts racial and ethnic minorities, particularly African Americans, emphasizing the need for targeted interventions.

While significant strides have been made in preventing vertical transmission, the stigma associated with HIV remains a major barrier to care and quality of life. Addressing HIV stigma, enhancing social support, and empowering individuals through increased internal LOC can significantly improve outcomes for those with perinatally acquired HIV. Research continues to emphasize the critical role of mental and behavioral health interventions in addressing the complex needs of this population. Focusing on the intersections of demographic factors, psychological health, social dynamics, and public health efforts can better support HIV-positive individuals in achieving improved health and well-being outcomes.

## Treatments

Adults with perinatally acquired HIV may face a multitude of challenges, including mental health disorders such as anxiety and depression, substance use issues, HIV stigma, and inadequate social support, compounded by varied LOC levels. Addressing these complex and interrelated issues requires a comprehensive treatment approach incorporating various effective interventions. The treatment interventions of psychoanalytic, psychodynamic, cognitive-behavioral therapy, mindfulness-based therapy, group therapy, psychotropic medications, psychoeducation, and hypnotherapy offer a robust framework for supporting the mental health and overall well-being of individuals living with perinatally acquired HIV.

## Psychoanalytic and Psychodynamic Therapies

Psychoanalytic and psychodynamic therapies both focus on unconscious processes and early experiences. These approaches assist in addressing mental health issues such as anxiety, depression, and HIV stigma in perinatally acquired HIV adults by delving into the unconscious mind to uncover and resolve deep-seated conflicts related to their diagnosis. This therapeutic approach posits that unresolved unconscious conflicts from childhood experiences significantly influence current behavior, emotions, and thought patterns. In the context of perinatally acquired HIV, individuals often face complex emotional challenges, including internalized stigma, fear of disclosure, and social isolation. Through techniques like free association, dream analysis, and transference, psychoanalytic therapy helps individuals bring these unconscious conflicts to the surface, allowing them to gain insight into their behavior and emotional responses. By understanding the root causes of their mental health issues, individuals can begin to address and resolve long-held internal conflicts, leading to a reduction in anxiety and depression.

Psychoanalytic therapy enhances individuals' internal LOC by fostering a deeper understanding of their motivations and behaviors. By working through unconscious conflicts, individuals can gain a stronger sense of self-awareness and self-efficacy, which is crucial for managing a chronic illness like HIV. This increased self-awareness enables one to recognize and challenge internalized negative beliefs and stigmas, fostering a more positive self-perception. Additionally, the therapeutic relationship in psychoanalysis provides a model for building trusting and supportive relationships outside of therapy, thereby addressing issues related to social support. As individuals learn to navigate and resolve their internal conflicts, they become more empowered to take control of their health and social interactions, leading to improved mental health and overall quality of life. Psychoanalytic and psychodynamic therapy thus offers a comprehensive approach to treating the multifaceted mental health issues faced by adults with perinatally acquired HIV.

### Cognitive-Behavioral Therapy

Cognitive-behavioral therapy (CBT), including cognitive restructuring, is a widely recognized and effective treatment for various mental health issues such as anxiety, depression, and HIV stigma. CBT operates on the premise that maladaptive thoughts and behaviors contribute to emotional distress and psychological disorders. Cognitive restructuring, a core component of CBT, involves identifying and challenging distorted cognitions and replacing them with more accurate and adaptive thoughts. In the context of anxiety and depression, cognitive restructuring helps individuals recognize negative thought patterns that perpetuate feelings of fear, hopelessness, and sadness. By reframing these thoughts, patients can reduce symptoms of anxiety and depression, improving their overall mental health. Regarding HIV stigma, CBT helps individuals confront and modify the internalized negative beliefs about themselves due to their HIV status, thereby alleviating associated stress and improving self-esteem and social functioning.

Furthermore, CBT, through cognitive restructuring, effectively addresses issues of increasing social support and internal LOC. Individuals with inadequate social support often experience heightened feelings of isolation and loneliness, exacerbating their mental health problems. CBT interventions can enhance social skills and encourage the development of more supportive relationships, thereby increasing perceived social support. Additionally, by fostering more positive and realistic thinking patterns, CBT can help individuals feel more capable of influencing their environment and outcomes, addressing lower internal LOC levels. This shift can empower individuals to take proactive steps to manage their mental health, improving psychological well-being. By targeting both cognitive and behavioral aspects, CBT provides a comprehensive approach to treatment, addressing the complex interplay of thoughts, behaviors, and social factors that contribute to mental health issues.

### Mindfulness-Based Cognitive Therapy

Mindfulness-based cognitive therapy (MBCT) is a clinically validated intervention designed to address mental health issues such as anxiety, depression, and HIV stigma by integrating principles of mindfulness with cognitive therapy techniques. MBCT teaches individuals to cultivate a non-judgmental awareness of their thoughts, feelings, and bodily sensations. This mindfulness practice helps individuals recognize and disengage from automatic negative thought patterns that often exacerbate anxiety and depression. By observing thoughts without immediate reaction or judgment, individuals can reduce the emotional impact of these thoughts and prevent the escalation of distressing emotions. For those dealing with HIV stigma, MBCT helps reduce the internalization of negative societal attitudes by fostering a compassionate and accepting attitude toward oneself. This self-acceptance diminishes the psychological burden of stigma and improves emotional well-being.

MBCT also addresses issues related to poor social support and lower levels of internal LOC. Mindfulness practices promote greater self-awareness and emotional regulation, which can enhance social interactions and relationships. Individuals become more attuned to their own needs and the needs of others, leading to more meaningful and supportive connections. Additionally, by fostering a present-focused awareness, MBCT helps individuals develop a stronger sense of agency and control over their reactions to life's challenges. This increased internal LOC empowers individuals to take proactive steps in managing their mental health and life circumstances. Through the combined benefits of mindfulness and cognitive restructuring, MBCT offers a holistic approach that not only alleviates symptoms of anxiety, depression, and HIV stigma but also strengthens social support systems and enhances personal agency.

### Group Therapy

Group therapy is an effective intervention for treating mental health issues such as anxiety, depression, and HIV stigma by providing a supportive environment where individuals can share experiences, learn from others, and receive feedback. In the context of anxiety and depression, group therapy helps participants understand they are not alone in their struggles, which can significantly reduce feelings of isolation and hopelessness. By discussing their challenges and coping strategies, individuals can gain new insights and develop healthier ways of thinking and behaving. For those facing HIV stigma, group therapy offers a safe space to express fears and experiences related to their condition, fostering a sense of community and mutual understanding. This shared experience can reduce the internalization of stigma and enhance self-acceptance, improving overall mental health.

Additionally, group therapy addresses poor social support and lower levels of internal LOC by enhancing interpersonal relationships and fostering a sense of empowerment. The group setting naturally provides social support as members offer empathy, encouragement, and practical advice to one another. This supportive network can alleviate feelings of loneliness and improve social connectedness. Through group interactions and clinical provider guidance, participants can develop better communication and social skills, which can be transferred to their relationships outside the therapy context. Regarding internal LOC, group therapy encourages individuals to take responsibility for their progress and actively participate in their recovery. By witnessing others' successes and challenges, participants can build confidence in their ability to effect change in their lives, thus increasing their sense of agency and control over their mental health. Group therapy, therefore, provides a comprehensive approach that not only addresses specific mental health issues but also strengthens social support systems and enhances personal empowerment.

### Psychotropic Medications

Psychotropic medications are a cornerstone in the treatment of anxiety and unipolar depressive disorders. These medications work to alter brain chemistry to stabilize mood and reduce symptoms. Selective serotonin reuptake inhibitors, for example, increase serotonin levels in the brain, which can help alleviate depressive symptoms and reduce anxiety. Benzodiazepines, another class of psychotropic drugs, are often used for their sedative properties to manage acute anxiety symptoms. Adults with perinatal-acquired HIV may experience a range of other mental health disorders, including post-traumatic stress disorder (PTSD) and mood disorders. By targeting the neurochemical imbalances associated with these disorders, psychotropic medications improve mood, decrease anxiety, and enhance overall functioning. These outcomes may provide significant relief and improve the quality of life for individuals dealing with complex mental health challenges alongside HIV.

### Psychoeducation

Psychoeducation is a valuable intervention for adults with perinatally acquired HIV, providing them with critical information and skills to manage anxiety, depression, HIV stigma, lack of social support, and an internal LOC. Through structured educational sessions, individuals learn about the psychological and physiological aspects of their condition, which can demystify symptoms and reduce anxiety and depression. By understanding the nature of HIV and its impact on mental health, individuals can challenge internalized stigma and develop a more positive self-image. Psychoeducation also fosters the development of coping strategies and resilience, enabling individuals to better manage stress and emotional challenges. Group-based psychoeducation can enhance social support by creating a community of individuals with shared experiences, reducing feelings of isolation. Additionally, by emphasizing the importance of personal agency and self-management, psychoeducation strengthens the internal LOC, empowering individuals to take active steps in managing their health and well-being. Overall, psychoeducation equips adults with the knowledge and skills necessary to navigate the complex interplay of HIV and mental health, promoting a more empowered and supported approach to their condition.

### Hypnotherapy

Hypnotherapy can be an effective adjunctive treatment for adults with perinatally acquired HIV, helping them manage anxiety, depression, HIV stigma, lack of social support, and issues with LOC. Through guided hypnosis, individuals enter a deeply relaxed state, which can facilitate the exploration and modification of unconscious thoughts and beliefs that contribute to anxiety and depression. By addressing these underlying cognitive patterns, hypnotherapy can alleviate negative emotional states and promote a more positive outlook. Additionally, hypnotherapy can help reduce internalized HIV stigma by fostering self-compassion and reinforcing positive self-perceptions. This therapeutic approach can also enhance social functioning by reducing social anxiety and increasing confidence in social interactions, thereby improving social support networks. Furthermore, hypnotherapy often incorporates techniques that bolster the internal LOC, such as visualizing success and developing problem-solving strategies, which empower individuals to take more active and effective roles in managing their health and lives. Overall, hypnotherapy provides a holistic and integrative approach to addressing the multifaceted psychological challenges faced by adults with perinatally acquired HIV.

In conclusion, addressing the multifaceted challenges faced by adults with perinatally acquired HIV requires a comprehensive and integrative approach. The aforementioned interventions provide unique benefits that collectively support the overall well-being of those living with a stigmatized chronic illness. These therapies help manage mental and behavioral concerns while enhancing social support and strengthening the internal LOC. By leveraging the strengths of these diverse therapeutic approaches, healthcare providers can create a robust and personalized treatment framework that empowers individuals to lead healthier and more fulfilling lives.

## Reflective Questions for Consideration

1  How might the observed gender differences in LOC and quality of life among adults with perinatally acquired HIV influence the design and implementation of gender-specific interventions to improve their overall well-being and HIV management?
2  How can the integration of various therapeutic approaches, such as psychoanalytic therapy, cognitive-behavioral therapy, and mindfulness-based therapy, provide a comprehensive treatment plan for individuals with perinatally acquired HIV?
3  In what ways do group therapy and psychoeducation specifically enhance social support and internal LOC for adults facing the combined challenges of perinatally acquired HIV and mental health disorders?
4  How might psychotropic medications and hypnotherapy complement other psychotherapeutic interventions to effectively manage the psychological and emotional impacts of HIV stigma, anxiety, and depression in this population?

## References

Brandon, C., Chakravarti, N., & Hemelaar, J. (2022). Retrospective analysis of preconception HIV diagnosis and vertical transmission rates from 2008–2019. *Journal of Infectious Diseases, 225*(6), 1123–1131. https://doi.org/10.1093/infdis/jiaa622

Bishop, M., Frain, M. P., Rumrill, P. D., & Rymond, C. (2009). The relationship of self-management and disease modifying therapy use to employment status among adults with multiple sclerosis. *Journal of Vocational Rehabilitation, 31*(2), 119–127.

Bishop, M., Smedema, S., & Lee, E. (2009). Quality of life and psychosocial adaptation to chronic illness and disability. In F. Chang, E. da Silva, & J. Chronister, *Understanding psychosocial adjustment to chronic illness and disability.* (pp. 521–558). Springer Publishing Company.

Centers for Disease Control and Prevention. (2008). Mother-to-child (perinatal) HIV transmission and prevention: CDC HIV/AIDS fact sheet. CDC. https://www.cdc.gov/hiv/

Centers for Disease Control and Prevention. (2017). *Preventing Pregnancy Related Deaths.* Retrieved from https://www.cdc.gov/mmwr/volumes/66/wr/mm6647e1.htm.

Centers for Disease Control and Prevention. (2019, February). HIV surveillance report, 2017 (Vol. 29). CDC. https://stacks.cdc.gov/view/cdc/85285

Centers for Disease Control and Prevention (CDC). (2020). HIV surveillance report, 2020. *CDC.* https://www.cdc.gov/nchhstp/director-letters/2020-hiv-surveillance-report.html

Cohen, R. F. (2004). Attitudes toward chronic illness. *Instruments for Clinical Health-care Research,* 315–334.

Earnshaw, V. A., & Chaudoir, S. R. (2009). From conceptualizing to measuring HIV stigma: A review of HIV stigma mechanism measures. *AIDS and Behavior, 13*(6), 1160–1177. https://doi.org/10.1007/s10461-009-9593-3

Goffman, E. (1963). *Stigma: Notes on the management of spoiled identity.* Prentice-Hall.

Hegazi, A., Rickenbach, M., & Pantelic, M. (2020). The psychosocial impact of HIV stigma: Examining the moderating role of gender and ethnicity. *Journal of Health Psychology, 25*(9), 1212–1225. https://doi.org/10.1177/1359105318779440

Jenkins, R. A., & Patterson, T. L. (1998). HIV Locus of Control and Adaptation to Seropositivity 1. *Journal of Applied Social Psychology, 28*(2), 95–108.

Kamau, C., Kuria, M. W., & Mathai, M. (2012). Psychiatric morbidity among HIV-infected children and adolescents in Kenya. *International Journal of Mental Health Systems, 6*(6), 38. https://doi.org/10.1186/1752-4458-6-6

Kamya, M. R. (2012). Assessing the effectiveness of HIV testing and counseling services in Uganda. *Journal of Social Aspects of HIV/AIDS, 9*(2), 59–69. https://doi.org/10.1080/17290376.2012.683586

Kimmel, M. S. (2000). *The gendered society.* Oxford: Oxford University Press.

Krist, A. H., & Crawford-Faucher, A. (2002). Management of HIV infection in children: Updates in epidemiology and antiretroviral therapy. *American Family Physician, 66*(7), 1113–1120.

Lampe, F., Gatell, J., & Porter, K. (2023). Historical trends in perinatal HIV transmission in the United States. *AIDS Research and Therapy, 20*(3), 145–157. https://doi.org/10.1186/s12981-023-00479-6

Malee, K. M., Tassiopoulos, K., Huo, Y., Siberry, G., & Mellins, C. A. (2011). Mental health functioning among children and adolescents with perinatal HIV infection and exposure. *AIDS Patient Care and STDs, 25*(7), 413–422. https://doi.org/10.1089/apc.2011.0026

Miners, A., Phillips, A., Kreif, N., Rodger, A., & Johnson, M. (2014). Health-related quality of life of people with HIV in the era of antiretroviral therapy: A comparison with the general population. *The Lancet HIV, 1*(1), e32–e40. https://doi.org/10.1016/S2352-3018(14)70018-9

Nachega, J. B., Marconi, V. C., & Uthman, O. A. (2020). HIV treatment adherence, retention, and related outcomes: A review of the evidence. *The Lancet Infectious Diseases, 20*(3), 157–170. https://doi.org/10.1016/S1473-3099(19)30469-3

Nesheim, S. R., Taylor, A., Lampe, F., Gatell, J., & Porter, K. (2017). Trends in perinatal HIV infections in the United States, 1978–2013. *Pediatrics, 139*(6), e20164272. https://doi.org/10.1542/peds.2016-4272

Pantelic, M., Ziauddeen, N., Boyes, M., O'Hara, M. E., Hastie, C., & Alwan, N. A. (2022). Long Covid stigma: Estimating burden and validating scale in a UK-based sample. *Plos one, 17*(11), e0277317.

Pozniak, A. (2014). HIV and life expectancy: Changes in quality of life and health outcomes. *The Lancet HIV, 1*(2), e44–e45. https://doi.org/10.1016/S2352-3018(14)70025-6

Santamaria, E. K., & Dolezal, C. (2011). The impact of HIV disclosure on depression and internalizing behavior problems in youth with perinatally acquired HIV. *Journal of Child Psychology and Psychiatry, 52*(8), 885–893. https://doi.org/10.1111/j.1469-7610.2011.02363.x

Selph, S. S., Bougatsos, C., Dana, T., Grusing, S., & Chou, R. (2019). Screening for HIV: Evidence summary for the U.S. Preventive Services Task Force. *Journal of the American Medical Association, 322*(8), 797–806. https://doi.org/10.1001/jama.2019.10425

Tadesse, A. W., Berhane Tsehay, Y., Girma Belaineh, B., & Alemu, Y. B. (2012). Behavioral and emotional problems among children aged 6–14 years on highly active antiretroviral therapy in Addis Ababa: a cross-sectional study. *AIDS Care, 24*(11), 1359–1367.

Taylor, A. W., Nesheim, S., Zhang, X., & Lampe, F. (2017). Reduction in perinatal HIV infections in the United States. *Pediatrics, 139*(4), e20160762. https://doi.org/10.1542/peds.2016-0762

Thoits, P. A. (1985). Social support and psychological well-being: Theoretical possibilities. *Journal of Health and Social Behavior, 26*(1), 53–79. https://doi.org/10.2307/2136759

Toth, L., Ross, J., & Ojikutu, B. (2018). Social support needs of perinatally HIV-infected youth. *AIDS Care, 30*(9), 1141–1152. https://doi.org/10.1080/09540121.2018.1472767

Turan, B., Budhwani, H., & Lerebours-Nadal, L. (2019). HIV stigma as a barrier to care: A decade of evidence from various settings. *Journal of the International AIDS Society, 22*(S3), e25383. https://doi.org/10.1002/jia2.25383

Ubbiali, A. L. E. S. S. A. N. D. R. O., Donati, D., Chiorri, C., Bregani, V., Cattaneo, E., Maffei, C., & Visintini, R. (2008). The usefulness of the Multidimensional Health Locus of Control Form C (MHLC-C) for HIV+ subjects: an Italian study. *AIDS Care, 20*(4), 495–502.

UNAIDS. (2020). Global HIV & AIDS statistics—2020 fact sheet. *UNAIDS.* https://www.unaids.org/en/resources/fact-sheet

United Nations Children's Fund. (2018). Women: At the heart of the HIV response for children. UNICEF

Williams, R. B., Barefoot, J. C., & Blumenthal, J. A. (2004). Psychosocial predictors of mortality in cardiac patients: The role of social support. *Journal of Psychosomatic Research, 56*(2), 169–176. https://doi.org/10.1016/S0022-3999(03)00077-4

Wood, S. M., & Shah, S. S. (2009). Psychiatric disorders in perinatally HIV-infected youth. *Journal of Acquired Immune Deficiency Syndromes, 52*(3), 316–322. https://doi.org/10.1097/QAI.0b013e3181b371f8

# 16 Human Services and Sexuality Consultation

## The Need to Move beyond Clinical Discomfort in Talking about Sex

*Anastasia Gorden*

## Introduction

There remains professional discomfort with talking about sex within a therapeutic context. One does not have to be a sex therapist to talk about sex issues with their clients. In fact, many sexual issues are common and can come in the form of sexual dissatisfaction, gender identity, sexual trauma, exploration, or working through shame of one's sexuality and are often linked to mental health issues such as depression and anxiety (Buehler, 2017). Sex can be related to a deeper core sense of self among clients served by practitioners. The list can go on and reflects a need to make space for clinical discussions around sex and sexuality as part of the overall mental health of clients. Clients, in fact, have a tendency to bring up sexual issues with therapists outside of sex therapy, often as a result of the rapport and therapeutic alliance gained throughout the process of therapy (Emond et al., 2024). However, it is important to note the responses some therapists may have when unprepared for what a client could say regarding sexual issues coming up for their clients outside of other reported mental health concerns. This stands as further research will show how sexual issues can have an overall impact on sexual and mental health.

Buehler (2017) discusses how sexual health can be a good and important part of one's overall mental health. Discussions about sexuality should not be treated as an unnecessary added piece of mental health that therapists can sidestep if uncomfortable with the topic. She also stated that sexual issues are quite common but that a majority of mental health professionals are unprepared to discuss or broach sexual concerns already expressed by their clients. This is due in part that many therapists still have not explored their own reservations about discussing sex and sexuality. In a society that still struggles with providing spaces for knowledge and insight around sexuality, therapists as well as clients can remain in the dark and adhere to a code of silence when it pertains to sex (Gorden, 2024). This code of silence and distancing around discussing sex can also be a result of sexual abuse and trauma experienced by therapists, or even vicarious trauma in hearing others' narrative of sexual trauma (Buehler, 2017).

Buehler also mentions how therapists may experience anxiety and distance from sex topics with clients due to strict training laws regarding law and ethics, and to ensure therapists are practicing with the utmost integrity. Although very important, it also creates a fear-based response that does not help therapists promote professional boundaries and mirror healthy discussions of sex with clients as part of their professional development.

How can therapists become more comfortable discussing sex topics? Reading about sexuality, receiving ongoing sex-positive education, learning of queer theory, sexual minority

DOI: 10.4324/9781003531258-19

models, and clinical training from sex educators, instructors, and supervisors could be a start (Constantinides et al., 2019).

It is important for therapists and other health professionals to address their worldview of sex and sexuality. These worldviews can embody an internalized narrative with many aspects of sexuality, including various beliefs, values, and attitudes revolving around sexual identities and sexual behaviors. These belief systems regarding sexuality can stem from social influences seen in communities such that are related to family, peers, and as it relates to specific or intersecting cultural identities, or in the form of institutions like school and religion (Belous et al., 2012). According to Buehler (2017), it is expected that practicing therapists be non-judgmental and empathic to clients to be effective in assisting clients with sexual issues. To do that, therapists must do the work of setting aside any biases they can and will experience related to their client and sexuality.

## Common Sexual Stereotypes among Therapists

Many therapists still hold a lot of stereotypes embedded with the social stigma of sex and sexuality. Some include more readily pathologizing clients who report having more recent sexual partners (i.e., sex addiction). Other therapists can also be less accepting of alternative sexual lifestyles (i.e., having open or poly relationships or engaging in kink practices).

There are also many therapists who hold homophobic and transphobic attitudes toward same-sex oriented and transgender individuals. For those who are challenging the aforementioned attitudes, there may be confusion regarding newer understandings of orientation and gender fluidity (i.e., men who have sex with men but do not identify as gay, identifying as queer so as not to ascribe to one gender and/or orientation). Constantinides and colleagues (2019) share how this shows up with binary thinking that limits the nuances and variations of sexual and gender minority stressors that can be unique and specific to sexual minority clients. Gender, as a social construct, can be seen as fluid and often overlaps with the binary thinking (either/or limitations) seen in sexual orientation. Sexual orientation is often seen according to the binary thinking of male and female genders and so limits how one can be understood in terms of sexual attraction (i.e., gay for two males attracted to one another or lesbian for two females sexually attracted to one another). Constantinides et al. further explore how the sexual orientation bisexual has come under fire in recent years due to how it can be assumed that "bi" only focuses on attraction to the male and female genders, even though from a socially constructive lens, "bi" can simply refer to sexual attraction to two genders. However, more terms to better include non-binary thinking have been reinforced, including the use of the term "pansexual," which encompasses an all-inclusive sexual attraction to others not specifically defined by two genders. Finally, there are other biases that can be present among therapists. In fact, there are recent reports that still show that many therapists think sex should only be for the young. However, recent data shows that in elderly-assisted living facilities have reported more older adults aged 65 and up are still engaging in sexual behaviors (Buehler, 2017).

There are many reasons why a mental health clinician could struggle with providing effective therapy services when either attempting to breach or avoid the topic of sex with their clients. However, it is also worth sharing why it is important to bring up or explore sexual issues in therapy. This can include culturally specific as well as intersecting issues tied to relevant identities, both sexual and nonsexual alike. In detailing specific common sexual issues that can come up for clients in different social locations, exploring how clinicians can manage their discomfort when discussing sex with their clients will be discussed moving forward.

### Culturally Specific Issues Related to Sexuality and Clients—Promoting Sex Positivity

Thorpe et al. (2022) discuss from a Black female lens how sex and sexuality are often discouraged or omitted from discussions in sexual health. Although important to emphasize sexual issues and oppression impacting Black women and Black communities at large, it is important that there is a balance that focuses on creating sex-positive spaces that speak to "resilience, strength, and 'good stuff' related to sex" (Hargons & Thorpe, 2022, p. 7). What does that mean? Examples include feeling satisfied emotionally, physically, and mentally during sexual moments that can include mind–body–soul awareness, sex-positive partnered interactions, and experiencing an orgasm, according to Thorpe and colleagues (2022). Such a study that embodies two primary intersecting identities can also be reflective of other communities of color and the need to provide safe spaces to explore sex-positive aspects of sexuality and address heavy sex-negative narratives often cloaking multifaceted experiences within communities regarding sexual expression.

As noted previously, it is important to talk about sexual issues, including preventive measures or management of sexual issues (i.e., sexually transmitted infections or STIs or pelvic floor pain). In addition, consideration must be given to revolving dialogues on safer sex practices and healing from sexual trauma. These are issues still impacting many communities in and outside the United States. For example, issues with discussing STIs, such as HIV, can be seen in a study based in South Africa with how "fear, discomfort, embarrassment ... limited knowledge about sensitive topics, and lack of self-confidence" made conversations difficult to discuss HIV with parents and their adolescents (Knight et al., 2023). This study goes on to provide suggestions that resulted in respondents from the study consider having conversations with adolescents around sexual health and HIV. Yet, it was noted how the limited conversation on sexual concerns had to be discussed to explore potentially different outcomes for future studies. Some of the topics of sexual health that may not be engaging or fun to talk about can be scary or involve communities that lack the knowledge and awareness to discuss, even among the youth.

However, what can be gained in moving past the discomfort of talking about sex with clients can include more self-awareness and acceptance as a clinician, as well as for clients, dismantling shame around discussing sex (Buehler), also building bodily awareness and function. Healthy and normalized conversations of sex and sexuality can also be mirrored in a consenting and safe environment in a therapeutic setting.

### Issues with the DSM

Often, sexual interest and practices are seen as odd, bizarre, or can be flat out pathologized. As noted in the current *Diagnostic and Statistical Manual* (DSM-5-TR version), some paraphilic disorders, although problematic in what can be seen as sexual behaviors causing high distress to non-consenting people and children, can be an issue. However, it seems important to make distinctions between what is harmful and what can involve adult consensual forms of fun and safe sexual play (like sadism, masochism, and fetishes). From a sex-positive perspective, intimate expression and relationships that regard all consensual sexual practices and activities as fundamentally healthy and pleasurable (Queen et al., 2015) invite human services and mental health practitioners to encourage clients to explore their sexuality, while promoting a safe space without shame or judgment. Being a sex-positive mental health professional means challenging societal taboos regarding sexuality with the aim of promoting sexuality as a natural and healthy part of life (Buehler, 2017). However, to do that, ongoing dialogue and safe spaces to have these discussions need to be in place for understanding consent, boundaries, and consequences. Without these discussions with clinicians and clients, this limits the means of engaging in consensual sexual practices and behaviors that can be fulfilling and meaningful to clients. This also inhibits or results in people hiding sexual desires, fantasy, interest, and expression for fear of judgment, including engaging or exploring sexual practices in secret (and possibly in questionable and unsafe spaces).

## Consent Is Sexy Campaign

A recent study by Hovick and Silver (2019) on the "Consent Is Sexy!" Campaign aligns with the notion that sexual communication is a skill often misunderstood and it is due to a lack of communication about sex. So not only was this campaign added to sexual violence prevention campaigns, but its specific focus also addresses the misperception that communicating sexual consent is not sexy and, instead, provides ways that can normalize what sexual communication with consent can look like. Part of the issue noted was a need for students on college campuses to gain more exposure to sexual communication tools that endorse consensual conversations about sex. What's amazing and ironic about this campaign is the fact that there is a focus on gaining awareness about a relevant piece regarding sexual health and communication that some mental health professionals are still very uncomfortable with.

In a couples' study by Machette and Montgomery-Vestecka (2023), the authors discuss how even interpersonal sexual communication (ISC), which include "the verbal and nonverbal exchange of messages containing educational, episodic, and/or relational content between intimate partners" (p. 124), is limited due to the risk of relational consequences such as conflict, judgment, and criticism from the other partner. However, when ISC discrepancies are low, couples can feel more connected, openly communicate needs and desires, and experience less judgment from partners. Yet Emond et al.'s (2024) recent work suggests that only 59% of relational therapists will focus on working through sexual issues as a goal in relationship therapy. This percentage may invite practitioners to think about why some therapists continue to opt out of addressing sexual issues with couples. This seems interesting if a party presents sexual issues while in relationship therapy. Some information in the study discusses other stressors outside of sexual issues impacting a couple's relationship, such as conflict management, and how many couple therapists will disregard sexual issues with the belief that a couple's expressed sexual issues are a symptom of larger communication and conflictual issues impacting the couple. Although research has shown that this could be possible, this perspective held by many couple therapists can result in sexual issues being avoided with the hopes that once the prioritized stressors are addressed, then sexual issues will resolve on their own (Machette & Montgomery-Vestecka, 2023). This perspective, although relevant, can be an oversimplified view of couples' sexual issues that can get in the way of effective treatment in relationship therapy.

**Sexual Minority Stressors**

There are several issues that impact the mental health of LGBTQ+ individuals and their intimate and sexual relationships, including the management of sexual minority stressors. As noted by Buehler (2017), these stressors can vary from covert and overt discrimination; management of being closeted due to unsafe spaces; limited emotional and physical public displays of affection due to fear of physical, emotional, and mental harm and harassment due to being open with queer relationships; the strain that aforementioned issues can have on intimate relationships; and internalized homophobia and transphobia. There is data revealing that a large percentage of gay and lesbian individuals will mask or hide their identities to avoid being heavily impacted by stigma linked to sexual minority stressors, information that many practicing therapists are not aware of. In fact, the magnitude of some of these stressors can include forms of double discrimination. For instance, those who would consider identifying as bisexual may face discrimination, judgment, and a lack of acceptance of their identity from both those who identify with different-sex (heterosexual) and same-sex (gay and lesbian) sexual orientations. This can be perpetuated by sexual stereotypes that bisexual people are more promiscuous for having attraction toward both genders and that it is assumed they are likely to engage in a romantic or sexual affair or be seen as unfaithful to their partners and in some cases are not really seen as an acceptable part of the LGBTQ+ communities. Similarly, those who identify as asexual face discrimination with disbelief that they may not experience sexual attraction or desire toward anyone or in very limited contexts. Activist Yasmin Benoit (Harden Bradford, 2022) has been known for her intersectional work on Black identities and asexuality, noting how she faces minority stressors of her sexual orientation, with both same and different sex often denying asexuality as a sexual orientation. In her interview with Dr. Joy Harden Bradford's podcast "Therapy for Black Girls" (2022), Benoit shares her journey of being a Black female model that is often not taken seriously for her sexual orientation, partly because of intersectional issues around racial and sexual stereotypes that convey hypersexuality and promiscuity among Black and Brown folks of color as well as saying that not having any type of sex would imply that something is wrong with someone who shows little to no sexual desire toward others. Asexual folks, or "ace" as an abbreviated term for this sexual identity, are often not seen as a true part of the LGBTQ+ communities, often being assumed that their sexual minority stressors are not comparable to other sexual minority stressors previously shared. These stressors can also be a primary reason why mental health issues such as depression and anxiety can impact LGBTQ+ folks. Unfortunately, clinicians who can be homophobic and transphobic may willfully ignore the primary concerns of their clients. There are also identity gaps based on intersecting sexual and relationship identities, according to Rubinsky (2021), that can provide a challenge in sexual communication. Therapists would need to become aware of those intersecting identities and how sexual issues in communication may impact how they navigate themselves across contexts and circumstances.

Other sexual minority stressors can occur among sex workers who face legal restrictions over the rights to their bodies, making it difficult to have safer and healthier practices revolving around sex work. Bloomquist and Sprankle (2019) highlight some of the stigma and criminalization of sex work that contribute to negative health outcomes for sex workers. Some of the criminalization can include "threats of arrest, imprisonment, and ... receiv[ing] criminal records for violating prostitution laws" (p. 394). As a result of such stigma and criminalization, some sex worker minority stressors can include identity concealment to avoid legal ramifications and shame, internalized whorephobia, and anticipatory rejection. Bloomquist and Sprankle (2019) also discuss a sex worker-affirmative therapy approach similar to the LGBTQ+ affirmative therapy model that outlines the following for mental health practitioners to provide better mental health care for sex worker clients:

- Acknowledging specific minority stressors as they relate to sex workers and their professional work
- Increasing the competency of sex workers and sex work and going beyond just accepting a client's identity without judgment or treating sex workers like a therapist would with any other client.
- Therapist connecting and becoming a supporter of sex worker communities and organizations
- Visibly identifying as a sex worker-affirmative mental health practitioner
- Highlighting sex workers' strengths; an example includes noting how sex workers are creative in running their business and are great sex educators
- Challenging internalized whorephobia
- Expanding on a support network for sex workers and engaging in a harm reduction approach that also addresses institutional oppression specific to sex workers

There are other foundational standards with the sex worker-affirmative approach; however, for the sake of this literature, the idea is to provide examples of how much awareness, knowledge, and action are needed when working with marginalized communities facing sexual minority stressors and the need for more mental health support regarding what are also mental health issues.

Other communities left out and often misunderstood by mental health professionals include those of different relationship orientations outside of cis-heterosexual monogamous relationships. Often, many of these relationship orientations are classified under consensual non-monogamy (CNM) or ethical non-monogamy (ENM) (Herbitter et al., 2024). There is often double discrimination that can be experienced from those in CNM/ENM relationships. The CNM umbrella term can involve more common terms that involve non-dyadic intimate relationships and interactions such as polyamory, polygamy, swinging. This is also a community that can be hypersexualized as it is assumed that they are practicing non-monogamy for sexual benefits (Herbitter et al., 2024). Stigmatizing are still assumptions around family building for those in CNM/ENM relationships, including receiving rejection and criticism from raising children from other family members (Girard & Brownlee, 2015). There is also double discrimination from other sexual minority groups that either have internalized larger societal messages of monogamy or will reject CNM relationships, who may believe that the sexual identity of those in CNM does not fit into the LGBTQ spectrum. Again, this emphasizes the need for mental health professionals to go just beyond being accepting and non-judgmental of their clients. Some clients may not even share information regarding sex work, their relationship orientation, or other sexual identities due to fear of being judged or not actively taken care of based on those identities with their therapist (Herbitter et al., 2024).

### Disabilities, Chronic Illness, and Perceived Sexlessness

Another community often left out in managing sexual concerns includes folks with disabilities and chronic illnesses. According to Enzlin (2014), most people facing one or more chronic illnesses and/or disabilities are viewed by larger society as "sexless" and experience a "waiting room culture" when even wanting to address sexual issues. Most are even denied in being seen as a sexual being (or on the other end can be very fetishized). Such issues detail the need for therapists and counselors to be aware of specific sexual issues that may vary from person to person, facing similar chronic illnesses and disabilities. Mental health clinicians should also be aware of larger societal stigma around disabilities and sexuality to better assist clients who may not talk about sexual concerns due to fear of being judged or shut down from other perceived biases that involve only focusing on treating and managing the chronic illnesses and/or disabilities (Enzlin, 2014).

### What Is Gained in Discussing Sex in Clinical Spaces: What Clients Take Away from Therapists Open to Discussing Sexuality

To conclude, it was detailed specifically why it is important for mental health clinicians to move past the discomfort in discussing sex because human sexuality is such a broad topic and one embedded with unique mental health issues that will come up in clinical settings with clients. Therefore, it helps to understand what sexual issues come up and within different populations and communities who are impacted in similar and very different ways. On a simpler note, some relevant points were provided below on what can be gained in moving past the discomfort in discussing sex with clients:

Less shame and stigma
Experiencing non-judgmental conversation of sex, reducing fear in discussing sex and sexuality
Understanding complexities and options in sexual identities, cultural identities, and sexual expression
Reduction in mental illness and other psychological concerns having a strong correlation to sexual issues
Culturally specific complexities around sexual pleasure and safety regarding sex and sexuality and understanding the importance of embracing both
More accurate education revolving around sex and sexuality

### What Mental Health Clinicians Can Do to Build Comfort in Talking about Sex

As is noted throughout, sexual communication is important in managing a myriad of sexually complex issues. As mental health clinicians, it is important to be open in building awareness of these issues, their intersecting complexities, and normalizing communication about sex with clients in session. Below are a few suggestions on how mental health professionals can begin building comfort in discussing sex with their clients:

– Practice saying sex-related words and phrases out loud when alone as a step toward building more comfort with saying them in front of a client (can be clinically related sex terms or everyday vernacular as well, if meeting clients where they are at in saying sex terms).
– Buehler (2017) recommends more self-reflection on why sexual issues are uncomfortable to talk about, being proactive in identifying biases and old messages coming up regarding sex and sexuality. This could also be a topic explored in a therapist's own personal therapy.

- Seeking consultation with a supervisor whom mental health clinicians see as a safe space to explore discomfort and negative attitudes toward sex and sexuality.
- Also being proactive in therapists continuing to educate themselves on sex and sexuality. This could be done by watching sex educational video tools, listening to audio tools, reading books on sex therapy and education, and including sex therapy as part of the training CEs required for a majority of mental health professionals to maintain licensure.

Some common sex-related topics that clients can explore in a mental health setting can revolve around sexual communication, sexual health and anatomy, sexual and gender identities, sexual issues, and trauma. Additionally, the more a mental health professional can become comfortable with discussing these topics of sex and sexuality with clients, the more effective they can be in their role as a mental health practitioner. Learning and unlearning about sex and sexuality should be an ongoing process as we continue to evolve and incorporate this in the field of therapy and counseling.

## Questions for Reflection

1  Since different sexual identities and various forms of sexual expression are here to stay and growing, is it possible to consider that our perception of professional development should also grow with more training linked to sexual and mental health?
2  Every human being has internalized biases, and sexual biases are not an exception; thus, would it not be important for mental health professionals to embrace this perspective and continue building awareness to better manage those biases so as not to continue the impact those biases can have on their clients?
3  Who can we also expand within our professional network to continue our professional growth? This can include connecting with sex educators, therapists/counselors, sexological body workers, partner surrogates, and more.

## References

Belous, C. K., Timm, T. M., Chee, G., & Whitehead, M. R. (2012). Revisiting the sexual genogram. *The American Journal of Family Therapy, 40*(4), 281–296. https://doi.org/10.1080/01926187.2011.627317

Bloomquist, K., & Sprankle, E. (2019). Sex worker affirmative therapy: Conceptualization and case study. *Sexual and Relationship Therapy, 34*(3), 392–408. https://doi.org/10.1080/14681994.2019.1620930

Buehler, S. (2017). *What every mental health professional needs to know about sex* (2nd ed.). Springer Publishing Company, LLC. https://search.ebscohost.com/login.aspx?direct=true&scope=site&db=nlebk&db=nlabk&AN=1413602

Constantinides, D. M., Sennott, S. L., & Chandler, D. (2019). *Sex therapy with erotically marginalized clients*. Routledge.

Emond, M., Byers, E. S., Brassard, A., Tremblay, N., & Péloquin, K. (2024). Addressing sexual issues in couples seeking relationship therapy. *Sexual and Relationship Therapy, 39*(1), 115–130. https://doi.org/10.1080/14681994.2021.1969546

Enzlin, P. (2014). Sexuality in the context of chronic illness. In Y. M. Binik, & K. S. Hall (Eds.), *Principles and practices of sex therapy* (5th ed., pp. 436–456). Guildford Press.

Girard, A., & Brownlee, A. (2015). Assessment guidelines and clinical implications for therapists working with couples in sexually open marriages. *Sexual & Relationship Therapy, 30*(4), 462–474. https://doi.org/10.1080/14681994.2015.1028352

Gorden, A. M., Seshadri, G., Glebova, T., & Nylund, D. K. (2024). Sensate focus: addressing potential preconceived notions of black sexuality. *Sexual and Relationship Therapy, 40*(2), 315–339. https://doi.org/10.1080/14681994.2024.2366506

Harden-Bradford, J. (Host). (2022, June 26). Exploring asexuality & aromanticism. [Episode 262]. Therapy for Black Girls. https://podcasts.apple.com/us/podcast/session-262-exploring-asexuality-aromanticism/id1223803641?i=1000566477237

Hargons, C., & Thorpe, S. (2022). #HotGirlScience: A liberatory paradigm for intersectional sex-positive scholarship. *Journal of Positive Sexuality, 8*(1), 3–11. https://doi.org/10.51681/1.811

Herbitter, C., Vaughan, M. D., & Pantalone, D. W. (2024). Mental health provider bias and clinical competence in addressing asexuality, consensual non-monogamy, and BDSM: A narrative review. *Sexual and Relationship Therapy, 39*(1), 131–154. https://doi.org/10.1080/14681994.2021.1969547

Hovick, S. R., & Silver, N. (2019). "Consent is sexy": A poster campaign using sex-positive images and messages to increase dyadic sexual communication. *Journal of American College Health, 67*(8), 817–824. https://doi.org/10.1080/07448481.2018.1515746

Knight, L., Humphries, H., Van der Pol, N., Ncgobo, N., Essack, Z., Rochat, T., & van Rooyen, H. (2023). 'A difficult conversation': Community stakeholders' and key informants' perceptions of the barriers to talking about sex and HIV with adolescents and young people in KwaZulu-Natal, South Africa. *Culture, Health & Sexuality, 25*(12), 1725–1740. https://doi.org/10.1080/13691058.2023.2178674

Machette, A. T., & Montgomery-Vestecka, G. (2023). Applying sexual scripts theory to sexual communication discrepancies. *Communication Reports, 36*(2), 123–135. https://doi.org/10.1080/08934215.2023.2175004

Queen, C., Rednour, S., & Lafrenais, A. (2015). *The sex & pleasure book: Good Vibrations guide to great sex for everyone.* Barnaby LTD, LLC. https://archive.org/details/sexpleasurebookg0000quee

Rubinsky, V. (2021). Exploring the relational nature of identity gap management in sexual communication. *Journal of Intercultural Communication Research, 50*(4), 352–370. https://doi.org/10.1080/17475759.2021.1893794

Thorpe, S., Malone, N., Hargons, C. N., Dogan, J. N., & Jester, J. K. (2022). The peak of pleasure: US southern Black women's definitions of and feelings toward sexual pleasure. *Sexuality & Culture: An Interdisciplinary Journal, 26*(3), 1115–1131. https://doi.org/10.1007/s12119-021-09934-6

# 17 The Impact of Loss, Death, and Bereavement across the Lifespan

*Michelle M. Pliske*

There may be no greater certainty in life than that of death. Death, grief, and anguish are pervasive and an inevitable human experience. Grief is our personal experience of loss, shaped by mourning or the psychological and physiological processing that occurs after the death or a significant loss. We grieve loss hundreds of times over during our lifespan. Loss of a relationship, separation from those we love, loss of a home, loss of a job, loss of a community or an ecosystem, loss of health or ability, loss of our dreams—these losses are in many ways deaths, invoking a sense of lost identity or membership or an end to a piece of ourselves. Social workers are commonly found at the intersection of suffering and loss. We serve postpartum units following pregnancy loss. We are in medical settings comforting families of patients who have lost their loved ones to illness or sudden death. We intervene and support parents who relinquished their child to adoption or foster care. Social workers serve in mental health clinics, providing psychotherapy services to those who are grieving. We hold the hands of the dying and comfort their surviving family members. Social workers create a holding space to nurture and care for those who are unable to make sense of the shattering they have experienced. Understanding the impact of loss requires providers to examine the context of that loss during the course of a client's life.

## Life Course Perspective

The life course perspective analyzes patterns of thought and behaviors for individuals, families, and communities. This theoretical approach attends to the impact of social and structural forces across the individual's lifespan and the impact of those forces on subsequent generations (Elder et al., 2003). The life course perspective challenges us to consider the effects of cohorts, historical timeframes, factors of development or age, environmental influences, cultural norms, and societal factors that catalyze a turning point in our story.

### Cohorts and History

The construct we form as a generation is based on characteristics and the timeframe for which a cohort of people is born. Typically, generations refer to about 20 years, but cohorts can develop within generations to encompass all or some of those 20 years, depending on the social history, shared identity, or events occurring within a specific timeframe. The attack on the World Trade Center in 2001 is one example of cohort development within a generation. Confusion and fear spread across the United States as millions of Americans watched the events unfold live on national television. Millennials (1981–1996) born earlier in the generation differ from those born later in the generation due to their developmental

DOI: 10.4324/9781003531258-20

age and life experience prior to the terrorist attack. Older millennials were undergraduates in college, part of the workforce, or members of the military living independently, of voting age, and ready to engage in critical thinking about the events and the response required. Younger millennials reflect on their experiences being picked up from school by terrified parents, brought home to be immersed in the anxiety of their families and the nation. They describe being too young to understand what was happening around them but carry memories of how that day felt. The terrorist attack is one example of how a generational cohort can fracture through significant life events. Providers often begin by examining the generational or cohort effects of a client. The next step typically shifts the analysis toward assessing major transitions and trajectories the client has experienced as their life has evolved.

### Transitions and Trajectories

Humans move through transitions as their lifespan evolves. The roles or status we hold may drastically change or transform as a result of a life event (Torres & Young, 2016). We cannot escape transition in life. We relocate to new communities, form unions, welcome new life, begin new jobs, enter the military, exit relationships or career choices, and find ways to carry on in life following a death. Rituals surrounding death and bereavement can mark one type of transition. The psychological impact of grief and loss will influence the behavior of a surviving loved one, yet we cannot ignore the collective process of culture and the patterns of relationships within social structures. These social structures provide insight regarding the loss, how the loss has been perceived within the community, and the social nuances of how to mourn (McCoyd et al., 2021). Social rituals are fundamental to the transition during the mourning process. These rituals may vary with individuals, depending upon life course, cultural or spiritual variables, and developmental factors. Trajectories can often best be understood as life in a rearview mirror. Life does not follow a straight line but takes on a new direction following a transition. The transition in life following death or a significant loss can fundamentally change the trajectory of someone's life.

### Life Events and Turning Points

Life events are specific and can become a predominant story in someone's life. The terrorist attacks of September 11 were a life event impacting every generation and cohort. The event was profound, serving as a turning point for countless individuals and families. A death can involve several life events intertwining; therefore, it is helpful to assess the perceived stress of the cluster of life events. Often, life events become the turning point or defining moment that creates a change in trajectory (Hutchison, 2022). Turning points can reveal a personal strength or identify for an individual a new viewpoint of the world they live in. The life course perspective provides support for a narrative context of loss, allowing a provider to shift toward the exploration of compounding factors contributing to grief reactions.

### Compounding Factors for Grief and Loss in the Life Course: Disenfranchised Grief

When survivors are not accorded the right to grieve, they experience disenfranchised grief. That grief may be an expression that is not acceptable within a community, the nature of the loss may influence the grief process, the loss of a relationship could be a factor, or the experiences of grief are not openly acknowledged, socially validated, or publicly observed (Doka, 2002). Grief experienced by children, adolescents, adults, and older adults may have overwhelming support (e.g., the death of a loved one as a result of cancer), while other grief can become disenfranchised when ignored or mocked (e.g., divorce, relinquishment of a child to foster care, loss of a friendship). Doka (1989) offered three classifications to disenfranchised grief: (1) the relationship is not recognized, meaning there is not a recognizable kin tie. These losses could be of friends, neighbors, colleagues, or stepchildren. The loss can have long-lasting impacts but is largely met with confusion by others or minimized as "just life." (2) The loss is unacknowledged, describing a grief process which is not socially defined as significant. This loss may be due to incarceration or institutionalization. It may be a loss associated with a sudden change in the ability or the loss of a parent due to Alzheimer's disease. (3) The griever faces exclusion. These situations of disenfranchised grief detail a griever with little to no social recognition. Persons with intellectual disabilities, young children, and older adults often fall into this classification. Later research by Doka (2008) built two more classifications into our knowledge of disenfranchised grief. (4) Circumstances of the death or the cause of death are stigmatized by society. Examples may be grief experienced due to a suicide or suicide attempt, loss associated with a tragic accident when substances were involved, when a loved one perpetrates a crime and is killed by police, or incarceration leading to execution. Finally, (5) the way an individual grieves can contribute to disenfranchisement. Cultural customs of grief may be viewed by the dominant society as odd or unusual, not following the rules dictated by the overarching societal structure.

### Compounding Factors for Grief and Loss: Trauma

Adverse childhood experiences (ACEs) were traditionally described by Felitti et al. (1998) as childhood abuse (physical, sexual, and psychological or emotional abuse) and household dysfunction (violence, substance abuse, mental illness, suicidal ideation, or incarceration of a family member). Finkelhor et al. (2015) expanded the conceptualization of ACEs to include community factors and environments. Pliske et al. (2022) built an assessment tool modifying the ACE assessment to revise gendered language and the limitation of language related to loss. The tool also took into consideration social determinants of health, discrimination, poverty, historical trauma, racism, and oppression. When an individual presents with grief and loss for any reason, it is prudent to examine the history of that client for adversity and trauma. The client may have experienced multiple losses or have unresolved losses or traumatic histories, complicating the current expression of grief. ACEs and disenfranchised grief can merge the grief and loss responses, complicating mourning. Grief assessment and intervention requires an understanding of developmental aspects influencing grief. Children, adolescents, and adults navigate the process of mourning and develop adaptation in response to loss in direct relation to their life course or lived experiences.

### Grief and Loss across the Lifespan

It hurts to live after someone has died. It just does. It can hurt to walk down a hallway or open the fridge. It hurts to put on a pair of socks, to brush your teeth. Food tastes like nothing. Colors go flat. Music hurts, and so do memories. You look at something you'd otherwise find beautiful—a purple sky at sunset or a playground full of kids and it only somehow deepens the loss. Grief is so lonely this way.

Michelle Obama (2021)

## Childhood Grief

Bowlby (1961) and his subsequent research captured a conversation about bereavement and the impact of loss on children. Prior to Bowlby's work and theory of attachment, many psychologists, analysts, and human service professionals didn't believe children were capable of grief or a mourning process. Bowlby posited that attachment to a caregiver during childhood was a universal phenomenon and children do grieve when separated from their attachment figures (Bowlby, 1980). When separated, children respond with shock, numbness, and disbelief, quickly moving to anger. There are urgent efforts by the child to recover what was lost to them. Over time, children experience despair and longing, moving toward withdrawal and in many cases misery (Bowlby, 1980). Prior to research on attachment and childhood bereavement, it was thought that a child would forget their loss and never face any consequences as a result of that loss. Children were perceived as resilient, and sadness over a loss was expected to be superficial and short-lived. We now know that children are greatly impacted by loss and carry those memories with them throughout their lives. Understandably, adults want to protect children from difficult emotions, including grief, and effectively try to shelter children from suffering. Attempts to protect children more often result in further isolation and exclusion, leaving children in a position to organize their own thoughts and emotions. That organization can become laden with guilt, self-blame, fear, or illogical thinking errors.

## Children's Comprehension of Death

Adults understand that death is irreversible, inevitable, and a universal experience for all living organisms. There is clarity in the knowledge that all things that live will eventually die. Children typically do not reach this knowledge until around the age of eight, due to cognitive developmental processes (Silverman, 2000). However, children who live through the death of a family member and subsequently see over time that the family member has not returned can begin to develop at an early age schematic frameworks around the finality of death. Children may grow observant following the death of a pet, noticing other deaths around them of plants or organisms. These experiences shape their conceptualization of death and dying, altering their knowledge of how death occurs and its implications.

## Preoperational Stage: Ages 2–7

Preschool-age and young school-age children are magical thinkers (Piaget, 1954). Children of this age do not differentiate causality and struggle to remove their own emotions from a logical thought process. A six-year-old child who presented to counseling following the death of her father eventually confessed in session that she was the cause of his death. Her aunt had kept her occupied while her mother made phone calls and funeral arrangements. She read the child her horoscope using a daily app on her smartphone. The aunt told her niece she was a cancer, which was identified by her birthdate. The child was convinced that because she was born a cancer, and her father died of cancer, she was to blame. Young children struggle to comprehend the irreversibility of death, often thinking in terms of what they know; therefore, folklore and fairy tales are applied to the construction of meaning. One five-year-old expressed with intense anger and disbelief that her mother wouldn't kiss her father at his funeral. The kiss would wake him, and he could come home. Another seven-year-old child wanted to visit her mother in heaven, just for the day. If she died too and went to heaven, she could see her mother and come home before dinner. Children attribute emotions and sensations to the dead during this developmental stage. One father described his seven-year-old daughter in a complete panic at the funeral. His wife, who died of breast cancer, had chosen the dress she wanted to be laid out in during the funeral. She wanted light colors and to be remembered for her bright personality, a woman who had loved life deeply. Her daughter saw this dress during the month of January and began screaming that her mother would be cold. She was desperate to give her mother a coat before they closed the casket and buried her in the ground. Children of this age are concrete in their thinking, often literal, and can distort reality to conform whatever data they are being presented with to their current understanding of the phenomenon, despite contradictions (Shaffer & Kipp, 2014). Children of this age may also struggle with worry about where their loved one has gone and be afraid that others will die too, leading to regression and separation anxiety. Young children may not present with typical reactions we often associate with grief or may experience their grief intermittently, confusing family members (Webb, 2010).

## Concrete Operations: Ages 7–11

Children of this age will master the understanding that death is final and permanent. Piaget (1954) reported his reasoning about children's use of language and symbolism, transforming their thinking and cognitive abilities toward greater complexity. Children can begin to understand perspective taking and identify others' emotions around them as being separate from their own. Children of this age are influenced by media and literature, developing concepts of ghosts, angels, and other cultural frameworks for imagery associated with death. A ten-year-old boy feared he would become haunted by his grandmother because she had died in their home. Cultural approaches to death and dying will significantly influence a child's perspective. An 11-year-old child described her family's Irish wake following the death of her uncle. She recalled the party of family and friends coming to celebrate his life. Her mother described laughter and sharing stories were the best way to honor the dead and medicine for the living to survive their loss. Another child, age nine, described her anticipation of día de muertos (Day of the Dead). She helped select photographs of her abuela (grandmother), candles, and food to place on her family's altar. The involvement in the ritual and event brought comfort and a sense of importance and belonging.

## Grief Therapy for Children

Clinical mental health professionals are required to complete a comprehensive psychological assessment not only to determine the nature of the loss and previous exposure to ACEs but also to gather information pertinent to diagnostic considerations of mental health-related illnesses. Children experiencing grief and loss are served well in generalist counseling practices, in non-clinical settings, or through grief and loss support centers. Some children will require clinical intervention due to meeting criteria for a mental health condition, or there is a greater risk and impairment to the child's well-being. Assessments should follow a comprehensive process to gather information holistically about the child, their environment, and grief-related factors and to determine the appropriate level of care, as shown in Figure 17.1.

Children entering grief counseling benefit from individual, group, and family evidence-based counseling interventions. Individual counseling provides an opportunity for

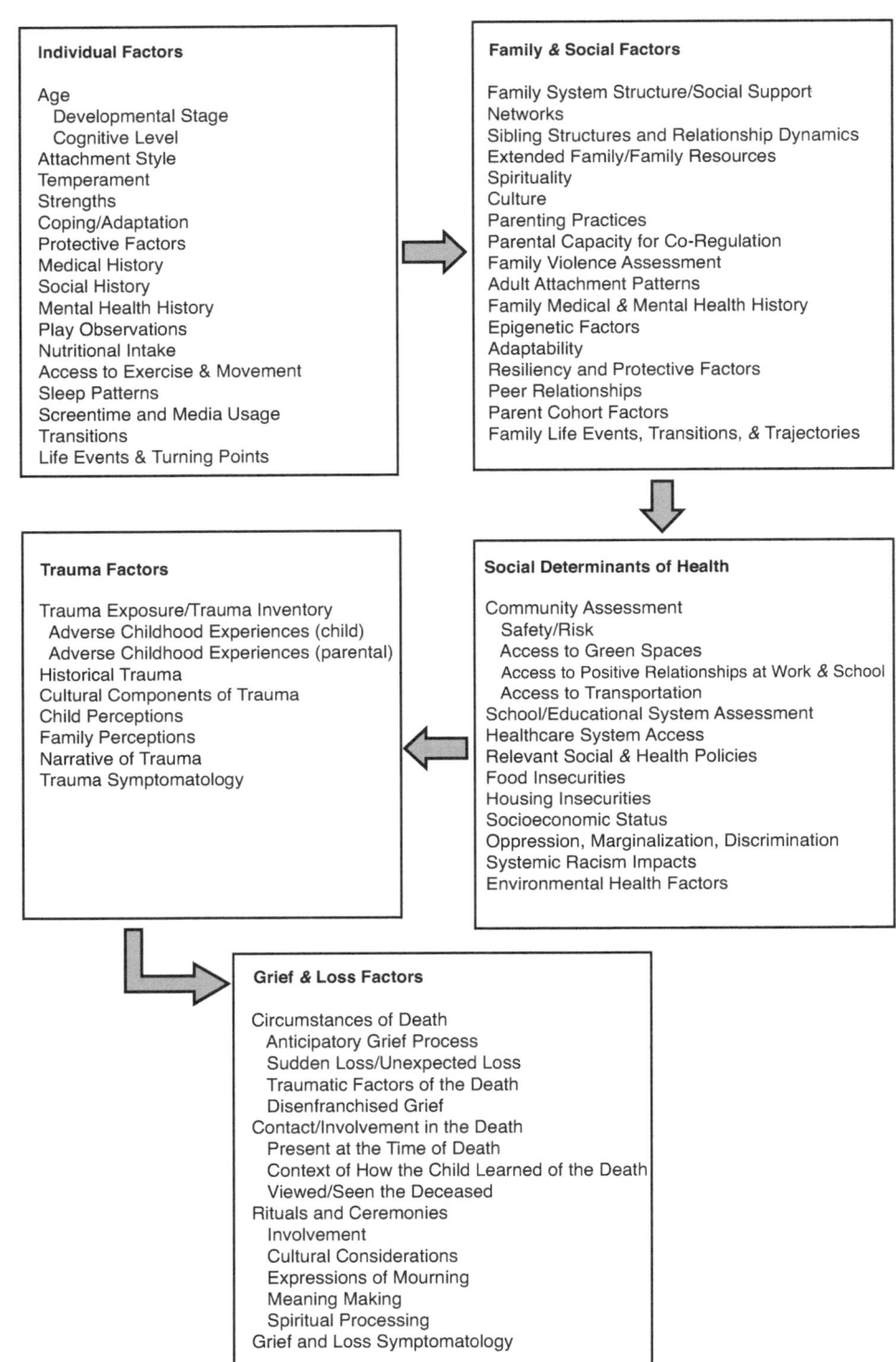

*Figure 17.1* Pentad assessment process for childhood bereavement.

a child to explore their emotions and grief story without needing to edit or adjust the story, depending upon who is in the room (e.g., family members, peers also experiencing grief). Providers create an environment with the space they welcome children into and through their own affect and engagement with the child. The environment plays a critical role in the child's ability to approach difficult content; therefore, the creation of a therapeutic holding space is a combination of the child's access to play with a provider who can co-regulate their experience (Ray, 2011; Winnicott, 1996). Materials are selected by the provider to thoughtfully provide options to children for the expression of positive and negative emotions. Children gain access to toys and art materials to support a range of behaviors and experiences from warm and nurturing play to aggressive play or play with themes of violence. Allowing children the ability to take the lead in what they play and how they play fosters non-verbal and verbal processing of grief.

Brea (age seven) and Anna (age five) entered into therapy one week prior to their mother's death. The hospice team admitted their mother, Jen, who was diagnosed with Amyotrophic Lateral Sclerosis (ALS). The hospice team was preparing to remove life support the following week. Jen and her husband, Mark, wanted to ensure Brea and Anna understood what was happening and were prepared for the loss. They didn't understand why so many hospital people were in their home and what was wrong with their mother. The family needed help facilitating a conversation with Brea and Anna to explain what was happening. Jen told them about the diagnosis, stating the disease had no cure, which meant the doctors couldn't make it go away. She assured her children the illness couldn't be caught (like a cough or a cold) and that it was not their fault she was ill. The hospice team described the death and dying process and what the family could expect to see the following week. Jen and Mark assured Brea and Anna that they were loved. They had a conversation about their philosophy of an afterlife. Jen told both girls she believed she would be in heaven with God.

The girls engaged in individual sessions over the course of the week leading up to their mother's death. Brea wanted to know everything she could about death, asking questions and using the materials in the play therapy room to understand what was happening. She revisited her mother's narrative repeatedly, finally deciding on creating an image of heaven. Brea painted an image of her mother under a rainbow surrounded by trees. She described that in this place no one was sick and that everyone was safe and loved.

Anna attended her individual sessions and, with a five-year-old's curiosity, explored the medical play toys, replicating much of what she had seen in her home. She checked vital signs and described how a medicine would taste or how a procedure would feel. Anna told me the puppet she cared for was very, very sick and he would die. She explained that when he died he would be gone and we wouldn't be able to see him anymore. Anna described how the puppet would go to heaven and then paused. Anna couldn't capture in words her thinking about heaven and instead turned to the sandtray and created an image in the sand of heaven. She used trees and plants to build her image, selecting a large rainbow which arched across the tray. She selected a queen and placed her under the rainbow, surrounded by gems and shining rocks. "This is heaven. It is a place where you are warm all the time and never sick. This is where mama is going."

Brea and Anna needed to create a concrete representation of the abstract concept of heaven presented to them. They independently made their images. Anna was given a picture of her sandtray, and when she shared her image with Brea they were amazed to see the similarities. They decided to bring their artwork to their parents and talk about their discovery together. The family therapy session that followed was one of shared insights and connection. Each family member was open about the magnitude of the loss and how they would remember Jen. They decided to plant a tree in their yard, similar to what the girls depicted in their artwork. This tree became a foundation of remembrance and a place where the girls could contribute painted stones and sit with the memory of their mother as a continued bond. Brea and Anna were both given a rainbow pendant to wear on the day their mother died. She wanted them to be able to keep her close to their hearts and know she was with the rainbows, safe and warm, no longer sick or in pain. Mark hung crystals in the window in the months following Jen's death. He recounted hearing the girls exclaim, "mommy!" from the living arriving to find them dancing among what appeared to be hundreds of rainbows. Their laughter and sheer joy in that moment was what he described as a knowing that there could be life after death. Brea and Anna's story demonstrated several protective factors, including stable and supportive relationships, open communication, encouragement, routine and structure, and emotional support, combined with positive memory and legacy building. Table 17.1 provides a list of protective factors which serve to reduce the impact of loss and support the psychological well-being of grieving children.

*Table 17.1* Protective Factors for Bereaved Children

| | |
|---|---|
| *Stable and Supportive Relationships* | Secure attachments and nurturing relationships with surviving family members and other supportive adults. These adult relationships provide consistent support without obligations from the child to earn their attention. |
| *Open Communication* | Transparency with age-appropriate conversations about death and dying, the loss, and emotions related to it. |
| *Encouragement* | Creating opportunities to express feelings and ask questions. Children may ask repetitive questions. Providers and caregivers can answer these questions consistently and without judgment. |
| *Routine and Structure* | Maintaining daily routines will provide a sense of normalcy and security. Predictable schedules help children feel more in control and reduce anxiety. |
| *Healthy Coping Strategies* | Encouragement in activities that promote relaxation and emotional expression, such as arts, sports, and hobbies, is beneficial. Children with access to creative arts have an outlet for self-expression or catharsis. Providers and caregivers can use direct and indirect teaching to promote and model healthy ways to cope with stress and emotions. |
| *Physical Health* | Focusing on pillars of health, including nutrition, sleep, and exercise, will support a stronger foundation for emotional regulation. |
| *Emotional Support* | Children need access to counseling or support groups specifically designed for bereaved children. Ideally, children connect to providers with additional training and expertise in grief and loss work. Expansion of emotional support to community resources (e.g., teachers, school counselors, and clergy) creates a larger availability of trusted adults who can provide emotional guidance and reassurance. |
| *Educational Support* | Involving the child's school will help develop an understanding and supportive school environment. Teachers and school counselors who are aware of the child's situation can provide additional support as needed. |
| *Peer Support* | Opportunities to interact with peers who have experienced similar losses create a like-me phenomenon. Children feel less isolated and alone. Peer-based group activities can promote social connections and shared experiences. |
| *Positive Memories and Legacy Building* | Children need to see their loved ones. Maintaining photos in their room or the home provides access to a visual memory. Children should be included in building activities that help the child remember and honor the deceased, such as creating memory books or participating in rituals. |

*Adolescent Grief*

Adolescence, occurring between childhood and adulthood, involves dramatic changes in physical development, cognitive development, and emotional development. Teenagers take on new roles and new responsibilities, and they begin to develop their identities, a framework for how they see themselves and the world they live in (Siegel, 2013). The grief process differs from that of children and adults. Teens may find themselves grappling with existential questions about religion or spirituality. They may not necessarily believe in the same faith structures as their parents or extended family. Adolescence serves as a time for spiritual inquiry, and many teens find themselves open to learning and exploring many religious or spiritual perspectives (McCoyd et al., 2021). There may be unresolved issues with the person who has died or is dying. Teens have access to information and technology at their fingertips. Social media resources, an abundance of messaging and knowledge, are shared on the internet, which can serve to support or hinder the grief process. Adolescents may struggle with the circumstances surrounding death and experience a significant transition because of the life event. Adolescents feel deeply and can experience intense emotions (Dorn et al., 2019). Loss experienced by teens can sometimes confuse parents. One parent of a 13-year-old child struggled to understand how the death of an acquaintance could evoke strong emotions that are more typically reserved for a family member. The still-developing prefrontal cortex limits executive functioning and judgments or decision-making (Siegel, 2013). Intensely felt emotions can lead to impulsive behaviors and risk-taking. Alternatively, teens may limit or mask their emotions ("I'm fine") in the presence of family or other adults. They may not want to burden others or simply want to present themselves as more adult-like, thinking adults should offer little emoting or expression.

*Grief Therapy for Adolescents*

Adolescents experiencing grief and loss benefit from environments which promote unconditional positive regard, mutual empathy, authenticity, integrity, and an ability to express thoughts and emotions through a variety of methods. Teens engage easily in talk-based therapies yet appreciate room for creativity and self-exploration through expressive arts (e.g., music, therapeutic art, movement, sandtray).

Assessment of the adolescent follows a comprehensive pentad model to support arriving at a diagnosis (if appropriate) and to guide interventions and care plans. Teens are squarely embedded in a complex environmental web of educational systems, healthcare systems, family systems, and, in some cases, legal systems. Creating plans which are multisystemic supports the teen within their environment. These plans typically entail individual, family, and group support with collaboration and advocacy at the community level as needed. The assessment and subsequent counseling process should allow for enough time and space for a teen to set the pace and have a sense of control over the process. The provider's process in building a trusting and secure relationship creates the necessary base to challenge thinking or offer alternative perspectives.

The concept of continuing bonds can be woven into the fabric of therapeutic storytelling for adolescents, giving room to piece together their narrative and find meaning as they navigate the next chapter. Creating a continuing bond posits that grief is a transitional process following a life event. The event shifted the individual's trajectory in life. While a teen adjusts to the loss of the relationship, they can simultaneously redefine and continue the relationship in a separate way (Klass et al., 1996). Providers can help teens adjust and transition their relationship toward memories, rituals, and thoughts as opposed to a physical presence. Teens can develop strategies to continue their relationship. These strategies might contain skills to have conversations with their loved one in their mind or through writing (journaling or letter writing). One teen wrote letters to her mother she kept in a journal. This gave her the ability to share her thoughts or simply talk about her day. Teens process loss through specific activities. A 17-year-old girl drove an hour each year on her best friend's birthday to sit by the ocean. They had "their spot" at the coast, and she would talk with her friend, sit, and relax, watching the waves roll in and out until dusk. Another avenue to continue bonds and the relationship is through honoring the legacy of that relationship. Teens can dedicate a performance or pay tribute to the deceased through a gesture before a big event or game. The goal is for teens to have ample space to explore who they are, develop their identity shaped by loss, and find pathways for continued connection.

Family therapy options for teens impacted by grief serve to build social support and strengthen relationships. Teens from families who have experienced loss within their immediate family can be helped by being invited to rewrite the script and transform an isolated grief experience into a shared grief experience. Allowing each family member an opportunity to share their own emotions, thoughts about the deceased, and the roles that loss vacated in the family bridges the conversation toward a new chapter for how the family will remember. Families can contribute to their expectations for how roles will be performed or handled as they rebalance or find a new equilibrium. The outcome is to help families find cohesion and unity through collaboration, mutual empathy, and communication. Protective factors, as described to support childhood bereavement, apply to adolescent populations and can be expanded to include adaptive coping unique to adolescent support of grief expressions.

### Adaptive Coping

Protective factors detailed within the section on childhood bereavement can be applied to adolescent well-being and serve to support adaptive coping. One 15-year-old teen described grief as feeling like a storm. Sometimes he would become drenched by emotions. His goal was to make sure his storm did not become a hurricane, something out of his control and overwhelming. Adaptive coping is a prevention plan for teens. Supporting adolescents in building adaptive coping strategies can provide assistance to weather the storm. Table 17.2 outlines adaptive coping mechanisms for adolescents experiencing disenfranchised grief or bereavement.

### Adult Grief

Adults experiencing grief differ from children and adolescents by the nature of their lived experiences, roles, and responsibilities occurring within the context of grief. Bereaved adults describe sadness as the most common feeling, sometimes resulting in shame or guilt because of the expression of that sadness. Brea and Anna's father left the bedside of his wife after the hospice team declared her death and walked outside. He described that he "lost it," collapsing on the front lawn, weeping. His daughters joined him, and they held one another in their grief. His recounting of the event and the intense shame associated with showing such emotion, as opposed to "being strong for my family" filled Mark with worry about how he had potentially damaged his children. The reality was that he provided a gift of modeling grief during a moment of human suffering. No one needs to suffer alone, and during the aftermath of profound loss, the family stayed connected in their shared

*Table 17.2* Adaptive Coping Skills for Adolescent Bereavement Support

| | |
|---|---|
| *Journaling* | Creative writing or journaling about emotions, thoughts, and memories of the deceased can serve to support a teen in developing their grief narrative. Providers can give prompts to help teens explore their emotions and process their grief more fully. |
| *Creative Expression* | Teens who develop strategies for using creative expression (modalities such as art, music, writing, or theater) create an outlet for expressing emotions. Simultaneously teens are building lifelong roadmaps for how to process adverse experiences over the trajectory of their lifespan (Pliske et al., 2021). |
| *Mindfulness and Relaxation Techniques* | Teens need structure and guidance for how to participate in mindfulness exercises, such as deep breathing, meditation, or progressive muscle relaxation. Providers can facilitate and demonstrate these exercises and guide teens toward appropriate media supports accessible through a phone or tablet. |
| *Physical Activity* | Teens should be encouraged to engage in regular physical activity, such as walking, running, yoga, or team sports. Exercise offers a release for pent-up emotions and reduces stress. |
| *Social Support* | Teens are social creatures and naturally want to gravitate toward peer support. Spending time with friends who provide emotional support and understanding serves as a resource during the grief process. Family and support groups serve a grieving teen, whether that is through talking or simply being in the presence of a person who cares about and supports them. Psychoeducation and skill-building can support teens in learning how to set boundaries with others or when they need time alone and are not ready to talk about their grief. |
| *Healthy Lifestyle Choices* | Teens can struggle with making good choices around nutrition and sleep. Providers help develop a lifestyle of good sleep hygiene habits, nutritious eating, and recreational time to reduce stress. |
| *Relaxation and Self-Care Activities* | Providers can help teens build a routine around activities that promote relaxation and self-care, such as taking baths, reading, or listening to music. Teens are busy and often under significant pressure to succeed. Scheduling regular "me-time" to unwind and recharge can not only serve them in their academic pursuits but also aid in preparation for when grief and loss resurface. |
| *Talking About the Deceased* | Storytelling and shared memories of the deceased support continued bonds. Providers can support families in creating rituals or traditions to honor the memory of a loved one. |
| *Engaging in Meaningful Activities* | Teens are in a cohort with an ethos of activism and community engagement. Providers can assist teens in discovering activities that give a sense of purpose and fulfillment, such as volunteering or helping others. Teens may find a connection to their loved one or find meaning by channeling grief into positive actions. These actions could include fundraising for a cause related to the deceased or the circumstances surrounding the loss. |

experience of intense pain. Bereaved adults report experiencing anger, often coming from one of two sources: a sense of frustration that nothing could be done to prevent the death or an anger, which is regressive in its experience following the loss (Worden, 2009). Adults describe an experience of a continued mixed bag of emotions: guilt and self-reproach, anxiety, loneliness, fatigue, helplessness, shock, yearning, emancipation, relief, and numbness (Walsh, 2023). They depict their emotions through words of physical pain. Eisenberger and Lieberman (2004) articulated research findings of the brain's response to pain. The anterior cingulate cortex did not distinguish between social pain and physical pain. Simply put, the brain registers pain as pain regardless of its origin. Connections are essential to life; therefore, the loss of a connection is typically captured in terms of pain and anguish: "I'm heartbroken," "this is gut-wrenching," or "I feel sick."

### Grief Therapy for Adults

A comprehensive biopsychosocial assessment will help determine whether a client meets criteria for a mental health condition comorbid with grief and bereavement or whether the client meets a prolonged grief diagnosis. Prolonged grief disorder is defined by the American Psychological Association (2022) as an identity disruption (e.g., feeling as though part of oneself has died) with a marked sense of disbelief about the death, avoidance of reminders, and intense emotional pain related to the loss. Adults report difficulty with reintegration into life following the loss (e.g., problems engaging with friends, pursuing interests, planning for the future), emotional numbness (e.g., absence or marked reduction of emotional experience), a feeling that life is meaningless, and intense loneliness (e.g., feeling alone or detached from others) (American Psychological Association, 2022). Assessment of the bereaved adult is structured and inclusive to understand community and cultural experiences, including those associated with death, and encompasses an inventory of the client's social determinants of health. Assessment processes evaluate ACEs, disenfranchised grief experiences across the lifespan, and protective factors.

Grief counseling with adults classically follows the specific goals of (1) helping the client accept the reality of the loss, (2) helping the client navigate the emotional pain and behaviors of grief, (3) helping the client readjust to new roles or expectations following transition, (4) helping the client find meaning following a loss, and (5) devising a method for maintaining a bond with the deceased (Worden, 2009). Grief counseling requires flexibility to adapt to these classic goals, depending upon the type of grief experience or the circumstance the client is facing. Disenfranchised grief may involve a grief process due to divorce, loss of ability, loss of a job, and invisible losses such as pregnancy loss. Goals can be adapted to best meet the needs of the client and then specifically tailored to the type of loss and circumstances leading up to the loss.

Therapeutic work with adults requires a relationship built on trust in an environment which can support complex processing of emotions. Adult clients expect authentic connections to allow small risks to be taken as more is revealed about the self in the process of therapy (Jordan, 2018). The goals or tasks before the bereaved adult benefit from conversation and unpacking the layers of loss. Grief is never just about the person who was lost but encompasses a loss of roles, identities, labels, futures, and fantasies. One client described the loss of her husband as "infinite losses." She lost her spouse, but she also lost her children's father, her identity as a wife, the fantasy they held together about building their dream home, and a future of retirement and growing old with one another. She lost her financial security. She lost her sense of direction as he served as the compass in their family. She lost her lover and best friend. She described her grief in terms of layers. She could only face the topsoil depth under the magnitude of so many interconnected losses. She described that at some point she would reach the bedrock of her grief, viewing therapy as someone handing her the shovel, standing alongside her in reassurance as she dug toward her pain.

Life-limiting and terminal illnesses give rise to questions of disbelief and uncertainty. Audre Lorde reflected on her diagnosis of breast cancer at age 44 as "I carry tattooed upon my heart a list of names of women who did not survive, and there is always a space left for one more, my own" (Gay, 2020, p. 101). Adults facing loss of ability and end of life need an opening to say what hasn't been said, bringing them closer to family, friends, or community. Adults want to avoid unresolved or unfinished business. Talking about what feels taboo or about an issue that hasn't been touched in years allows the dying to continue participating in their life with control (Kessler, 2007). Providers can bridge communication-scaffolding support for their adult clients to share what needs to be said while there is time to process past events or old wounds. The needs of adults at the end of life are to control pain; provide humane, comfortable living conditions; preserve the dignity and worth of the individual; and offer unconditional love with continued affection.

## Conclusion

The experience of being human and living life wholeheartedly also means we cannot escape loss. Grief is experienced over the course of a lifespan because we are social beings wired to connect and love deeply. To love another person and have a passion for a career, a home, and a way of being is a risk we take in leading a full life. No one is immune to social problems or suffering. Life events, whether they are expected or unexpected, will shift our worldview and perspective as we adjust and approach life in a new way. Grief counseling shines a light into what otherwise feels like a landscape of darkness. We cannot offer a cure to grief, only illuminate a path toward living with the loss. We guide our clients toward how to repair and rebuild their lives around the loss, remembering the significance of the loss and the legacy we leave behind.

## Reflective Questions for Consideration

1 Thinking about the life course perspective, what experiences of loss have created a transition or new trajectory in your life? How did the loss impact you and your family? Does that experience influence your work as a helping professional?
2 How do cultural attitudes toward death and mourning influence a child's or adolescent's grief experience?
3 What role does the family unit play in supporting a grieving child or adolescent, and how can family dynamics complicate or assist the grieving process?
4 What roles do social support systems (e.g., family, friends, and community groups) play in supporting grieving adults, and how might these systems change as individuals age?
5 How does the cumulative nature of loss (e.g., loss of peers, physical abilities, independence) affect the grief process in older adults?

## References

American Psychological Association. (2022). *Diagnostic and statistical manual of mental health disorders* (5th ed., Text Revision). American Psychological Association.
Bowlby, J. (1961). Childhood mourning and its implications for psychiatry. *American Journal of Psychiatry, 118,* 481–498. https://doi.org/10.1176/ajp.118.6.481
Bowlby, J. (1980). *Attachment and loss volume III: Loss, sadness, and depression.* Basic Books.
Dorn, L. D., Hostinar, C. E., Susman, E. J., & Pervanidou, P. (2019). Conceptualizing puberty as a window of opportunity for impacting health and well-being across the life span. *Journal of Research on Adolescence, 29*(1), 155–176. https://doi.org/10.1111/jora.12431
Doka, K. J. (1989). *Disenfranchised grief: Recognizing hidden sorrow.* Lexington Books.

Doka, K. J. (2002). Theoretical overview. In K. J. Doka (Ed.), *Disenfranchised grief: New directions, challenges, and strategies for practice* (pp. 1–22). Research Press.

Doka, K. J. (2008). Disenfranchised grief in historical and cultural perspective. In M. S. Stroebe, R. O. Hansson, H. Schut, & W. Stroebe (Eds.), *Handbook of bereavement research and practice: Advances in theory and intervention* (pp. 223–240). American Psychological Association. https://doi.org/10.1037/14498-011

Eisenberger, N. I., & Lieberman, M. D. (2004). Why rejection hurts: A common neural alarms system for physical and social pain. *Trends in Cognitive Sciences, 8,* 294–300. https://doi.org/10.1016/j.tics.2004.05.010

Elder, G. H., Johnson, M. K., & Crosnoe, R. (2003). The emergence and development of life course theory. In J. T. Mortimer, & M. J. Shanahan (Eds), *Handbook of the life course. handbooks of sociology and social research* (pp 3–19). Springer. https://doi.org/10.1007/978-0-306-48247-2_1

Felitti, V. J., Anda, R. F., Nordenberg, D., Williamson, D. F., Spitz, A. M., Edwards, V., Koss, M. P., & Marks, J. S. (1998). Relationship of childhood abuse and household dysfunction to many of the leading causes of death in adults: The adverse childhood experiences (ACE) study. *American Journal of Preventive Medicine, 14*(4), 245–258. https://doi.org/10.1016/S0749-3797(98)00017-8

Finkelhor, D., Shattuck, A., Turner, H., & Hamby, S. (2015). A revised inventory of adverse childhood experiences. *Child Abuse and Neglect, 45,* 13–21. https://doi.org/10.1016/j.chiabu.2015.07.011

Gay, R. (2020). *The selected works of Audre Lorde.* Norton.

Hutchison, E. D. (2022). The human life journey: A life course perspective. In E. D. Hutchison, & L W. Wood (Eds.), *Essentials of human behavior: Integrating person, environment, and the life course* (3rd ed., pp. 329–357). Sage.

Jordan, J. V. (2018). *Relational-cultural therapy.* American Psychological Association.

Kessler, D. (2007). *The needs of the dying: A guide for bringing hope, comfort, and love to life's final chapter.* Harper.

Klass, D., Silverman, S., & Nickman, S. (1996). *Continuing bonds: New understandings of grief.* Taylor & Francis.

McCoyd, J. L. M., Koller, J. M., & Walter, C. A. (2021). *Grief and loss across the lifespan: A biopsychosocial approach* (3rd ed.). Springer.

Obama, M. (2021). *Becoming.* Crown.

Piaget, J. (1954). *The construction of reality in the child.* Basic Books.

Pliske, M., Stauffer, S., & Werner-Lin, A. (2021). Healing from adverse childhood experiences through therapeutic powers of play: "I can do it with my hands." *International Journal of Play Therapy, 30*(4), 244–258. https://doi.org/10.1037/pla0000166

Pliske, M., Werner-Lin, A., & Stauffer, S. (2022). Posttraumatic growth following adverse childhood experiences: "My creative arts teacher got me through it." *Psychology and Behavioral Sciences, 11*(4), 102–115. https://doi.org/10.11648/j.pbs.20221104.11

Ray, D. C. (2011). *Advanced play therapy: Essential conditions, knowledge, and skills for child practice.* Routledge.

Siegel, D. J. (2013). *Brainstorm: The power and purpose of the teenage brain.* Tarcher Penguin.

Silverman, P. R. (2000). *Never too young to know: Death in children's lives.* Oxford University Press.

Shaffer, D. R., & Kipp, K. (2014). *Developmental psychology: Childhood and adolescence* (9th ed.). Cengage.

Torres, J., & Young, M. (2016). A life-course perspective on legal status stratification and health. *SSM—Population Health, 2,* 141–148. https://doi.org/10.1016/j.ssmph.2016.02.011

Walsh, F. (2023). *Complex and traumatic loss: Fostering healing and resilience.* Guilford Press.

Webb, N. B. (2010). The child and death. In N. B. Webb (Ed.), *Helping bereaved children* (3rd ed., pp. 3–21). Guilford Press.

Winnicott, D. W. (1996). *Thinking about children.* Karnac Books.

Worden, J. W. (2009). *Grief counseling and grief therapy: A handbook for the mental health practitioner* (4th ed.). Springer.

# Section III

# Leading Conversations

Cultural Considerations and Social Justice

# 18 Edge Dancers

## Mixed Heritage Identity Negotiation of Multiracial/Ethnic Students in Higher Education—Are They Welcome in Human Services Departments?

*Mikel Hogan*

## Introduction

The academic discipline of Human Services operates as a microcosm of the larger societal context in which the ideology of monoracism, white supremacy, and hypodescent still prevail as part of a long legacy of colonization. The attempted insurrection on January 6, 2021, was to stop the certification of the 2020 election. Alongside this, the dire impact of the COVID-19 pandemic on Black, Indigenous, and People of Color (BIPOC) and other vulnerable communities, the public murder of George Floyd in 2020, and the ongoing killing of people of color by police propels the current racial justice movement. These events clearly demonstrate that the United States has not effectively resolved its political, economic, educational, and social system failures in crafting an inclusive democracy. These social system failures are embedded in our denial and avoidance of the long legacy of racism and the interrelationship of racism, sexism, and economic and other forms of oppression that form the social fabric of this country dating back to colonial days and even earlier in the interest of power and property (Alim et al., 2020; French, 2022; Hill, 2017; Horne, 2017, 2020; Wijeyesinghe, 2021; Wolf, 1999).

For this chapter on the experience of mixed-race/ethnic people in academic programs inclusive of human services and recommendations for change, I underscore the deep-seated and prevailing beliefs in monoracism, white supremacy, and the rule of hypodescent that form the ideological foundation of U.S. academic programs nationally and underpin a global power system in which whiteness is central to the construction of our racialized unequal world (Annamma & Booker, 2020; Beliso-De Jesús & Pierre 2019; Beliso-De Jesús et al., 2023; Demerath, 2022; French, 2022; Horne, 2017, 2020).

Flowing from this historical ideological context and in the interest of power and property, the U.S. national culture defines race in essentialist terms of a Black/white binary monoracial, hierarchical classification system called the "monoracial imperative." Monoracism is defined by Johnston and Nadel as "a social system of psychological inequality where individuals who do not fit monoracial categories may be oppressed on systemic and interpersonal levels because of underlying assumptions and beliefs in singular discrete racial categories" (2010, p. 125). Additionally, Hamako defines monoracism as "the systemic privileging of things, people, and practices that are racialized, as a single race and or racially pure" (2014, p. 81). U.S. social devices, such as laws, policies, and institutions, are all informed and crafted according to the monoracial imperative (persons only fit into one race category) and rule of hypodescent (also called the "one-drop rule") in which mixed-race persons are defined as belonging to the race considered as subordinate within the U.S. racial classification system. Such as a person of Black and white heritage would be considered

DOI: 10.4324/9781003531258-22

Black. The "one-drop rule" aligns blood to racial advantages and disadvantages, which relate to power and property, as enslaved Black people in the past could not own property and that legacy lives on in current disparities in housing and homeownership (Hill, 2017, pp. 13–22). People of mixed race are therefore perceived and rendered invisible through the monoracial imperative and rule of hypodescent in which they are assigned to one racial category that is subordinate or inferior (Houston & Hogan, 2009, p. 55; Johnston-Guerrero et al., 2021). Moreover, the constructs of monoracism, white supremacy, and the rule of hypodescent normalize how multiracial people are forced to identify with one race rather than their multiple heritage identity. White supremacy is an aspect of monoracism in that it reinforces the concept of "monorace" as a biological category in which whiteness is defined as the top of the racial classification system, conferring purity, status, and privilege as inherent to anyone with white skin. Recent claims by white nationalists that their DNA ancestry tests demonstrate their racial purity and superiority due to their European roots are a current example of the interrelationship of biological notions of racial superiority, monoracism, and white supremacy that have a cumulative negative impact on mixed-race/ethnic people, as this chapter will show.

## Background Research Literature on Mixed-Race/Ethnic Persons and the Term "Edge Dancers"

Individuals identifying as multiracial/ethnic are currently one of the fastest-growing minoritized groups in the United States (Misa-Escalante et al., 2022). The terms "multiracial/ethnic," "mixed race/ethnic," and "multiple/mixed heritage" will be used interchangeably throughout this chapter. Social factors that underlie the increase in mixed-race/ethnic persons include the changes in U.S. immigration law during the 1960s that allowed an influx of non-European immigrants into the United States (Koppelman, 2020, pp. 160–161). Two other developments are the landmark 1967 civil rights case of *Loving vs. the Commonwealth of Virginia* that ended all race-based legal restrictions on marriage and the globalization of the world's economy in which there is the rapid flow of information, trade goods, natural resources, finance capital, human labor, and international and national inter-marriages leading to the inevitable birth of mixed-race, mixed ethnic-heritage children (Houston & Hogan, 2009, pp. 50–51; Koppelman, 2020, pp. 160–161).

A consequence of the increase in mixed-race/ethic persons within academic institutions is that scholars and researchers did not recognize or articulate the lived experiences and identities of mixed-race/ethnic persons until the 1980s with such publications as Paul Spickard's *Mixed Blood: Intermarriage and Ethnic Identity in Twentieth-Century America* (1989) and Maria Root's anthology *Racially Mixed People in America* (1992).

The term "Edge Dancers" coined in 2009 by Houston and Hogan in their publication "Edge Dancers: Mixed Heritage Identity, Transculturalization, and Public Policy and Practice in Health and Human Services" was inspired by the ethnographic study in 2001 of multiracial white-Vietnamese Americans by K. Valverde. In the ethnography, for example, Valverde describes the dynamic identity-defining efforts of mixed-white/Vietnamese Americans as doing "the mixed-race dance." Houston and Hogan describe further, "Within a community context of class hierarchy rife with gross generalizations and stereotypes about multiracial individuals" [Valverde]

> adeptly documents how multiracial Vietnamese negotiate and create a social space for themselves. The ability of these individuals to maneuver this classification system varies

by person and situation, but Valverde perceptively refers to their performance and agency as, "doing the mixed-race dance."

(Houston & Hogan, 2009, p. 49)

Houston and Hogan draw from Valverde's metaphor and coin the term "edge dancers" to present their research on the lived experiences and identity negotiations of mixed-race/ethnic individuals in the United States, calling their model the "Dynamic, Emic Agency Model of Mixed Heritage Identity Construction" (2009, p. 66).

Houston and Hogan describe mixed-race/ethnic individuals as "edge dancers" whose dance of identity construction is fluid, multidirectional, and dynamic, not at all static nor linear (2009, p. 66). Furthermore, the interviewees' racial and ethnic identity "dance" revealed three experiential themes of *alienation, complexity, and celebration. Alienation* is the emotional pain experienced in relation to bullying and constant "subtle acts of exclusion" or microaggressions (Jana & Baran, 2020). For example, the following case of a Japanese/Black interviewee illustrates microaggressions about the racial and ethnic differences within mixed-race/ethnic families. The Japanese/Black interviewee described the anger and frustration she felt when several of her father's Black family members told her she was "too Japanese," and her maternal Japanese grandmother told her she was "too Black" in relation to her physical appearance, her hair, and the way she danced (Houston & Hogan, 2009, p. 58). Another Japanese/white interviewee described the cruel double standard imposed on her and her siblings by her maternal white grandparents because she had whiter skin than her siblings. Yet, the privilege over her siblings stopped when she went to school and was continually harassed about being a "chinaman," even though she is a woman and is mixed. She said her white grandparents treated her "awful, terrible almost every day," but they treated her siblings worse because of their darker skin (2009, p. 58).

*Complexity* is another theme discerned by Houston and Hogan in which their interviewees embrace the liminal complexity of their multiple heritages from a position of strength, not from confusion. They recognize and articulate their feelings of betwixt and between as strength, claiming it is other people's narrow thinking that is wrong. One interviewee said, for example, in relation to the term "Afro-Asian" that she crafted as a young adult to describe herself:

> arriving at this label (Afroasian) has been an evolution—I can't even say when it began. My first recollection is that you deal with the labels given to you—like hypodescent which would say I am African American. When I was growing up it was "Black." That was the label, and I was at a level of awareness that didn't allow me to critically question the label given to me.

The interviewee then describes how, through self-reflection, she grew to accept her mixed essence "I always knew I was different. I am not Black and I am not Japanese American. I am both—a different category altogether" (2009, p. 62). Another Black/Japanese/Native American interviewee said as she grew up and experienced the different versions of living Japanese American from her Japanese relative's different lifestyles such as home decorations and ways to cook Japanese food, from visiting Japan and immersing in its version of Japanese ways, followed by visiting her father's family in Alabama made her realize: "All these different family members on both sides living in different places has really exposed me to my ethnic identity—all of it. Absorbing these experiences in different places increased and strengthened my personal ethnic identity" (2009, p. 61).

*Celebration* is the third theme, "perhaps sustained by their trademark resilience, informants fused the inherent pain of alienation with the social reality of their respective complex backgrounds to celebrate their mixed heritage identities" (2009, p. 62). Participants in the study repeatedly said that their mixed heritage gave them "more love, more holidays, more diversity of experiences, and more fun." One participant talked about her "chameleon effect," in which she "is able to move creatively in and out of her Japanese and Italian American cultures with considerable ease and grace" (p. 62). She says further, "a part of me really likes being mixed. It gives me a foothold on many perspectives. The best part is that I know there is no right way to be. There are many very legitimate ways of being" (p. 63).

The significance of Houston and Hogan's conceptual framework is that the identity construction process for edge dancers involves multiple ways of using their creative agency to perceive, define, reframe, and reinvent themselves while maintaining identities that push against U.S. national culture's hegemonic monoracial categorization. Edge dancers do this with intentionality, creative agency, dynamic reframing, and resilience. *Intentionality* is demonstrated with linguistic and cultural code switching that aligns culturally appropriate communication to the cultural dynamics of the situation (e.g., switch from speaking English to Spanish when Mexican grandfather visits, kiss Mexican grandfather on both cheeks yet bow to Japanese grandmother). Edge dancer *creative agency* is demonstrated in the above case of the Japanese/Black/Native American who realized and proudly embraced her multiple identities after visiting different relatives of both ethnicities, saying, the experience "increased and strengthened" her ethnic identity. *Dynamic reframing* of earlier lived experiences is another characteristic, as in the above case of the Japanese/white grandchildren whose white grandparents were so cruel and who made her "feel awful" most days. Reflecting on her childhood abuse, she said, "I didn't realize it at the time, but they were the worst of all racists" (2009, p. 58). Edge dancer's *resilience*, the ability to recover, readjust, and spring back from a challenge or conflict, is clearly articulated in the following quote, "What is also apparent ... is the remarkable resilience informants exhibit as they construct their respective mixed heritage identities," ... their "learned ability to either ignore or to pity the inability to understand their mixed heritage existence," ... and "the way edge dancers use experiences of alienation to re-formulate the experience into positive identity constructions," such as the interviewee who called herself "Afro-Asian" as she got older (2009, pp. 60, 55–67).

## Edge Dancer Experience in Higher Education

Recently, the Houston and Hogan's edge dancer model has been applied to the lived experience and identity negotiations of college students. In "Edge Dancing: Campus Climate Experiences and Identity Negotiation of Multiracial College Students of Multiple Minoritized Ancestry," the researchers Kim Misa-Escalante et al. (2022) explain that, although individuals identifying as multiracial/ethnic are currently one of the fastest-growing minoritized groups in the United States, before the 2000 census, mixed persons were not counted in the census and the proportion of mixed-race/ethnic persons in the U.S. population, therefore, could not be quantified. Given the prediction that by 2050 one in five Americans will identify as mixed-race/ethnic persons; the number of mixed-race/ethnic college students is predicted to rise as the number of mixed people increases. The goal of the 2022 study, hereafter called, Misa-Escalante et al. study, attempts to increase, enrich, and deepen the understanding of the lived experiences of the multiracial/ethnic student population by examining their perceptions in relation to two key questions: First, how do mixed-race/ethnic students negotiate their identities while on campus and, second, how are they treated by the campus institutions, particularly in terms of whether the overall campus climate is inclusive and welcoming to this student population?

## Findings in Relation to Identity Negotiations on Campus

### *General Findings about Edge Dancers on Campus*

The Misa-Escalante et al. study compares the experiences of multiracial/ethnic persons with two minoritized parents (TMPs) and those with one white parent (OWP). By exploring if there are differences in perceptions and experiences of TMP students versus OWP students, the researchers articulate nuances in the lived experiences and identity negotiation of mixed students on campus. (2022, pp. 42–43).

While the identity processes for all multiracial/ethnic persons may be characterized as contextual, dynamic, and fluid, the processes for TMP multiracial students are often qualitatively different from OWP multiracial students. Issues experienced by TMP individuals differ from those of OWP individuals because the TMP individuals are more likely to be perceived as minorities within U.S. society due to the monoracism imperative and rule of hypodescent (2022, pp. 51–56). The case of an OWP Irish Mexican American student from California, going to college in New York, serves as an example. In California she experienced being "other" because of her Spanish surname, yet in New York she was commonly perceived as unique and exotic because of her blond hair and Spanish surname.

Two simultaneous identity processes are distinguished by Misa-Escalante et al.: a racial identity process and a cultural (ethnic-heritage) identity process. *Racial identity processes* involve how the TMP is racially perceived by each constituent group to which they belong (e.g., family, friends, colleagues), how they are racially perceived by members of the national U.S. society (e.g., teachers at school), and how they racially perceive themselves (either by "blood" and/or phenotype characteristics in line with U.S. monoracist imperative that they internalized growing up). In contrast, *cultural or ethnic-heritage identity processes* entail the possession (or not) of cultural knowledge or heritage learning: knowing about and acting according to the sociocultural rules of their heritages, such as the values, customs, rituals, behaviors, and verbal and non-verbal languages. Therefore, individuals with multiracial/ethnic identity must continually negotiate several levels of racial and cultural knowledge: (1) racial and cultural knowledge that allows them to negotiate and navigate their minoritized groups (e.g., Afro-Asian student who speaks Japanese to her Japanese American church parishioners and wears corn-row braided hair taught by her Black cousins on her dad's side of the family) (Houston & Hogan, 2009); (2) racial and cultural knowledge that allows them to negotiate and navigate majority U.S. society (e.g., Afro-Asian student who speaks and writes "proper" English in her classes); (3) racial and cultural knowledge that allows them to negotiate and navigate in multiracial/ethnic spaces, both formal (e.g., church membership) and informal (e.g., family events); (4) racial and cultural knowledge that allows them to negotiate and navigate their family spaces, both nuclear (e.g., at home) and extended (e.g., an Irish Mexican American interviewee knowing to speak Spanish to his Mexican American elders at a family reunion to show respect). At the same time, TMP and OWP individuals, as all persons, must continually negotiate the intersecting vectors of U.S.

hegemonic oppressions of sexuality, gender, class, age, and physical ability identities as well (2022, p. 45; Annamma & Booker, 2020; Collins & Bilge, 2016).

### Specific Findings about the Identity Negotiations of Edge Dancers on Campus

The findings in relation to the first question of how multiracial/ethnic students negotiated their identities on campus revealed four identity negotiations: *Bridging, Contextualizing, Sitting, and Homesteading. Bridging* is when mixed-race/ethnic individuals act as a bridge with their membership in both groups and can be a bridge across racial/ethnic groups such as African American and Native American. *Contextualizing* is when mixed-race/ethnic individuals match their identity expression to the current context, for example, "I find myself identifying differently depending upon the situation" (2022, pp. 53–55). *Sitting* is when individuals decisively and intentionally sit on the border of their mixed-race/ethnic identity, for example, "I am able to challenge stereotypes about my racial identity" or "I am able to empathize with others more easily" (p. 55). Last is *Homesteading*—when mixed-race/ethnic individuals create a home in one identity camp for an extended period of time before possibly shifting to another camp if psychological, emotional, and social needs necessitate (p. 56).

### Specific Findings about Perceptions of Campus Climate and Institutional Support for Multiracial/Ethnic Identity Development

The results of the second question about student perceptions of campus climate revealed that social spaces on campus were often not warm and welcoming to OWP or TMP. A student with OWP and a Black parent, for example, said that when he was admitted to the college, he was eager to join the Black Student Union, because he had grown up in a majority white city. At the initial meeting of the club in which parents were invited, the student said it was

> a very isolating experience, especially for his parents: ... because my mom's white and my dad's black and they were both there ... and people don't talk to you and they avoid you and especially for my parents, it was a very weird thing. It left a bad taste in my mouth, and I was like, great, I don't fit in here, what am I to do at this point?
>
> (2022, p. 56)

Results of the second research question revealed an overall lack of institutional support for mixed-race/ethnic students. One student said, for example: "There are no mixed student associations. There is no mixed student class .... And it would just be nice to know more about me and know other people like me" (p. 56). The student also said that within the college, she cannot identify "with those other colors of me because I am supposed to identify with just one color" (p. 56). Mixed students with TMP and OWP also reported that, although their university did encourage minoritized students to explore their monoracial/ethic identity, such as Ethnic Studies classes, *there was no encouragement to explore their multiple-race/ethnic identities* (p. 57). One example,

> I'm also a part of the Latino Alumni Association, which is a great program and I also go by (Ethnic Student) services quite often. ... They are both great resources, but I definitely don't think they help me be multiracial, specifically. They help me being a Latino or they help me being African American, but there's never all of me, in that sense.
>
> (p. 57)

The on-campus research of edge dancers by Miso-Escalante et al. thus adds much depth and richness to our understanding of the alienation, complexity, and celebration themes reported in the 2009 Houston and Hogan research on edge dancers.

## How Academic Departments, such as Human Services, Can Become More Welcoming and Supportive of Mixed-Race/Ethnic Students

Two recent volumes, *Multiracial Experience in Higher Education*, edited by Johnston-Guerrero and Wijeyesinghe (2021) and *Preparing for Higher Education's Mixed-Race Future: Why Multiraciality Matters*, edited by Johnston-Guerrero et al. (2022), present numerous chapters that enhance and broaden our understanding of the nuance and complexities of the lived experiences of edge dancers on campuses. The two volumes also include strategies for human services and other departments in higher education to transform their policies, programs, and processes to include and support mixed-race/heritage students, faculty, administrators, and staff. Given the page limit for this chapter, however, the following section will focus on the theory and recommendations of three researchers featured in the two volumes. The research of Prema Chaudhari, V.K. Malaney-Brown, and Orkideh Mohajeri is featured because their aim is to create inclusive and welcoming learning environments for mixed-race/ethnic students in higher education. The research and recommendations for change of these three scholars serve as examples of what we can do going forward.

Prema Chaudhari emphasizes that students with multiple-race/ethnic identities need to develop a "sense of belonging" within their college/university experience because it is a vital part of a student's overall psychosocial development and learning. The current monoracial context of higher education, however, creates barriers at the macro- and micro levels that impact the sense of belonging of multiple identity students. *Macrolevel barriers* derive from monoracist structures and programs that place mixed-identity students on the periphery of campus initiatives designed to support diverse students. The case of the student quoted above, who felt he "did not fit in at all" when he, his white mother, and Black father were ignored at the Black Student Union Welcome event, is one example.

In relation to *microlevel exclusion*, Chadhari describes Johnston and Nadel's taxonomy of five campus-wide microaggressions that multiracial/multiethnic students experience. Johnston and Nadel define "multiracial microaggressions" as "daily verbal, behavioral, or environmental indignities, whether intentional or unintentional, enacted by monoracial persons and communicate hostile, derogatory, or negative slights toward multiracial individuals or groups" (2010 p. 126). The microaggressions are (1) Exclusion/Isolation, in which multiracial/multiethnic students experience their authenticity is questioned, "you are not Mexican enough because you don't speak Spanish"; (2) Eroticism/Objectification, being asked, "what are you?" or being told, "oh, you're so exotic being part Thai"; (3) Assumed Monoracial Identity or Mistaken Identity, saying, "You don't act white"; (4) Denial of Multiracial Reality, "You say you are part white because you reject that you are really Black"; (5) Pathologizing of Identity and Experience, saying, "Are you adopted as you can't be mixed, that's wrong" (Chadhari, 2022, pp. 108–109).

Some recommendations that Chaudhari suggests for transforming monoracist campus culture include *intentional and purposeful planning* to become more mindful and inclusive of multiracial/ethnic students. *Assessments of campus climate* may be useful to identify issues and areas of exclusion for planning programs in various campus domains such as residential halls, curricula development, investing in identity-affirming events and resources, promoting multiracial/ethnic student organizations and conferences geared toward multiracial/ethnic topics, organizing ongoing intergroup dialogues, modifying campus race/ethnic data gathering to recognize fluid identities, and offering these programs to the whole campus to reduce adherence to the monoracist imperative (Chaudhari, 2022, pp. 121–122).

The second example is V.K. Malaney-Brown's research suggests that, becoming less oppressive, higher education programs need to promote *multiracial/ethnic consciousness development* based on Paolo Freire's critical consciousness concept developed in his work with Brazilian peasants (1974/2013). Freire suggested there are three levels of consciousness: a "pre-level consciousness" or "massification" in which people do not recognize systemic oppression because they are manipulated by a hegemonic elite to remain passive and silent and to focus on survival, simplify problems, and not question status quo power relations. Consciousness level two recognizes racism and oppression through reflective education and practice, yet these persons still doubt themselves in relation to their social justice activism because of the effects monoracism on them, such as internalizing the belief that they are "other." The third level involves social justice activism. Brown says, multiracial consciousness is defined

> as a heightened level of self-awareness where the student self-reflects on their multiple racial identities, has the ability to describe how monoracism affects daily life experiences, and influences their decisions and choices to engage or disengage from ethnic, cultural, or racial justice causes.
>
> (Malaney-Brown, 2022, p. 132)

Malaney-Brown recommends four ways to create a welcoming, inclusive college environment. First, colleges need to *create learning opportunities* for student self-reflection to understand the oppressive nature of the campus's white supremacist monoracist culture. Understanding one's oppressive life conditions through critical consciousness is the foundation for institutional change. Second, engage multiracial/ethnic student population in *social justice programming* by creating spaces and using library resources for student self-reflection and learning about the history and cultures of their multiple identities. Third, promote opportunities for multiracial/ethnic students to *create college communities*, such as student clubs where they can learn from each other and feel a sense of belonging; and, fourth, provide consistent opportunities for multiracial/ethnic students *to share their ideas and opinions about policy and program development throughout their college years* (Malaney-Brown, 2022, pp. 140–142).

The last exemplar addressing a path forward is the research of Orkideh Mohajeri who proposes *five essential race "discourses"* to learn about and to understand for reversing the monoracial white supremacy imperative of higher education, saying that white supremacy operates through structures, systems, and the prevailing "white supremacist discourses active in current U.S. society" (p. 146). Specifying the five discourses on white supremacy, which overlap and reinforce each other, is important because the discourses create internalized subjectivities of unwantedness and lack of belonging. First is the approximately 500-year-old discourse of the *essentialist anti-Black racism*, which is structured around the mythological race concept. Some of this discourse focuses on biology; others focus on measuring head size, or measuring intelligence or IQ, for creating the racial hierarchy that envisions whites at the top and Blacks at the bottom of the racial classification of all humans (Beliso-De Jesús & Pierre, 2019; Beliso-De Jesús et al., 2023; Mohajeri, 2022, p. 148).

Second is *the racial binary discourse* that divides the U.S. population into just two broad racial categories of Black or white and omits or glosses over other people of color. This relates to the one-drop rule (or hypodescent) discourse in which "one drop" of Black blood relegates an individual to the lower status in the racial binary system, and it is a system that has been encoded in U.S. laws. In the binary discourse, whites are perceived and defined as desirable and Blacks as "Other" (Mohajeri, 2022, p. 149). The *discourse of normative whiteness* is the third. Whiteness is defined and broadly perceived as "normal" to the extent that it is experienced as common sense, average, correct, modern, and universal and is not even consciously thought about by whites (p. 149). Mohajeri says, "The aim of this discourse is to normalize and make visible the unexamined current power relations" (p. 149). The fourth *discourse of color blindness* occurs when an individual says, "I do not see race," implying that race does not matter. This response shifts blame away from themselves and onto the person who initially brought up the issue of race. "Thus, the identification of oppression and the call to address it are summarily dismissed as personality flaws. Politeness and kindness are used to silence real talk around race, and thus, uphold white supremacy" (Mohajeri, 2022, p. 150).

Lastly, the fifth *discourse of denial* is closely related to the colorblind discourse. Whereas colorblind discourse stops discussion of racism at the individual level, the discourse of denial operates at the institutional and societal level. Analyses of this discourse demonstrate three semantic expressions that deny racism: saying it is "an isolated incident" or "it is not a racial issue," or the minoritized person is said to be "overly sensitive" (2022, pp. 150–151).

For transforming higher education, Mohajeri recommends *direct education of the race discourses* with an emphasis on critiquing and self-reflecting about the power of the white supremacist discourses on students' sense of self and well-being. Student affairs could create spaces for dialogue of these discourses, create student organizations that span undergraduate and graduate years for mixed-race ethnic students, and create networks of these organizations in the community. Mohajeri concludes, "Study and practice which aims to name, delineate, and trouble these discourses and their enactments constitute one core means of dismantling white supremacy and creating postsecondary environments that are more critically conscious" and inclusive of diversity (p. 161).

## Human Services Departments and Edge Dancers

Although human services departments are a microcosm of a white supremacist, monoracist, and neo-liberal academy, its interdisciplinary nature is a strength and the variety of theoretical and praxis frameworks embedded in its faculty training, pedagogy and curricula can be a resource for promoting institutional transformation (Dávila, 2006; Demerath, 2022; Giroux, 2014; Hyatt, 2017; Lazzari, Larsen, & Orlandi, 2024; Parekh, 2022, pp. 11–12; Shear & Zontine, 2017). Human service faculty and students are especially prepared to engage in social justice, decolonizing activities on campus because of their student-centered, dialogic, and praxis-infused education models. Over the past few years, for example, faculty in my department developed a course on multiple heritage identity for human services and other majors. Human service faculty and students readily partner with other departments to promote social justice programs, such as participating in the library's speaker program. Each semester, an HUSR faculty member presents training on inclusive teaching strategies for edge dancers on campus, including faculty, students, staff, and administrators.

Other plans include promoting student and faculty participation in the Chicano Studies Department of the Social Justice and Story Telling Institute, which centers academic healing as a path to personal healing with the goal of broad social healing. Collaborating with local high schools, a feeder-school source for human service majors, by participating in an art contest in which students draw their multiracial/ethnic identities, is another current project. Centering a discussion of edge dancer pedagogical issues and practice at the bi-annual faculty retreat, and possibly the annual retreat of the College of Health and Human Development, are two other actions that will raise awareness of the edge dancer campus experience. Lastly, working with our accreditation organization, the Council on Standards for Human Service Education includes mixed-race/ethnic curricula issues in our self-study, which is used for assessing the quality of our Human Services program. Infusing issues of students' multiple heritage identity in the accreditation process is another way to promote awareness, understanding, and skills for working with edge dancers.

## Conclusion

The focus of this chapter was to illuminate the experience of mixed-race/ethnic students on campus by first presenting the initial research that coined the term "edge dancers" in 2009. More recent studies were then described that further deepen and enrich our understanding of edge dancers' lived experiences in higher education institutions that treat them as invisible and "other" because of the prevailing monoracist white supremacist "imperative." Each current study presented aptly promotes understanding and recommends practical actions aimed at transforming our current institutional practices to include and welcome mixed-race/ethnic college/university students. Researching the lived experience of edge dancers for over 20 years evokes for me the truth of C.D. Lee's words,

> How do we resist simplistic assumptions about the meaning of group membership and develop more nuanced and complex research agendas that work from a basic assumption that human beings always have agency, always have resources, and make meaning of their experiences in varied ways?
>
> (Lee, 2003, pp. 3–5)

The chapter ended with an array of suggested inclusive actions taken by the author's human services department in recent years to promote the essence of C.D. Lee's words.

## Questions for Reflection

1  What is your sense of the experience of multiracial/ethnic students on your campus?
2  Are there inclusive strategies your college/university is already implementing to make multiracial/ethnic students feel safer, to improve policy, and to establish networks for them?
3  What additional strategies might your college/university consider to create an inclusive campus climate?
4  Who might be the focus of your energy if you are going to reach out to others who are not engaged in this issue? What would be compelling to them?
5  How might you leverage your skills and/or knowledge in this outreach effort to promote inclusivity on your campus?

## Bibliography

Alim, H. S., Paris, D., & Wong, C. P. (2020). Culturally Sustaining Pedagogy: A critical framework for centering communities. In N. S. Nasir, C. D. Lee, R. Pea, & M. M. De Royston (Eds.), *Handbook of the cultural foundations of learning* (pp. 261–276), Routledge, Taylor & Francis. New York and London. https://doi.org/10.4324/9780203774977

Annamma, S. A., & Booker, A. (2020). Integrating intersectionality into the study of learning. In N. S. Nasir, C. D. Lee, R. Pea, & M. M. De Royston (Eds.), *Handbook of the cultural foundations of learning* (pp. 297–313), Routledge, Taylor & Francis. New York and London. https://doi.org/10.4324/9780203774977

Beliso-De Jesús, A. M., & Pierre, J. (2019). Special section: Anthropology of white supremacy. *American Anthropologist, 122*(1), 65–75. https://doi.org/10.1111/aman.13351

Beliso-De Jesús, A. M., Pierre, J., & Rana, J. (2023). White supremacy and the making of anthropology. *Annual Review of Anthropology, 52*(1), 417–435. https://doi.org/10.1146/annurev-anthro-052721-040400

Brenneis, D., Shore, C., & Wright, S. (2005). Getting the measure of academia: Universities and the politics of accountability. *Anthropology in Action, 12*, 1–10. https://doi.org/10.3167/096720105780644362

Chaudhari, P. (2022). A mixed sense of belonging: Fluid experiences for multiracial and multiethnic college students. In M. P. Johnston-Guerrero, L. D. Combs, & V. K. Malaney-Brown (Eds.), *Preparing for higher education's mixed race future* (pp. 105–124). Palgrave Macmillan.

Collins, P. H., & Bilge, S. (2016). *Intersectionality*. John Wiley & Sons.

Dávila, A. (2006). The disciplined boundary: Anthropology, ethnic studies, and the "minority" practitioner. *Transforming Anthropology, 14*(1), 35–43. https://doi.org/10.1525/tran.2006.14.1.35

Demerath, P. (2022). Decolonizing education: Roles for anthropology. *Anthropology & Education Quarterly, 53*(3), 196–214.

Foner, E. (2023, December 7). *The complicity of the textbooks*. The New York Review of Books. https://www.nybooks.com/articles/2022/09/22/the-complicity-of-the-textbooks-teaching-white-supremacy/

Freire, P. (1974/2013). *Education for critical consciousness*. Bloomsbury.

French, H. W. (2022). *Born in blackness: Africa and the making of the modern world*. Norton.

Giroux, H. (2014). *Neoliberalism's war on higher education*. Haymarket Books.

Grzanka, P. R. (2014). *Intersectionality: A foundations and frontiers reader*. Westview Press.

Hamako, E. (2014). *Improving antiracist education for multiracial students*. [unpublished doctoral dissertation, University of Massachusetts Amherst].

Hill, M. L. (2017). *Nobody: Casualties of America's war on the vulnerable, from ferguson to flint and beyond*. Simon and Schuster.

Hogan, M. (2013). *Four skills of culture diversity competence, a process for understanding and practice*. Brooks/Cole Cengage Learning.

Horne, G. (2017). *The apocalypse of settler colonialism: The roots of Slavery, White supremacy, and capitalism in 17th century North America and the Caribbean*. NYU Press.

Horne, G. (2020). *The dawning of the Apocalypse: The roots of slavery, White supremacy, settler colonialism, and capitalism in the long sixteenth century*. Monthly Review Press.

Houston, H. R., & Hogan, M. (2009). Edge dancers: Mixed heritage identity, transculturalization, and public policy and practice in health and human services. *The Applied Anthropologist, 29*(2), 49–76.

Hyatt, S. (2017). Using ethnographic methods to understand universities and neoliberal development in north central Philadelphia. In S. B. Hyatt, B. W. Shear, & S. Wright (Eds.), *Learning under neoliberalism* (pp. 56–76). Bergahn.

Jana, T., & Baran, M. (2020). *Subtle acts of exclusion: How to understand, identify, and stop microaggressions*. Berret-Koehler. https://doi.org/10.4324/9780203774977

Johnston, M. P., & Nadel, K. L. (2010). Multiracial microaggressions: Exposing monoraciam in everyday life and clinical practice. In D. W. Sue (Ed.), *Microaggressions and marginality: Manifestations, dynamics, and impact* (pp. 123–144). Wiley.

Johnston-Guerrero, M. P., Combs, L. D., & Malaney-Brown, V. K. (2022). *Preparing for higher education's mixed race future, why multiraciality matters*. Palgrave Macmillan.

Johnston-Guerrero, M. P., & Wijeyesinghe, C. (2021). *Multiracial experiences in higher education*. Stylus.

Johnston-Guerrero, M. P., Wijeyesinghe, C., & Combs, L. (2021). Intergenerational reflections and future directions. In *Multiracial experiences in higher education* (pp. 233–247). Stylus.

Koppelman, K. L. (2020). *Understanding human differences*. Pearson.

Lazzari, M., Larsen, P. B., & Orlandi, F. (2024). Introduction—The heritage and decoloniality nexus: Global exchanges and unresolved questions in sedimented landscapes of injustice. *American Anthropologist, 126*, 311–316. https://doi.org/10.1111/aman.13951

Lee, C. D. (2003). Why we need to rethink race and ethnicity in educational research. *Educational Researcher, 32*(5), 3–5.

Malaney-Brown, V. K. (2021). On the path to multiracial consciousness: Reflections on my scholar-practitioner journey in higher education. In M. P. Johnston-Guerrero, & C. Wijeyesinghe (Eds.), *Multiracial experiences in higher education* (pp. 88–97). Routledge.

Misa-Escalante, K., Takada Rooks, C., & Shimako Abe, J. (2022). Edge dancing: Campus climate experiences and identity negotiation of multiracial college students of multiple minoritized ancestry. In M. P. Johnston-Guerrero, L. D. Combs, & V. K. Malaney-Brown (Eds.), *Preparing for higher education's mixed race future* (pp. 41–59). Palgrave Macmillan.

Mohajeri, O. (2022). The "Unwanted, Colored Male": Gendered contested white subjectivity hailed through contemporary racial discourse. In M. P. Johnston-Guerrero, L. D. Combs, & V. K. Malaney-Brown (Eds.), *Preparing for higher education's mixed race future* (pp. 145–161). Palgrave Macmillan.

Parekh, G. (2022). *Abelism in education, rethinking school practices and policies*. W.W. Norton.

Root, M. (1992). *Racially mixed people in America*. Sage.

Shear, B. W., & Zontine, A. I. (2017). Reading neoliberalism at the university. In S. B. Hyatt, B. W. Shear, & S. W. Wright (Eds.), *Learning under neoliberalism* (pp. 103–128). Bergahn.

Spickard, P. (1989). *Mixed blood: Intermarriage and ethnic identity in twentieth-century America*. University of Wisconsin Press.

Sue, D. W., & Spanierman, L. (2020). *Microaggressions in everyday life*. John Wiley & Sons.

Wijeyesinghe, C. (2021). Monoracism: Identifying and addressing structural oppression of multiracial people. In M. P. Johnston-Guerrero, & C. Wijeyesinghe (Eds.), *Multiracial experiences in higher education* (pp. 57–72). Routledge.

Wolf, E. R. (1999). *Envisioning power: Ideologies of dominance and crisis*. Univ of California Press.

# 19 Health Equity

## Addressing a Social Justice Imperative for Black, Indigenous, and People of Color (BIPOC) through a Population Health Framework

*Darrin E. Wright*

## Glossary of Terms

| Terms | Definition |
|---|---|
| *Social Determinants of Health (SDOH)* | The social determinants of health (SDOH) are the non-medical factors that influence health outcomes. They are the conditions in which people are born, grow, work, live, and age, and the broader set of forces and systems shaping the conditions of daily life. These forces and systems include economic policies and systems, development agendas, social norms, social policies, and political systems (World Health Organization). |
| *Black, Indigenous, People of Color (BIPOC)* | BIPOC is an acronym that acknowledges the distinct histories, cultures, and struggles of Black and Indigenous peoples alongside other people of color. It emphasizes the interconnectedness of these communities in the fight against systemic racism and oppression. By specifically naming Black and Indigenous peoples, BIPOC highlights their often-overlooked experiences within discussions of racial inequality (Watson-Singleton et al. 2023). |
| *Health Equity* | Health equity is the state in which everyone has a fair and just opportunity to attain their highest level of health (Centers for Disease Control). |
| *Systemic Racism* | Systemic racism refers to the totality of ways in which societies foster racial discrimination through mutually reinforcing systems of housing, education, employment, earnings, benefits, credit, media, healthcare, and criminal justice. These patterns and practices, in turn, reinforce discriminatory beliefs, values, and distribution of resources, according to Zinzi Bailey et al. |
| *Social Justice* | Social justice is the view that everyone deserves equal rights and opportunities, including the right to good health (American Public Health Association). |
| *Population Health* | Population health is "the health outcomes of a group of individuals, including the distribution of such outcomes within the group" (American Public Health Association). |
| *Socioeconomic status* | Socioeconomic status refers to the absolute or relative levels of economic resources, power, and prestige closely associated with the wealth of an individual, community, or country. Socioeconomic status is a multidimensional construct comprising multiple factors such as income, education, employment status, and other factors (Centers for Disease Control). |

*(Continued)*

DOI: 10.4324/9781003531258-23

| Terms | Definition |
|-------|-----------|
| *Health disparities* | Health disparities are preventable differences in the burden of disease, injury, violence, or opportunities to achieve optimal health that are experienced by socially disadvantaged populations (Centers for Disease Control, 2002). |

## Introduction

Health disparities persist among Black, Indigenous, and People of Color (BIPOC), stemming from various factors such as socioeconomic status (SES), access to healthcare, and systemic racism (Bell & Lee, 2011; Ndugga et al., 2024). This chapter explores the importance of employing population health models tailored to communities of color to address these disparities and promote health equity. According to the Institute of Medicine (2013), the United States is among the wealthiest nations in the world and spends far more per person on healthcare than any other industrialized nation. However, its population's health is rapidly deteriorating. Over the past three decades, on average, Americans have died sooner and experienced higher rates of comorbid diseases and injury when compared to populations in other high-income nations. A recent study by the Commonwealth Fund assessed the healthcare systems of 11 high-income nations, including the United States, and identified the following patterns related to poor health outcomes.

1  The United States ranked last among the 11 countries for health outcomes, equity, and quality despite having the highest per capita health expenditures.
2  The United States also had the highest rate of mortality amenable to healthcare, meaning more Americans die from inadequate care quality than any other country involved in the study.
3  Poor access to primary care in the United States has contributed to inadequate chronic disease prevention and management, delayed diagnoses, and safety concerns, among other issues (Commonwealth Fund, 2018).

This pervasive pattern of poorer health and health outcomes across the life course, from birth to old age, raises concerns about the social determinants of health, as well as health disparities between groups in the United States in general, and particularly among BIPOC, as a result of the historical legacy of systematic racial and ethnic discrimination. (IOM, 2017; Riley, 2012). For example, African Americans are less likely to seek medical care at the same rate as their Caucasian counterparts due to their mistrust of the healthcare system (Office of Minority Health). This mistrust dates back to the Tuskegee Experiment in the 1930s, when African American males were recruited into a study under the guise of "bad blood" in which the researchers were studying the effects of syphilis, and treatment was purposefully withheld, resulting in the death of many. "It destroyed the trust many African Americans held for medical institutions—a legacy that persists today (Washington Post, 2017)." Other examples include Henrietta Lacks, an African American woman from East Baltimore, treated for cervical cancer; without her knowledge or consent, the surgeon snipped a sample of her tumor for a research team down the hall. Those cells thrived in the lab and became the famous "HeLa" line of cells that would transform medical research, even as her children struggled to understand their mother's fate (Sloot, 2010). These examples provide context for African Americans' mistrust of the healthcare system, which frequently comes at the expense of their overall preventive health practices, with African Americans reporting greater mistrust than their white counterparts (Arnett et al., 2016).

## Social Determinants of Health

According to the Office of Disease Prevention and Health Promotion-Healthy People 2020 Report, social determinants of health are a range of personal, social, economic, and environmental factors contributing to individual and population health. For instance, people with a quality education, stable employment, safe homes and neighborhoods, and access to preventive services tend to be healthier throughout their lives. Poor health outcomes are often made worse by the interaction between individuals and their social and physical environment, where one or all are absent (Healthy People, 2020). These societal factors are often influenced by policies that impact the distribution of money, power, and resources nationally and internationally (World Health Organization, 2018). These social determinants are primarily responsible for health inequalities between groups in a nation.

## What Are Health Inequalities?

Health inequalities are the unjust and avoidable differences in people's health across the population and between specific population groups, including differences that occur by gender, race, ethnicity, education, income, disability, or living in various geographic localities (Healthy People, 2020). Health inequalities go against the principles of social justice because they are avoidable (Dahlgren & Whitehead, 2008). They do not occur randomly or by chance; instead, they are socially determined by circumstances beyond an individual's control. Additionally, these circumstances disadvantage people and limit their chances of living longer, healthier lives. The existence of health inequalities means that everyone's right to the highest attainable standard of physical and mental health is not being enjoyed equally across any given population (Dahlgren & Whitehead, 2008).

In the United States, health inequalities related to race, ethnicity, disability, and SES still pervade the American healthcare system (Palacio et al., 2009). As such, BIPOC communities are often excluded from receiving appropriate healthcare due to cost. Such inequalities exist in areas concerning the quality of healthcare, access to healthcare, levels and types of care, and many other clinical factors. Moreover, factors such as vulnerability, SES, and inadequate and fractured systems help contribute significantly to differences in health status and health outcomes (Palacio et al., 2009). SES is a critical component that should be factored into the discourse related to health inequality. Because of its significant implications for health and health outcomes, SES impacts one's ability to access healthcare; low SES is directly associated with many health risks and lack of access to care (Agency for Healthcare Research and Quality, 2015).

## Disparities in Access to Healthcare among Americans

Access to healthcare among vulnerable populations is often a challenge and even more so for at-risk populations of color in comparison to most white Americans. As such, centering whiteness in discussions of health disparities and access to healthcare places a focus on how white dominance in societal structures, including healthcare systems, affects the distribution of resources, access to care, and health outcomes. By centering whiteness in discussions about health disparities, we critically examine how racial privilege impacts both healthcare systems and patient outcomes. This lens helps dismantle systems of oppression, foster a more equitable distribution of healthcare resources, and improve the health of marginalized communities (Churchwell et al, 2020). A recent study identified several distinct socioeconomic determinants of health, social, economic, physical environment, income level, and social support network, to name a few, that have an impact on BIPOC populations' ability to receive proper healthcare.

The report indicated that African Americans, Hispanics, and some Asian populations such as Korean Americans, Native Hawaiians, and Pacific Islanders, when compared to whites, appear to have lower levels of health insurance coverage, with Hispanics facing more significant barriers to health insurance than any other group (Office of the Assistant Secretary for Planning and Evaluation, U.S. Department of Health and Human Services, 2024). Likewise, among Hispanics, uninsured rates are much higher for Mexicans and Central Americans than for Puerto Ricans. Among Asians, Chinese, Japanese, Filipinos, and East Indians have uninsured rates that are comparable to or lower than those of whites.

In contrast, Koreans and Vietnamese have higher uninsured rates than African Americans. Among all the population groups of color, African Americans and Hispanics are less likely to have insurance coverage from a private employer, whether directly or through a spouse. They are more likely to have public health insurance coverage. African Americans and Hispanics are also more likely than whites to receive care in non-optimal healthcare settings (such as emergency rooms) and often lack continuity in healthcare after being discharged.

Findings from a recent report that assessed racial and ethnic differences in access to and the use of healthcare services in the United States indicate that, between 2014 and 2020, disparities with whites narrowed for Blacks and Hispanics on three key access indicators:

1  The percentage of uninsured working-age adults
2  The percentage who skipped care because of costs
3  The percentage of those who lacked a usual care provider

Findings seem to suggest that disparities were narrower on average rates on each of the three indicators for whites, Blacks, and Hispanics and were lower in 2014 through 2017 in states that expanded Medicaid under the Affordable Care Act (ACA) than in states that did not. Among Hispanics, disparities tended to narrow more between 2014 through 2017 in expansion states than in non-expansion states. Further, the ACA's coverage expansions were associated with increased access to care and reduced racial and ethnic disparities in access to care, with generally more significant improvements in Medicaid expansion states (Glied & Weiss, 2023; Hayes et al., 2017).

Challenges relating to access to adequate healthcare can range from inadequate insurance due to cost and limited availability of medical providers for people with a specific type of insurance (Medicaid and Medicare). There has been a significant difference in the types of care provided to people with high-end insurance, such as Kaiser, and those with state-funded insurance, like Medicaid. The geographic location and zip code that one resides in have affected and will continue to affect the population. BIPOC and the types of care they receive can also be affected by stereotypes. Stereotypes are prevalent in our society as one or more groups tend to see themselves as superior to the other. There is a disparity in how healthcare professionals view different ethnic groups. Unhealthy relationships abound among races, and this adversely affects healthcare and services provided to a population that needs to access healthcare. Stereotypes have direct adverse effects on the general well-being of the population, physically, psychologically, and emotionally. Stereotypes about BIPOC in healthcare practices contribute to disparities in treatment, misdiagnosis, and a lack of trust between communities of color and healthcare providers. These stereotypes often stem from historical racism, implicit bias, and cultural misunderstandings, leading to inequitable care and worse health outcomes for BIPOC individuals (Washington, 2006). Here are some common stereotypes and their impacts.

### Stereotypes about Pain Tolerance

- **Black patients** are often stereotyped as having higher pain tolerance, leading to the under-treatment of pain. This false belief is rooted in slavery-era justifications for the brutal treatment of Black people, and it continues to affect medical care today. Studies have shown that Black patients are less likely to receive adequate pain medication for the same conditions as white patients (Washington, 2006).
- **Indigenous and Hispanic patients** may also face assumptions that they exaggerate or underreport their pain, resulting in either dismissiveness or mistrust from healthcare providers (Kabir & Zaidi, 2002).

### Stereotypes of Non-Compliance

- **Hispanic and Black patients** are often stereotyped as being "non-compliant" or "unco-operative" in following medical advice or taking prescribed medications. This can result in doctors offering less detailed or thorough care, assuming patients won't adhere to treatment plans. These stereotypes overlook structural issues, such as language barriers, financial constraints, or mistrust of the healthcare system, that can impact compliance rather than patient willfulness (Kabir & Zaidi, 2002).

### "Strong Black Woman" Stereotype

- Black women are often viewed through the lens of the "strong Black woman" stereotype, which assumes they can endure more physical and emotional stress. This stereotype can lead to the dismissal of legitimate health concerns and a lack of empathy from health-care providers. This has contributed to **higher rates of maternal mortality** among Black women, who may report pain or complications during pregnancy or postpartum, only to have their concerns ignored (Saluja & Bryant, 2021; Washington, 2006).

### Model Minority Myth and Mental Health

- **Asian Americans,** particularly East and South Asian communities, are often stereotyped as the "model minority," which assumes that they are uniformly successful, healthy, and free of mental health issues. As a result, this stereotype can lead to healthcare providers overlooking or minimizing mental health struggles, like depression or anxiety, among Asian American patients. These myths or stereotypes also erase the struggles of Southeast Asian, Pacific Islander, and other subgroups within the Asian American community, who may experience significantly higher rates of poverty and health issues (Lee et al., 2009).

**In sum,** a balanced critical analysis is needed to assess the impact of stereotypes on the minority population's ability to access quality healthcare.

### Intersectionality of Social Justice Concerns in Healthcare Inequality

The bias and discrimination that lead to differences in access to resources and opportunities for health between social groups are unfair. Social justice touches on the intersectionality that public health and social work hold for social justice's core value. Social justice is the view that everyone deserves equal rights and opportunities; this includes the right to good health. Health is necessary for well-functioning societies. A population needs a decent level of health to ensure economic prosperity, political participation, collective security, and other social and civil aspects of daily living (WHO, 2010). Below, the authors describe a corrective approach through the population health model, which assesses how we think about population-based healthcare.

### Population Health Model

Population health has been described as:

1   A conceptual framework for thinking about why some populations are healthier than others, as well as the policy development, research agenda, and resource allocation that flow from it (Young, 1998)
2   The health outcomes of a group of individuals, including the distribution of such outcomes within the group (Kindig & Stoddart, 2003; Kindig, 2007; Kindig et al., 2008)
3   A population's health is determined by health status indicators, which are impacted by various factors, including personal health practices, individual capability, coping skills, early childhood development, human biology, social, economic, and physical settings, and health services (Dunn & Hayes, 1999)

Based on the prior definitions presented, Figure 19.1 provides a conceptual example of aspects to consider while creating a population health model.

### *The Fundamentals of Population Health Models*

Population health focuses on improving the health outcomes of entire populations by addressing the underlying determinants of health and implementing preventive measures. Population health models emphasize collaboration across sectors, community engagement, and data-driven decision-making to identify and address health disparities. However,

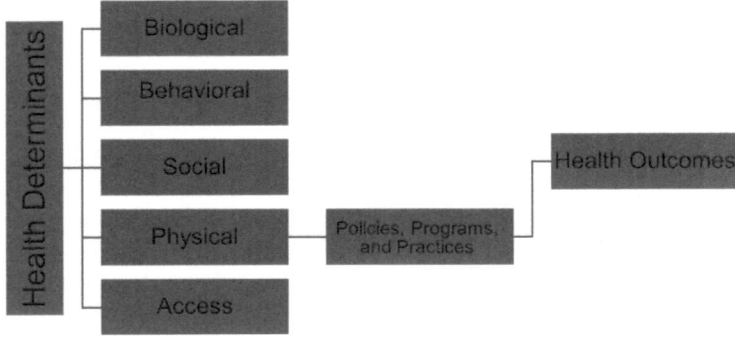

*Figure 19.1* Population health model overview.

generic population health approaches may need to be revised to adequately meet the needs of BIPOC communities, highlighting the importance of tailored models (Friedman & Starfield, 2003).

### Importance of Tailored Population Health Models

BIPOC communities often have unique healthcare needs and cultural considerations that must be addressed to improve health outcomes effectively. Tailored population health models recognize and incorporate these nuances, promoting culturally competent care, community empowerment, and equitable access to resources and services. By addressing the social determinants of health specific to BIPOC communities, these models can mitigate disparities and improve overall health outcomes (Bell & Lee, 2011).

### Strategies for Implementation

Implementing population health models tailored to BIPOC communities requires collaboration among healthcare providers, community organizations, policymakers, and other stakeholders. Strategies include building trust and partnerships with communities, investing in culturally competent healthcare providers, leveraging technology for targeted interventions, and advocating for policies that address systemic inequities (Bell & Lee, 2011).

### An example of Effective Strategies to Promote Health Equity for BIPOC Communities

1 **Culturally Competent Care:** Healthcare providers should receive training in cultural competency to better understand and address the unique healthcare needs and preferences of BIPOC patients (Holden et al., 2014).
2 **Community Engagement:** Involving BIPOC communities in designing, implementing, and evaluating healthcare programs and policies ensures that interventions are responsive to their needs and priorities.
3 **Addressing Social Determinants of Health:** Investing in education, affordable housing, employment opportunities, and access to healthy food in BIPOC communities can improve overall health outcomes.
4 **Anti-Racism Initiatives:** Implementing anti-racism policies and practices within healthcare organizations and institutions can help address implicit bias and discrimination in healthcare delivery.
5 **Healthcare Access:** Improving access to affordable healthcare services, including preventive care, mental health services, and chronic disease management, is essential for reducing health disparities among BIPOC populations (Raider et al., 2021).

## Success Stories and Best Practices

Several successful population health initiatives have demonstrated the effectiveness of tailored approaches in improving health outcomes for BIPOC communities. Examples include community health worker programs, culturally tailored health education campaigns, and interventions addressing social determinants of health, such as housing and food insecurity, as highlighted in a recent resource guide developed by the California Department of Public Health in 2021 on best practices in population health strategies. These success stories highlight the importance of understanding and addressing the specific needs of diverse populations (Raider et al., 2021).

### Possible Challenges Associated with a Population Health Program with BIPOC Communities

Recent research by Spencer Ohene-Ntow (2022) states that launching a population health program emphasizing BIPOC communities involves several essential issues that must be considered appropriately. Here are some challenges to think about:

1 Building trust: Many communities of color have experienced historical and ongoing discrimination in healthcare, leading to distrust of medical institutions. Overcoming this requires sustained community engagement, cultural competence, and transparent communication.
2 Addressing social determinants of health: BIPOC communities disproportionately face socioeconomic barriers like poverty, lack of transportation, and food insecurity. An effective program must go beyond clinical care to address these underlying factors.
3 Cultural competence: Healthcare providers and program staff need training to understand and respect diverse cultural beliefs, practices, and communication styles. This helps ensure appropriate, respectful care.
4 Language barriers: Providing culturally and linguistically appropriate services and materials in multiple languages and qualified interpreters is crucial for serving diverse populations.
5 Data collection and analysis: Collecting accurate, disaggregated data on race and ethnicity is essential but challenging. Some individuals may be reluctant to share this information due to privacy concerns or fear of discrimination.
6 Intersectionality: Recognizing that individuals may face multiple, overlapping forms of disadvantage (e.g., race, gender, SES) is essential for developing nuanced, effective interventions.
7 Funding and sustainability: Securing long-term funding for programs targeting underserved populations can be difficult, especially if immediate results are not apparent.
8 Workforce diversity: Recruiting and retaining a diverse healthcare workforce that reflects the community being served is crucial but can be challenging due to systemic barriers in education and professional advancement.
9 Addressing implicit bias: Healthcare providers and program staff may hold unconscious biases that affect care quality. Ongoing training and self-reflection are necessary to mitigate this.
10 Navigating political and policy landscapes: Population health programs may need more support from policymakers or institutions prioritizing health equity.

Successfully addressing these challenges requires a multifaceted approach involving community partnerships, cultural humility, and a commitment to addressing systemic inequities. By carefully considering these factors, population health programs can work toward improving health outcomes and reducing disparities for BIPOC communities.

### Conclusion

In conclusion, the integration of a population health model explicitly tailored for BIPOC communities is necessary and urgent. This model aims to bridge the health disparities gap and promote equitable health outcomes by addressing the unique social determinants of health that disproportionately affect these groups. Throughout this chapter, I have explored the multifaceted challenges faced by BIPOC communities, including socioeconomic inequities, environmental factors, and systemic racism. I have also examined how a population health model can be strategically implemented to address these issues through community engagement, culturally competent care, and policy advocacy (Holden et al., 2014).

The evidence presented underscores the importance of a comprehensive approach that includes preventive care, chronic disease management, and mental health services. By leveraging data and community insights, healthcare providers can develop targeted interventions that are both effective and culturally relevant. Furthermore, the role of policymakers, healthcare institutions, and community leaders is crucial in driving systemic change. Collaborative efforts can lead to the creation of policies and programs that not only improve health outcomes for BIPOC communities but also foster a more inclusive and just healthcare system (IOM, 2017; Riley, 2012).

In sum, a population health model that prioritizes BIPOC communities is a vital step toward achieving health equity. By addressing the root causes of health disparities and implementing tailored strategies, the human services profession can move toward a future where everyone can attain their highest level of health. This holistic approach not only benefits BIPOC communities but also strengthens the overall health and resilience of our society.

## Questions for Reflection

1  How does the population health model differ from traditional approaches to healthcare? What are its key components?
2  In what ways can the population health model help address health disparities among BIPOC communities?
3  What are some specific social determinants of health that disproportionately affect BIPOC communities? How do these impact overall health outcomes?
4  How might implicit bias and systemic racism contribute to health inequities for BIPOC individuals?
5  What strategies can healthcare systems implement to improve cultural competence and reduce barriers to care for BIPOC patients?

## Bibliography

Agency for Healthcare Research and Quality. (2015). *2014 National healthcare quality and disparities report*. U.S. Department of Health and Human Services. https://www.ahrq.gov/research/findings/nhqrdr/nhqdr14/index.html

Arnett, M. J., Thorpe, R. J., Jr, Gaskin, D. J., Bowie, J. V., & LaVeist, T. A. (2016). Race, medical mistrust, and segregation in primary care as usual source of care: Findings from the exploring health disparities in integrated communities study. *Journal of Urban Health: Bulletin of the New York Academy of Medicine*, 93(3), 456–467. https://doi.org/10.1007/s11524-016-0054-9

Bell, J., & Lee, M. M. (2011). *Why place and race matter: Impacting health through a focus on race and place*. Policy Link.

Benjamin, G. (2016). Ensuring population health: An important role for pharmacy. *American Journal of Pharmaceutical Education, 80*(2), 1–3.

Churchwell, K., Elkind, M. S. V., Benjamin, R. M., Carson, A. P., Chang, E. K., Lawrence, W., Mills, A., Odom, T. M., Rodriguez, C. J., Rodriguez, F., Sanchez, E., Sharrief, A. Z., Sims, M., Williams, O., & on behalf of the American Heart Association. (2020). Call to action: Structural racism as a fundamental driver of health disparities: a presidential advisory from the American Heart Association. *Circulation, 142*, e454–e468. https://doi.org/10.1161/CIR.0000000000000936.

Clarke, C. (2020, September 19). BIPOC: What does it mean and where does it come from? *CBS News*. https://www.cbsnews.com/news/bipoc-meaning-where-does-it-come-from-2020-04-02/

Commonwealth Fund. (2018). *Mirror, Mirror 2017: International Comparison Reflects Flaws and Opportunities for Better U.S. Health Care.* Retrieved from https://www.commonwealthfund.org

Dahlgren, G., & Whitehead, M. (2008). *European strategies for tackling social inequities in health: Leveling up Part 2.* World Health Organization. https://www.euro.who.int/__data/assets/pdf_file/0018/103824/E89384.pdf

Dunn, J. R., & Hayes, M. V. (1999). Toward a lexicon of health equity—Some social policy implications. *Canadian Journal of Public Health, 90*(Suppl 2), S7–S10. https://www.jstor.org/stable/41992584

Friedman, D. J., & Starfield, B. (2003). Models of population health: Their value for US public health practice, policy, and research. *American Journal of Public Health, 93*(3), 366–369. https://doi.org/10.2105/ajph.93.3.366

Glied, S. A., & Weiss, M. A. (September 2023). *Impact of the medicaid coverage gap: Comparing states that have and have not expanded eligibility.* Commonwealth Fund. https://doi.org/10.26099/vad1-s645

Hayes, S. L., Riley, P., Radley, D. C., & McCarthy, D. (August 2017). *Reducing racial and ethnic disparities in access to care: Has the affordable care act made a difference?* The Commonwealth Fund.

Holden, K., McGregor, B., Thandi, P., Fresh, E., Sheats, K., Belton, A., Mattox, G., & Satcher, D. (2014). Toward culturally centered integrative care for addressing mental health disparities among ethnic minorities. *Psychological Services, 11*(4), 357–368. https://doi.org/10.1037/a0038122

Institute of Medicine. (2013). *U.S. health in international perspective: Shorter lives, poorer health.* National Academies Press. https://doi.org/10.17226/13497

Kindig, D., & Stoddart, G. (2003). What is population health? *American Journal of Public Health, 93*(3), 380–383. https://doi.org/10.2105/AJPH.93.3.380

Kindig, D. A. (2007). Understanding population health terminology. *Milbank Quarterly, 85*(1),https://doi.org/10.9741/2766-7227.1014

Kindig, D. A., Asada, Y., & Booske, B. (2008). A population health framework for setting national and state health goals. *JAMA, 299*(17), 2081–2083. Agency for Healthcare Research and Quality; October 2022. AHRQ Pub. No. 22(23)-0030.

Kabir, R., & Zaidi, S. T. (2022). Implicit bias against BIPOC patients in clinical settings: A qualitative review. *Spectra Undergraduate Research Journal, 2*(1), 28–46.

Kindig, D. A., Booske, B. C., & Remington, P. L. (2008). Mobilizing action toward community health (MATCH): Metrics, incentives, and partnerships for population health. *Preventing Chronic Disease, 5*(4), A114. https://www.cdc.gov/pcd/issues/2008/oct/08_0239.htm

Lee, S., Juon, H. S., Martinez, G., Hsu, C. E., Robinson, E. S., Bawa, J., & Ma, G. X. (2009). Model minority at risk: Expressed needs of mental health by Asian American young adults. *Journal of Community Health, 34*(2), 144–152. https://doi.org/10.1007/s10900-008-9137-1

Ndugga, N., Hill, L., Pillai, D., & Artiga, S. (May 28, 2024). Race, Inequality, and health. In D. Altman (Ed.), *Health Policy 101.* KFF. https://www.kff.org/health-policy-101-race-inequality-and-health/.

Office of the Assistant Secretary for Planning and Evaluation, U.S. Department of Health and Human Services. (2024). *Health insurance coverage and access to care among Asian Americans, native Hawaiians, and Pacific Islanders: Recent trends and key challenges* (Issue Brief No. HP-2024-13). U.S. DEPARTMENT OF HEALTH AND HUMAN SERVICES. https://aspe.hhs.gov/reports/health-insurance-coverage-among-aanhpis

Office of Disease Prevention and Health Promotion. (2020). Healthy People 2020: Social determinants of health. U.S. Department of Health and Human Services. https://www.healthypeople.gov/2020/topics-objectives/topic/social-determinants-of-health

Palacio, A. M., & Shiboski, C. H. (2009). Socioeconomic status, health, and health disparities. In L. P. Boult (Ed.), *Cultural competence in health care* (pp. 57–72). Springer Publishing.

Petroka, K. F. (2015). *Facilitators and barriers to healthy eating and disease management among low-income seniors residing in subsidized housing: A case study.* https://core.ac.uk/download/190322168.pdf

Raider, F., Copan, L., & Smith, A. (2021, August). *Engaging communities for health equity and environmental justice*. California Department of Public Health. https://www.cdph.ca.gov/EHIB

Riley, W. J. (2012). Health disparities: Gaps in access, quality, and affordability of medical care. *Transactions of the American Clinical and Climatological Association, 123,* 167–172; discussion 172–174.

Saluja, B., & Bryant, Z. (2021). How implicit bias contributes to racial disparities in maternal morbidity and mortality in the United States. *Journal of Women's Health (2002), 30*(2), 270–273. https://doi.org/10.1089/jwh.2020.8874

Skloot, R. (2010). *The Immortal Life of Henrietta Lacks.* New York: Crown Publishing Group.

Smith, D. L. (2012). Health care disparities for persons with limited English proficiency: Relationships from the 2006 Medical Expenditure Panel Survey (MEPS). *Journal of Health Disparities Research and Practice, 3*(3), Art 4. https://digitalscholarship.unlv.edu/cgi/viewcontent.cgi?article=1043&context=jhdrp

Spencer, A., & Ohene-Ntow, A. O.-N. (2022). *Engaging communities of color to promote health equity: Five lessons from New York-based health care organizations* (Issue Brief). New York Health Foundation.

*The future of the public's health in the 21st century.* (2003). National Academies Press.

Washington, H. A. (2006). *Medical apartheid: The dark history of medical experimentation on Black Americans from colonial times to the present.* Doubleday.

Washington Post. (2017, May 16). *Why the Tuskegee Study still matters.* https://www.washingtonpost.com/news/to-your-health/wp/2017/05/16/why-the-tuskegee-study-still-matters/

Watson-Singleton, N. N., Lewis, J. A., & Dworkin, E. R. (2023). Toward a socially just diversity science: Using intersectional mixed methods research to center multiply marginalized Black, Indigenous, and People of Color (BIPOC). *Cultural Diversity and Ethnic Minority Psychology, 29*(1), 34. https://psycnet.apa.org/record/2021-69654-001

World Health Organization. (2010). *A conceptual framework for action on the social determinants of health.* World Health Organization. https://www.who.int/publications/i/item/9789241500852

World Health Organization. (2018). *Closing the gap in a generation: Health equity through action on the social determinants of health.* Final report of the Commission on Social Determinants of Health. https://www.who.int/publications/i/item/WHO-IER-CSDH-08.1

Young, T. K. (1998). *Population health: Concepts and methods.* Oxford University Press.

# 20 Death Customs

## Cross-Cultural Issues of Grief and Bereavement

*Rolanda L. Ward, Isiah Marshall Jr.,*
*Pedro M. Hernandez, and Patrice R. Jenkins*

Although death and dying is a commonality of the life course perspective shared by all populations, persons of varied ethnic backgrounds and beliefs celebrate, honor, and grieve (e.g., death customs) their dead in various ways, combining faith and cultural practices during services, family gatherings, and community celebrations. For example, in African cultures, death rituals can continue for periods that last long after the burial of the deceased; in addition, bereaved families and mourners are not allowed to socialize or leave the house (Baloyi & Makobe-Rabothata, 2014; Mabunda & Ross, 2022).

For the most part, cultural norms and practices within the context of death customs may be misunderstood and/or misconstrued by another group; additionally, due to xenophobia, implicit bias, lack of education, and/or pure ignorance, these norms may not be recognized or incorporated within varying cultural contexts. Researchers suggest that those who are assigned to care for the bereaved must understand these cultural traditions and beliefs; moreover, they must understand the problems that occur when they are unable to carry out specific cultural practices due to medical regulations, bureaucracy, or lack of adequate religious or social support (Clements et al., 2003; Firth, 2000; Gire, 2014; Haider, 2024; Kersey-Matusiak, 2024).

Similar to dominant cultures, those from various ethnic and cultural backgrounds may struggle with what is appropriate and accurate to maintain their practices in grief group settings. Even more impressive, there appears to be a lack of literature and research linked to cultural grief recovery and faith (Burns, 2007; Shaw & Min, 2017).

This study uses Critical Race Theory (CRT) and Ecological Systems Theory as a dual theoretical framework to examine the intersection of culture, faith, and grief. While intersectionality was introduced as a heuristic term to emphasize the distinct marginalization of American Black women in the workplace (Crenshaw, 1989), its use has gained prominence to include other oppressed, socially constructed identities (Cho et al., 2013). Atewologun & Mahalingam (2018) suggests, "Intersectionality is a critical framework or approach that provides the mindset and language to examine interconnections and interdependencies between social categories and systems" (p. 2). Furthermore, CRT can be used to analyze how systemic racial characteristics impact grieving experiences, whereas the Ecological Systems Theory offers a multilevel environmental perspective. This integrated approach provides a comprehensive understanding of cross-cultural grieving experiences, acknowledging individual and societal influences. Furthermore, this chapter details the lived experiences of culturally diverse community members in urban and Caribbean settings and their experiences seeking and finding support. Specifically, this chapter allows the respondents to explain how their faith and cultural practices converge and diverge with dominant practices. It is critical to understand respondents'

DOI: 10.4324/9781003531258-24

perspectives as a mechanism to better comprehend how dominant practices, at times, are not inclusive of all persons involved and could be damaging at such a sensitive time (Clements et al., 2003; Silverman et al., 2020). Examples would include the immediate aftermath of death; the period immediately following a death is emotionally charged and culturally significant; vulnerability of the bereaved; cultural and religious significance, community support; decision-making under stress; potential for conflict; and long-term impact on the grief process. These examples were recently observed during the COVID-19 pandemic, which disproportionately impacted Black and Latinos in the United States, exposed inequalities based on race, and forced many Black and Latino families to bury their dead outside of their normal death customs (Andraska et al., 2021; Corpuz, 2021; Tai et al., 2022). Additionally, this study serves as a tool to educate and provide helpful strategies to those who may provide direct care services to families, such as human service workers, healthcare practitioners, and case managers, during grief and sorrow for people of color.

## Literature Review

Grief has been described as a process that involves a range of feelings, emotions, and experiences. Early theorists suggest grief involves movement through stages (Kubler-Ross, 1969). Yet, this universal experience of loss is processed in many ways depending upon the culture and context in which one has been raised. For example, individuals may move between grief and moving forward or, as Stroebe and Schut (1999) suggest, a restoration-orientation grief. It has also been suggested recently that bereavement does not involve movement through stages when factors such as social experiences, networks, and spiritual needs of those grieving are considered (Worden, 2018). Some would suggest that grieving is socially constructed (Brabant, 2011; Neimeyer et al., 2014; Rosenblatt, 2008; Walter, 2006; Wambach, 1986). In faith communities, the grief of a church member is always marked with support from pastoral leaders and the church family through assistance with burial ceremonies. However, this informal caregiving is not known to move a person past Stroebe and Schut's (1999) grief oscillation, or these informal practices help or, at minimum, do not harm the bereaved. This is an important area of inquiry, as Stroebe et al. (2005) suggest that early and unsolicited interventions are not helpful. Furthermore, Abrahams (2007) argues that women who have experienced domestic violence follow a similar pattern that mirrors bereavement. The author proposes that women initially encounter shock, numbness, and disbelief. This is followed by mourning, disorganization and adjustment, depression, and lack of confidence. Lastly, they find time to reorganize and then recover. The authors term this "Reception, Recognition, and Reinvestment." Much like what Stroebe and Schut (1999) called oscillation.

Metcalf and Huntington (1991) suggest grief is variable. One aspect of variability that is relevant for social workers is the impact of culture on grief. Goodwyn (2013) argues that when additional dynamics, such as culture, are introduced to the bereavement process (e.g., urban, ethnic, SES, and no faith tradition), recovery from loss becomes complex. Though complex, disregarding the importance of one's culture during the bereavement process increases the likelihood of professional error during treatment. As practitioners, it is important to consider the relevance of culture as a contributing factor to one's grief and recovery process. Silverman et al. (2020) explain that, since death differs across cultures, its impact on grieving will also differ.

## Cultural Contexts

In understanding the complexities associated with those of varying ethnic and cultural backgrounds, grief groups, and the care that follows the death of a loved one, it is essential first to consider the cultural context associated with participating in such groups. Culture remains a significant factor in the success of services provided to this particular population and how well one responds to services rendered during bereavement. Though experienced by everyone, dying, death, and/or grief vary from one culture to the next, and the overall response to death or bereavement is based on cultural norms, beliefs, and traditions (Anderson, 2010).

Schreiber (1995) highlights the experience of grief and bereavement in an Ethiopian female refugee who was forced to relocate; symptoms of grief were exacerbated by her inability to perform her culturally sanctioned purification rituals. Due to the lack of knowledge regarding Ethiopian ritualistic practices and being culturally insensitive to the needs of this patient, clinicians further compounded the patient's grief by misdiagnosing her on numerous occasions; they failed to consider her personal beliefs and cultural practices as they related to death and bereavement. On several occasions, clinicians utilized "Western-derived diagnostic" criteria to treat the patient, thus resulting in symptoms regarding cultural bereavement being misdiagnosed. Cultural bereavement can be described as loss within the context of background/heritage (Eisenbruch, 1991). As clinicians, it is important to consider language barriers, cultural ritualistic practices, and beliefs when treating those of various ethnic and cultural backgrounds for grief or bereavement. According to Schreiber (1995), Westernized practices of healing, coupled with purification rituals and supportive psychotherapy, were essential in the treatment of this patient's presenting problem.

While existing literature has explored cultural variations in grieving, limited studies have applied CRT or Ecological Systems Theory to this context. Studies such as Rosenblatt and Wallace (2005) have begun to investigate how systematic racism affects minority bereavement experiences, but more research is needed. Similarly, Bordere (2016) applied Ecological Systems Theory to explore how different environmental conditions impact grieving, indicating that this paradigm has the potential to help explain cross-cultural grief.

## Theoretical Framework

This study uses two complementary theories to examine the intersectionality of culture, faith, and grief: CRT and Ecological Systems Theory. These theories provide a comprehensive framework for understanding how cultural and environmental factors shape grief experiences in diverse communities.

### Critical Race Theory

According to CRT, racism is woven into the fabric of society and institutions (Delgado & Stefancic, 2023). The theory, when applied to grief and bereavement, can help explain how dominant Western approaches to mourning may marginalize or invalidate the feelings and practices of racial and ethnic minorities (Rosenblatt & Wallace, 2005). CRT promotes a critical examination of how grief support services and bereavement practices might reflect and perpetuate white Western values (Granek, 2010). This perspective is crucial for our study, as it allows us to critically analyze how cultural practices in grief may be misunderstood or undervalued in mainstream bereavement support systems.

Western constructs regarding bereavement may have limited value when applied to ethnic and cultural minority groups if they fail to incorporate beliefs and norms from other cultures. CRT proponents argue that incorporating diverse cultural practices is crucial for "the rewriting of dominant groups' history to include the narratives of minimized, silenced, and excluded groups" (Lipscomb & Ashley, 2018, p. 54). By integrating these varied perspectives, professionals can honor and consider cultural constructs across the lifespan, fostering an appreciation for cultural diversity, particularly concerning bereavement norms, practices, and beliefs (Burns, 2007; Hooyman & Kramer, 2006). As racial, ethnic, and cultural diversity increases in the United States, clinicians must develop and maintain cultural competence in all aspects of care delivery, especially when providing bereavement services to grieving patients who also practice a faith tradition. Grief group educators, therefore, must intentionally expand their cultural knowledge and become more accepting of diverse cultural norms and beliefs (Sunoo, 2002).

*Ecological Systems Theory*

Ecological Systems Theory, developed by Bronfenbrenner (1979), provides a framework for understanding how multiple levels of environmental influence shape individuals' grief experiences. This includes the microsystem (i.e., immediate family and friends), mesosystem (i.e., connections between microsystems), exosystem (i.e., indirect environment), macrosystem (cultural context), and chronosystem (i.e., changes over time) (Bronfenbrenner & Morris, 2006). When applied to bereavement, this theory helps explain how cultural practices, community support, and broader societal norms influence the grief process (Balk, 2011).

In the context of grief and bereavement, this theory helps us understand how cultural practices at the macrosystem level may influence individual grief experiences and how changes in the environment (such as immigration) may impact grief processes over time (Balk, 2011).

## Integration of CRT and Ecological Systems Theory

Together, these theories provide a robust framework for our study. CRT offers a lens to examine how racial and cultural factors influence grief experiences and how dominant practices may marginalize minority experiences. Ecological Systems Theory allows us to consider how these experiences are shaped by various environmental levels, from immediate family to broader cultural contexts. This integrated theoretical approach guides us to examine individual grief experiences and how these experiences are situated within and influenced by wider cultural and systemic factors.

Using this theoretical framework, we aim to offer a comprehensive understanding of cross-cultural grieving experiences that recognize the role of systemic racial factors and the multifaceted contextual impacts on bereavement processes. This approach will enable us to interpret our findings in a way that can inform more culturally sensitive and effective bereavement support practices.

*Methods*

This study used a two-tier data collection strategy (focus groups and face-to-face interviews) to collect information from community members and clergy leaders about their views of grief, culture, and religion.

## Sample

Participants across three northeast metropolitan communities and one Caribbean community were recruited to participate in focus groups. A diverse pool of participants from various faith communities was recruited through professional, faith-based relationships (e.g., urban centers, immigrant communities, and Caribbean settings were the primary targets). A total of six focus groups and nine face-to-face interviews were conducted. For the sake of this analysis, five focus groups were used. Forty-four people participated in five focus groups. Self-reported racial identities included Black, Native American, African American, and Latino. In addition, participants from the Caribbean and those living in the northeast metropolitan areas reported national and tribal identities (e.g., African and Asian countries). Only three participants reported a Caucasian racial identity. Those participants were excluded from this analysis. Twenty-four participants reported a faith leadership role in their places of worship. Participants ranged in age from 20 to 78. Nine face-to-face interviews were completed. Of those, six were female, and three were male; all were Black. All face-to-face participants reported a racial or ethnic identity.

## Recruitment

A non-experimental, purposive, snowball sampling strategy was used to recruit clergy and community members. Focus groups consisted of individuals who had experienced the loss of a loved one, as well as clergy members who served as leaders in their faith communities. Informed consent was read aloud to make sure participants understood the aim, benefits, voluntary nature, risks, and confidentiality. Focus groups lasted between 60 and 90 minutes. At the end of the focus groups, participants were asked to participate in a follow-up interview. Individuals who consented to a face-to-face interview were contacted to arrange an interview that was convenient for them. Before beginning the interviews, informed consent was read to make sure participants understood the aim, benefits, voluntary nature, risks, and limits of confidentiality. Individual interviews lasted between 30 and 60 minutes. Both focus groups and individual interviews were conducted in English, audio recorded, and transcribed. In addition, participants were given a local resource sheet since grief memories can unsettle prior emotions surrounding the deceased loved one.

## Instrument

Face-to-face interviews and focus group guides were constructed using semi-structured, open-ended questions. Since grief is a topic that can elicit emotional responses well beyond the immediate months after a loss, it was important to structure the focus group and interview guides to allow participants to tell their stories. Interviewers allowed participants to talk freely and used follow-up prompts to clarify what was being discussed. The primary interview questions were developed to stimulate conversations about personal experiences involving the death process of a loved one and what faith practices surfaced during this process. Scholarly literature was examined to develop the interview guides.

## Data Analysis

Braun and Clarke (2006) suggest that the identification of patterns and themes in qualitative data is a viable method for analyzing data. Riessman (2008) argues that thematic analysis allows for the examination of emergent themes across multiple cases. Thematic analysis is interpretive and not just data summarization (Clarke & Braun, 2013). Latent thematic analysis involves moving beyond summarization (Braun & Clarke, 2006). Data was analyzed using latent thematic analysis to identify the intersectionality of participants' faith, culture, and grief experiences across cases.

CRT and Ecological Systems Theory provided the framework for our investigation. We categorized data not just for individual experiences but also for signs of systemic racial impacts and evidence of how various environmental levels (i.e., micro, meso, exo, macro, and chronosystems) influenced participants' mourning experiences. This approach allowed us to situate individual narratives within broader sociocultural contexts.

## *Findings*

A review of the data found that participants had apparent examples of cultural practices linked to grief and recovery. Some participants described processes that had very distinct cultural and ethnic expressions of grief. Some practices were linked to religious practices, and others were linked to cultural practices. Three themes emerged as examples of the intersectionality of grief, faith, and culture: religious and cultural practices at death, theology and grief containment, and varying practices of those who grieve. Grief containment can be described as holding one's emotions during periods of bereavement and loss.

## Religious and Cultural Practices at Death

Most participants were very descriptive about the intersectionality of time-of-death grief practices (i.e., those that involve religious and cultural practices). For some, cultural practices at death centered around named rituals that include different practices of hosting family and friends. Others experienced similar activities but did not formally name communal grief practices. Lastly, the intersection of religion and culture included certain expectations of faith leaders.

For most respondents, bereavement was a communal faith expression.

> For Puerto Ricans in Puerto Rico and even Puerto Ricans here, depending I think on the religion, if you are Catholic, they have what you call las nueve novenas ... they meet in that person's house for nine days straight, and they pray and they talk, and you know they eat food and stuff. ... But for the first nine days, there's always people in the house and prayer going on after the person dies.
>
> (Maria)

Furthermore, for most respondents, cultural practices at death were illuminated through marked responsibilities after a short period of time.

> After that the couple days, like a week after, they remember the person ... So that's a week later, and then they come together and socialize. They get together again, the family and the neighbors and the people who are close. They cook, and they eat, and they drink.
>
> (Monifa)

Hollie's recollection of sitting and talking with family and friends about the deceased was like others' stories. The practice of sitting did not need to happen in the family home, but it was also welcome at the place of death.

> So right away I got on the telephone, started calling relatives, and told them what was going on, and people came up there to the nursing home, they were there, about a few hours, just sitting there and talking about how she has affected our lives.

Family and friends were the primary people present at the time of death. In addition, the data showed that faith leaders had a role during this transition time. For almost all respondents, they discussed the role of pastors and/or church leaders during the initial bereavement stages at the place of death. In many cases, leadership was called to offer a prayer or other expressions of spiritual support.

> The pastor was there to be an intercessor prayer, for his support, my father was, at the time, he was chairman of the deacon board and just to be with the family, show love, support, pray with us, for us.
>
> (Millie)

> Sometimes you don't even have to call them. They're already there before you get there.
>
> (Wit)

Among this theme, one participant even hypothesized about the role of her pastor during his absence.

> If my pastor was in town, he definitely would have come because he's just one of those people that really shows support and he would have come up and at least pray[ed], probably wouldn't stay a long [time] but he would at least pray[ed] with the family and let them know that he cares and let them know that if there was anything that he could do to call him and he would do that.
>
> (Hollie)

Many agreed that pastoral presence was not just an act of support but an important pastoral duty or a true expectation of parishioners.

> I would expect them to be there ... that was like one of the first calls I made that day, that morning, you know, within a few hours, so yeah, I think it's expected.
>
> (Dawn)

The cultural traditions of bereaved individuals are essential during the initial moments of the grief process. For most focus group participants, the time immediately following the death of a loved one involved the practice of religious rituals: singing, praying, and communing with loved ones. Participants in this study also indicated that religious comfort was found in the actions of the faith leaders. In fact, the analysis showed that parishioners have expectations about when and what faith leaders should do during these communal gatherings. This finding provides insight into the antecedents of religious engagement with those who grieve.

### Theology and Grief Containment

Family members who experience the loss of a loved one use theology and faith references to express their grief. The second finding that participants expressed had to do with their understanding of grief through a faith lens and how faith helps them cope. More specifically, their expression of grief, at times, helps them contain the outward expression of their grief. Respondents discussed emotional responses that appeared to mute and validate their grief, as well as responses that measured their sense of being Christian.

Fatima's struggle to self-manage her grief appears to be connected to being a good Christian example for other family and church members. Fatima's containment appeared to be a mutation of her grief, and this mutation of her emotional response is grounded in her belief in the Word of God.

> Oh, when I cry [it] is like I [am] full of emotion, I [am] full of emotion, but like now I want to resist it, but I can't, yes. I want to resist it but I can't … I don't like [for people] to know that I suffer. I am a leader in the church. I can give a good example for my son, for my friend, for the men who I preach. I must accept [death] because I believe that the second life exists when you receive Jesus … [It] is our way. We must believe that word.

Like Fatima, Dawn's containment appeared to be a validation of her faith. Her description of death appears to describe how death made her a stronger believer. She connects the experience of death to an increased sense of strength.

> I'd got to see the full transition of death and it's not as scary as a lot of people imagine and I think I guess it depends on what your belief system [is], but since my belief system is God, I felt Him like never before and He just, you know, like, you were talking about the strength, where you get your strength from, and he gives you just unbelievable strength.

In contrast to Fatima and Dawn, Wit's containment of grief resulted in a sense of numbness: "I found that I couldn't call anybody. I was completely numb." For Wit, containment of grief meant self-isolation. He goes on to describe his sense of numbness:

> But to be totally numb to where you didn't know your name, couldn't write, couldn't even look at a phone and remember anybody—any number to call, the only number you remembered was her birthday, her social security number, that was the only thing I could remember. The date of our marriage. I couldn't remember anything else. It seemed as if Suzie was passing right before me and the final chapter was closed.

Also, although Wit shared a connection to Fatima, serving as a minister/leader in his church, Wit's sense of numbness and isolation prevailed, even though, as he says, "[Jesus Christ] is the most important thing." Even though he expressed a great connection to Jesus, he rejected the help of his church members.

> They were asking am I okay? Did I eat? and Most of the time I hadn't, so they were checking up to make sure I was taking care of myself, which I wasn't doing and so I basically shut them all out. I didn't want to be bothered. I guess I was going through a bout

of depression and that's a long way to go. It took a while before I was to get out of it, you know? I was angry … I was upset … I didn't know which way to go … and so I just shut everybody out.

Furthermore, grief containment also appeared to be an indication of one's magnitude of faith. Dawn talked about how death created instances of doubt, even though she shared earlier in the conversation about her strong faith commitment. This sense of doubt seems to be conquerable, and it has a strong connection to pastoral leadership. Furthermore, it appears as if pastoral leadership has to create spaces for doubt while also validating faith. This balance, at the intersection of faith and grief, provides support and validation of one's emotional response to grief.

Yeah, that point is spiritual support and like you said, to confirm who He really is, because in the face of death, whether it's expected or not expected, I think of the natural process of grief you still have questions about God, and one of the people that called me after was Elder Summers, who would always come over, I mean, come to the hospital and once I remember being so upset because I was upset that I questioned God and she confirmed to me that He wants you to question him sometimes, but had she not been there on that other line, you know, on the other end of the phone, I would have went crazy cause I was finally questioning God, but she was able to confirm Him, and she was able to go through scripture and listen to me cry and talk, but yeah they're there to be that support.

Dawn's experience of grief appears to have had a long-lasting implication, even with a strong faith in God. She seems to allude to how faith provided her strength to get through her grief and how, during her bereavement, she comforted others who did not have a strong sense of faith. Caring for others, muting her grief, and drawing upon her understanding of faith for the sake of others seem to have impacted her bereavement process.

Some people don't know God like I did and I think that it was Him that you had to, you know, had to be strong for everybody else because while they're breaking down, you can't break down too. If you're breaking down then, you know, so I just had to be, felt like I had to be strong for everybody. Looking back 6.5 years later, I don't know if that was the best thing, but at the time I guess it was.

Dealing with one's sense of faith while grieving is an important aspect of managing one's outward expressions of grief. Faith seems to offer comfort during this difficult time. Even though faith provides comfort, it also appears to have an impact on how grief is expressed. For most respondents, faith managed or muted their emotional response. For most, mutation was not always negative. Interestingly, even those with a strong sense of faith or who held leadership positions in the church struggled to manage grief, found themselves in isolation, or shared how they questioned God. Even though theological references provide comfort, the experience of grief can shake even the most grounded believer.

### Varying Practices of Those Who Grieve

All participants born outside of the mainland United States discussed differences between their experiences of grief in their home nations/territories and their observations of grief practices on the mainland. Many had stories about how their cultural norms were very different from the customs on the mainland. In addition, they discussed the impact of these practices on their grief process.

Monifa described the level of support the bereaved received in Africa. Support in Africa meant a long-term physical presence of family, friends, and community members.

> I was going to say, really, in Africa, there is nothing that a person can wish for because they have a lot of support. Support from their neighbors, support from people you don't even know, support from the family, there's a lot of support, like, even if you're losing someone, the only time you will be alone will be the night, or maybe a couple of weeks later, or month later, but even that you will always have someone around to call close to you.

In contrast, in the United States, she described a sense of aloneness in the grief process.

> In the U.S., I was just remembering, we lost a mother-in-law to my brother, she passed away, here, in the U.S., in the mainland. When she passed away, we didn't know what to do. It was hard for us. We didn't know the cost of the funeral, and we found out that everything was really, really tough, really, really hard. It was just our family, nobody else, no neighbors.

Not only did participants describe a difference between levels of community support, but they also described distinct differences between death practices and rituals. Many of the death practices were connected to their expression of faith. Individuals who are not familiar with these practices may, in fact, interfere with the grief process of those who are culturally different. In one instance, families felt like the funeral home attendants were surprised to learn the family wanted to take part in the burial process.

> [T]he cemetery and they were surprised at how our family was handling everything, they were very surprised, so when the time came to put the body in the grave, my brothers and those two people and her sons, the deceased sons, they came together, and said "okay, it's time, so now let's put her down." The two people came by, and they were like "Oh, that's our job." and we say "No, it's okay." So we did that ourselves, and we kept singing while we're doing that and my father prayed, and we prayed enough that we took them, what is that thing they use, (Interviewer: the shovel?) yeah, the shovel, before we did the shovel we did the, what, everything we do, the song and the flowers and everything and my brothers again and her sons, they put them, they covered, and the two people who worked at the cemetery they just, they are looking like this and again "That's our job." and we say "no, we gotta do this." So we did everything, and they are so surprised, and they are appreciated, they thanked us afterwards, they say "thank you for doing that." We say, "this is our person." It's our duty to do this.

Cultural grief practices are essential to those who practice them. Many of these practices are communal and performed in the community. These types of practices provide support to families. Even though participants came from different racial and ethnic groups, many expressed the need for communal faith support. Monifa shared, "I hope that at that time we had enough support from other people, support from the church, support from the community, that's what I wished we could have. Wish for more support."

The impact of not being able to grieve the way Rosa is used to or the impact of encountering individuals who do not understand her grief is striking. Rosa's thoughtful sentiments in the group's discussion capture the unique needs of cultural bereavement:

[I]t brings tears to my eyes as I hear you, well, first of all, describing the grief that you've experienced but then also the strangeness that you felt when your family member felt away in the U.S., and we didn't seem to pay attention to it enough.

Participants' recollections of their cultural grief practices in their home nations are very different from the grief practices on the mainland. These different practices are a natural support during a difficult time. However, when participants are unable to practice these traditions, there is a breakdown in the way cultural faith communities help each other process and heal their grief. As Rosa illuminated, strangeness leads to not paying attention to the needs of community members who need support at a difficult time.

## Discussion and Conclusion

As stated earlier, three themes emerged as examples of the intersectionality of grief, faith, and culture: religious and cultural practices at death, theology and grief containment, and varying practices of those who grieve. The intersection of religion and culture definitively incorporates the community (or communal) aspect of this time of grief. "Eulogies" (i.e., stories about the soon-to-be departed or departed) do not only take place inside religious settings or during religious events. People gather around recollecting, that is, telling stories, sometimes referred to colloquially as "war stories," honoring the deceased.

Community, in other words, lay people, offer those grieving support and a sense of alleviation. Communal healing, more specifically, the communal nature of grief, has been observed and documented by many cultural anthropologists (see, for example, Heart & DeBruyn, 1998; Robben, 2017). For instance, in many African countries as well as in many American Indian tribes, it is common that the community partakes in grief rituals to alleviate and help nurse those hurt before the "pain" gets worse and causes long-term "damages." The writer Sobonfu Some (2019, par. 14) wrote: "Communal grieving offers something that we cannot get when we grieve by ourselves. Through acknowledgment, validation, and witnessing, communal grieving allows us to experience a level of healing that is deeply and profoundly freeing." She also writes: "Unexpressed hurt and pain injures our souls, and can be linked directly to our general sense of spiritual drought and emotional confusion, not to mention the many illnesses we experience in our lives" (par. 7). The writer refers to this "unexpressed hurt and pain" as toxins, that is, emotional and spiritual toxins, and as with any toxins it can make us sick, both physically and mentally.

Faith leaders, faith healers, and/or clergy are part of this communal healing so much that they do not even have to be invited; they are a fixture in these times of need. The role of faith leaders, for some, may be to remind us that our loved one has only transitioned from one world to another, and he/she is still "watching over us."

Viewing our findings through the lenses of CRT and Ecological Systems Theory allows for a more comprehensive understanding of cross-cultural grieving experiences. The various activities of persons who grieve, for example, can be understood as a reflection of both cultural traditions (macrosystem) and immediate family dynamics (microsystem). Meanwhile, the challenges encountered by immigrants in carrying out their grieving rituals underscore the effect of systemic racial issues, as theorized by CRT.

Since grief is common, several behaviors cross language and cultural differences. Grief combines beliefs, values, experiences, traditions, customs, habits, religious and non-religious practices, and rituals. For some, following grieving and bereavement rituals will offer and bring a sense of security, strength, understanding, acceptance, relief, and, finally, normality and closure. It is difficult to know what to say to those who grieve. The foundation of understanding any culture is asking questions to inform our understanding of anyone's grief and our own. Learning can be achieved by listening and observing.

## Limitations of the Study

While our study provides valuable insights into cross-cultural grief experiences, it is important to acknowledge several limitations that may impact the interpretation and generalizability of our findings. The limited sample size of 44 focus group members and nine face-to-face interviews, while diverse, may only reflect part of the range of cultural grieving experiences. Furthermore, our geographic focus on selecting northeast urban neighborhoods and one Caribbean community restricts our findings' application to other regions or nations with distinct cultural settings.

Our recruitment method, which relied on professional and faith-based relationships, may have introduced a self-selection bias. Participants who volunteered to participate in the study may have had unique experiences or perspectives that are not indicative of the larger population. While the qualitative aspect of our research provides rich, in-depth data, it does not lend itself to statistical analysis or the comparison of different groups or behaviors, thereby constraining our ability to make far-reaching conclusions.

Comparing grieving experiences across cultures presented inherent challenges due to each culture's distinct circumstances and meanings. Our interpretations should keep this constraint in mind. The retrospective character of participants' accounts may be susceptible to memory biases or shifts in viewpoint over time.

While we aimed to examine intersectionality, our findings may not fully represent how different dimensions of identity (such as race, class, and gender) interact to influence grieving experiences. Our study gives a snapshot of grieving experiences but needs to account for how these feelings may evolve due to the lack of longitudinal data.

## Implications for Human Services Practice

Even though many beliefs and behaviors do cross the language and cultural border, one should never make assumptions or take for granted our cultural differences. One significant concern of human service professionals attending to the needs of foreign national and urban ethnic clients at the time of grief may not be the culture of the clients but the reaction (i.e., how they deal) with the dominant culture.

Human service professionals who help grieving clients from diverse backgrounds should consider both systemic racial characteristics and multilevel environmental variables. This might include advocating for more inclusive policies at funeral homes (exosystem), as well as assisting clients in navigating family dynamics (microsystem) and broader societal expectations (macrosystem).

As human service professionals, we should be aware that most of the time, people will take their culture for granted. The grieving period (or time) is a time of conflict, chaos, confusion, perplexity, and transition. However, cultural beliefs and faith traditions may provide essential comfort, which allows for the expression of emotions. Since no human service professional or even a human being can be aware of the hundreds of different cultural practices, it is imperative to be an active listener; maintain proper, respectful, and professional boundaries; and integrate a clinical understanding of human behavior through a cultural and faith lens.

## Future Research

In exploring the complexities of grief and faith, researchers should delve into contemporary issues such as fatalistic death (i.e., gang violence), death connected to incarceration, complex disease, and kidnappings. People of faith live in an ever-changing society, and some of the situational factors mentioned here are experienced and understood differently. Furthermore, since the United States has become heterogeneous, contexts such as geography (i.e., rural, urban, Caribbean) and logistics must be explored to determine how clinicians and those who practice grief care incorporate concerns into faith and grief practices. Other venues to further explore would be bicultural families, that is, families where the couple (or partners) are from different cultural backgrounds. Future deductive studies should examine the relevance of cultural assessment tools that measure the intersectionality of faith and culture in grief recovery. Future findings within this realm can be used to educate social workers, clergy, and lay leaders about the importance of culturally supporting community members during times of grief.

## Questions for Reflection

1  How can social workers and other helping professionals better integrate the religious and cultural practices at death described in this study into their support for bereaved clients from diverse backgrounds?
2  How can social workers balance evidence-based practice with respect to diverse cultural grieving practices that may not align with Western psychological models?
3  How might social workers collaborate more effectively with faith leaders to provide comprehensive support during the grieving process, as highlighted by participants in this study?

## References

Abrahams, H. (2007). *Supporting women after domestic violence: Loss, trauma and recovery*. Jessica Kingsley Publishers.

Anderson, H. (2010). Common grief, complex grieving. *Pastoral Psychology, 59*, 127–136. https://doi.org/10.1007/s11089-009-0243-5.

Andraska, E. A., Alabi, O., Dorsey, C., Erben, Y., Velazquez, G., Franco-Mesa, C., & Sachdev, U. (2021). Health care disparities during the COVID-19 pandemic. *Seminars in vascular surgery, 34*(3), 82–88. https://doi.org/10.1053/j.semvascsurg.2021.08.002

Atewologun, D., & Mahalingam, R. (2018). Intersectionality as a methodological tool in qualitative equality, diversity and inclusion research. In *Handbook of research methods in diversity management, equality and inclusion at work* (pp. 149–170). Edward Elgar Publishing. https://doi.org/10.4337/9781783476084.00016

Balk, D. E. (2011). Adolescent development and bereavement: An introduction. *The Prevention Researcher, 18*(3), 3–9.

Baloyi, L., & Makobe-Rabothata, M. (2014). The African conception of death: A cultural implication. *ScholarWorks*. https://scholarworks.gvsu.edu/cgi/viewcontent.cgi?article=1018&context=iaccp_papers.

Bordere, T. (2016). Social justice conceptualizations in grief and loss. In D. L. Harris, & T. C. Bordere (Eds.), *Handbook of social justice in loss and grief: Exploring diversity, equity, and inclusion* (pp. 9–20). Routledge.

Brabant, S. (2011). Death: The ultimate social construction of reality. *OMEGA - Journal of Death and Dying, 62*(3), 221–242. https://doi.org/10.2190/OM.62.3.b

Braun, V., & Clarke, V. (2006). Using thematic analysis in psychology. *Qualitative Research in Psychology, 3*, 77–101. https://doi.org/10.1191/1478088706QP063OA

Bronfenbrenner, U. (1979). *The ecology of human development: Experiments by nature and design.* Harvard University Press.

Bronfenbrenner, U., & Morris, P. A. (2006). The bioecological model of human development. In W. Damon, & R. M. Lerner (Eds.), *Handbook of child psychology: Theoretical models of human development* (pp. 793–828). John Wiley & Sons Inc.

Burns, C. B. (2007). The challenge for Christian chaplains: To provide spiritual care to all. *ETD Collection for AUC Robert W. Woodruff Library.* 326. https://digitalcommons.auctr.edu/dissertations/326

Clarke, V., & Braun, V. (2013). Teaching thematic analysis: Overcoming challenges and developing strategies for effective learning. *The Psychologist, 26*(2), 120–123.

Clements, P. T., Vigil, G. J., Manno, M. S., Henry, G. C., Wilks, J., Das, S., Kellywood, R., & Foster, W. (2003). Cultural perspectives of death, grief, and bereavement. *Journal of Psychosocial Nursing and Mental Health Services, 41*(7), 18–26. https://doi.org/10.3928/0279-3695-20030701-12

Corpuz, J. C. (2021). Beyond death and afterlife: The complicated process of grief in the time of COVID-19. *Journal of Public Health, 43*(2), e281–e282. https://doi.org/10.1093/pubmed/fdaa247

Crenshaw, K. (1989). Demarginalizing the intersection of race and sex: A Black feminist critique of antidiscrimination doctrine, feminist theory and antiracist politics. *The University of Chicago Legal Forum, 140*, 139–167.

Cho, S., Crenshaw, K. W., & McCall, L. (2013). Toward a field of intersectionality studies: Theory, applications, and praxis. *Signs, 38*(4), 785–810. https://doi.org/10.1086/669608

Delgado, R., & Stefancic, J. (2023). *Critical race theory: An introduction.* New York University Press.

Eisenbruch, M. (1991). From posttraumatic stress disorder to cultural bereavement: Diagnosis of Southeast Asian refugees. *Social Science Medicine, 33*, 673–680.

Firth, S. (2000). Cross-cultural perspectives on bereavement. In D. Dickerson, M. Johnson, & J. S. Katz (Eds.), *Death, dying, and bereavement* (pp. 338–345). Sage Publications.

Gire, J. T. (2014). How death imitates life: Cultural influences on conceptions of death and dying. *Online Readings in Psychology and Culture, 6*(2), 1–22. https://doi.org/10.970712307-0919.1120

Goodwyn, E. (2013). Recurrent motifs as resonant attractor states in the narrative field: A testable model of archetype. *Journal of Analytical Psychology, 58*, 387–408. https://doi.org/10.1111/1468-5922.12020

Granek, L. (2010). Grief as pathology: The evolution of grief theory in psychology from Freud to the present. *History of Psychology, 13*(1), 46–73. https://doi.org/10.1037/a0016991

Haider, S. (2024). Breaking the silence: Understanding the complexities of bereavement and grief among Syrian refugee fathers. In K. Jones, & M. Robb (Eds.), *Men and Loss* (pp. 188–200). Routledge. https://doi.org/10.4324/9781003333999

Heart, B., & DeBruyn, L. M. (1998). The American Indian holocaust: Healing historical unresolved grief. *American Indian and Alaska Native Mental Health Research, 8*(2), 56–78.

Hooyman, N. R., & Kramer, B. J. (2006). *Living through loss: Interventions across the life span.* Columbia University Press.

Kersey-Matusiak, G. (2024). *Delivering culturally competent nursing care: Working with diverse and vulnerable populations.* Springer Publishing.

Kubler-Ross, E. (1969). *On death and dying.* McMillan.

Lipscomb, A. E., & Ashley, W. (2018). Black male grief through the lens of racialization and oppression: Effective instruction for graduate clinical programs. *International Research in Higher Education, 3*(2), 51–60.

Mabunda, Y. P., & Ross, E. (2022). Experiences of Black South African widows regarding mourning rituals following the death of their spouses: Upholding cultural practices or violating human rights? *Death Studies*, 47(3), 328–338. https://doi.org/10.1080/07481187.2022.2065708

Metcalf, P., & Huntington, R. (1991). *Celebrations of death: The anthropology of mortuary ritual.* Cambridge University Press.

Neimeyer, R. A., Klass, D., & Dennis, M. R. (2014). A social constructionist account of grief: Loss and the narration of meaning. *Death Studies*, 38(6–10), 485–498. https://doi.org/10.1080/07481187.2014.913454

Riessman, C. K. (2008). *Narrative methods for the human sciences.* Sage Publications.

Robben, A. C. (Ed.). (2017). *Death, mourning, and burial: A cross-cultural reader.* John Wiley & Sons.

Rosenblatt, P. C., & Wallace, B. R. (2005). *African American grief.* Routledge.

Rosenblatt, P. C. (2008). Grief across cultures: A review and research agenda. In M. S. Stroebe, R. O. Hansson, H. Shut, & W. Stroebe (Eds.), *Handbook of bereavement research and practice: Advances in theory and intervention* (pp. 207–222). American Psychological Association Press.

Schreiber, S. (1995). Migration, traumatic bereavement and transcultural aspects of psychological healing: Loss and grief of a refugee woman from Begameder county in Ethiopia. *British Journal of Medical Psychology*, 68(2),135–142. https://doi.org/10.1111/j.2044-8341.1995.tb01820.x

Shaw, R. (2017). How to develop an effective grief recovery ministry. In T. Clinton & J. Pingleton (Eds.), *The struggle is real: How to care for mental and relational health needs in the church* (pp. 213–228). WestBow Press.

Silverman, G. S., Baroiller, A., & Hemer, S. R. (2020). Culture and grief: Ethnographic perspectives on ritual, relationships and remembering. *Death Studies*, 45(1), 1–8. https://doi.org/10.1080/07481187.2020.1851885

Some, S. (2019). Embracing grief: Surrendering to your sorrow has the power to heal the deepest of wounds. https://www.sobonfu.com/articles/writings-by-sobonfu-2/embracing-grief/

Stroebe, M., & Schut, H. (1999). The dual process model of coping with bereavement: Rationale and description. *Death Studies*, 23(3), 197–224. https://doi.org/10.1080/074811899201046

Stroebe, M., Schut, H., & Stroebe, W. (2005). Attachment in coping with bereavement: A theoretical integration. *Review of General Psychology*, 9(1), 48–66. https://doi.org/10.1037/1089-2680.9.1.48

Still B. (2011, December). Cultural grief. https://stillbirthday.com/2011/12/cultural-grief/

Sunoo, B. P. (2002, March–April). Cultural diversity and grief. *The Forum newsletter, Association for Death Education and Counseling*, (March–April), 1–4.

Tai, D. B. G., Sia, I. G., Doubeni, C. A., & Wieland, M. L. (2022). Disproportionate impact of COVID-19 on racial and ethnic minority groups in the United States: A 2021 update. *Journal of Racial and Ethnic Health Disparities*, 9(6), 2334–2339. https://doi.org/10.1007/s40615-021-01170-w

Walter, T. (2006). What is complicated grief? A social constructionist perspective. *OMEGA - Journal of Death and Dying*, 52(1), 71–79. https://doi.org/10.2190/3LX7-C0CL-MNWR-JKKQ

Wambach, J. A. (1986). The grief process as a social construct. *OMEGA - Journal of Death and Dying*, 16(3), 201–211. https://doi.org/10.2190/XBB0-LHXE-FDLH-8Q9M

Worden, J. W. (2018). *Grief counseling and grief therapy: A handbook for the mental health practitioner.* Springer Publishing Company.

# 21 A "Real-World" Social Work Analysis of Child and Family Welfare

## Implications for Culturally Competent Interventions to Address 21st-Century Issues

*Irma J. Gibson*

## Introduction

One of society's most important functions is the socialization of children (Traver, 2021). From birth, individuals are socialized via the primary agents of socialization: family, school, peers, media, social media, religion, and employers. While school, peers, and the media belong to the primary socialization category, the workplace and the government are secondary means of socialization that are also considered specialized statutes as we move through the life course. Socialization is the process of learning how to function in a group or society over time. It is a set of paradigms, rules, procedures and principles that govern perception, attention, choices, learning and development (Saras & Perez-Felkner, 2018). Early socialization is thought to occur primarily within the family (Grusec, 2011).

Macionis (2009) defines socialization as a process by which the cultural heritage of a society is transmitted to the next generation. Crucial to the socialization of children is the family.

In most societies, the family is the primary world for young children's first few years of life. Families transmit cultural and social values from infancy and are the primary source of emotional support and social position. Family is the first agent of socialization. Mothers and fathers, siblings and grandparents, and members of an extended family teach a child what he or she needs to know. Families, of course, come in all sorts of formations. Whether the young child is living with a biological parent, adopted by their parents, or exclusively raised by a sibling or a grandparent, this unit of family is what socializes the young child to the world first. Sociologists recognize that race, social class, ethnicity, religious preference, regional location, and other societal factors also play an important role in socialization (Rothschild, n.d.).

The degree to which children learn how to participate and be accepted by society has significant consequences for their development and future lives. Equally important, Perez-Felkner (forthcoming) posits that "the social codes that children and adolescents learn are specific not only to nation-states and regions of the globe but also to historical periods and social groups within larger societies." The socio-historical context is a critical dimension of the socialization of children and adolescents, both concerning their status within society (compared to adults) as well as their social role (Perez-Felkner, forthcoming)

Although the family has been slated as the most influential among these socialization agents, the first "school" experience for young children under the early education component, whether it be daycare, preschool, or kindergarten, generally serves as the second socialization agent for young children. This factor is crucial. "Most US children spend about seven hours a day, 180 days a year, in school, which makes it hard to deny the importance

DOI: 10.4324/9781003531258-25

school has on their socialization" (U.S. Department of Education 2004). Students are not in school only to study math, reading, science, and other subjects (the manifest function of this system) (Lumen Learning, n.d.); schools also serve a latent social function by social-izing children into behaviors like practicing teamwork, following a schedule, and using textbooks. School and classroom rituals, led by teachers serving as role models and leaders, regularly reinforce what society expects from children. Sociologists describe this aspect of schools as the hidden curriculum, the informal teaching done by schools (Rothschild, n.d.).

> As the most important agent of socialization for children, parents' values and behavior patterns profoundly influence those of their daughters and sons. Families are so influen-tial, for better or worse, because our families are such an important part of the socializa-tion process.
>
> (Barkan, 2012)

When we are born, our primary caregivers are almost always one or both of our parents or guardians. For several years, we have had more contact with them than with any other adults. Because this contact occurs in our most formative years, our parents' interaction with us and the messages they teach us can profoundly impact our lives (ELSI, 2016).

The point is that family is a critical aspect of socialization, and family socialization begins a process through which children learn to be the adult persons they become. For some, the effects of family socialization are evident and long-lasting; for others, there is lit-tle apparent effect.

And, for others, it still looks like there's no relationship. With scrutiny, one can observe that some evolving adults adopt behaviors and values that are entirely opposite to those of their families. Socialization is just as intense, but it has a different effect. Some adults' interactions with family continue in such a close relationship that the family maintains a dominant role in their ongoing socialization (Driscoll & Nagel, 2008). The socialization established during those crucial first seven years of life serves as a precursor to what could be a tumultuous or progressive future that impacts every facet of the lifespan, including adolescence and young adulthood.

### The Importance of Theories in Comprehending and Addressing Culturally Based Interventions

The main agents of socialization in social work lingo equate to the person in the environ-ment theoretical framework or the ecological/systems and ecosystems theoretical perspec-tive. Theories are generalized sets of ideas that describe and explain our knowledge of the world in an organized way (Swelindawo, 2019). They help us understand and contest ideas and the world around us, offer a framework for practice, and allow us to be accountable, self-disciplined, and professional (Payne, 2014, p. 3). Theories are overall explanations of the person-in-environment, as we are all products of our environment from birth to the present.

Bronfenbrenner's ecological systems theory views an individual's development within the context of the system of relationships that form his/her environment. Bronfenbrenner's the-ory has been historically applied to child development. By defining complex layers of envi-ronment, each influencing children's development, this theory emphasizes that children's interaction between factors in their maturing biology, their immediate family/community environment, and the societal landscape fuels and steers their development. Furthermore, changes or conflicts in any one layer will ripple throughout other layers. To study a child's development, then, we must look not only at the child and his/her immediate environment but also at the interaction of the larger environment (Kuna, 2014). Through their early experiences with primary caregivers and siblings, children learn the rules of relationships and begin to construct their views of the world (APA, 2009), which is why the nature versus nurture framework also deserves attention as a critical theory in comprehending human development and the importance of child and family relationship dynamics.

According to Gibson (2019), the nature versus nurture theory addresses the relative influence of an individual's innate attributes as opposed to the experiences from the environment in which one is brought up, determining individual differences in physical and behavioral traits. In layman's terms, we are all born with specific genetic characteristics that shape who we are from birth to the present, including but not limited to our personality, mannerisms, drive, and physical appearance.

Sir Francis Galton argued that intelligence and character traits come from hereditary factors and was in clear opposition to earlier scholars such as philosopher John Locke, who is well known for the theory that children are born a "blank slate," with their traits developing entirely from experience and learning (Honeycutt, 2019; Manouchakian, 2018). Both gentlemen believed that the environment and a person's unique experiences, i.e., nurture, were the prevailing forces in development (Rettew, 2017). Thus, the environment we are exposed to and projected as we progress throughout our lifespan provides opportunities to learn, grow, mature, and change accordingly. Through these experiences and via this exposure to a plethora of negative and positive encounters, risk and protective factors emerge and saturate the environment daily, beginning from birth (Gibson, 2019). "Children are like wet cement. Whatever falls on them makes an impression" (Haim Ginott, as cited in NYARCP, 2011).

Sociodemographic factors and environmental influences, including healthcare, family, and community factors, in early childhood have been demonstrated to have a significant impact on development, mental health, and overall health throughout the lifespan and have been associated with increased risk for mental, behavioral, and developmental disorders in children (Bitsko et al., 2016), which is why the state of child and family welfare mandates crucial attention in the 21st century more than ever.

"Maslow's hierarchy of needs is a theory of motivation and personality developed by the psychologist Abraham H. Maslow (1908–1970)". Maslow's hierarchy explains human behavior in terms of basic requirements for survival and growth. These requirements or needs are arranged according to their survival importance and power to motivate the individual. The most basic physical requirements, such as food, water, or oxygen, constitute the lowest level of the need hierarchy. Needs at the higher levels of the hierarchy are less oriented toward physical survival and more toward psychological well-being and growth. These needs have less power to motivate people and are more influenced by formal education and life experiences. The resulting hierarchy of needs is often depicted as a pyramid, with physical survival needs located at the pyramid's base and needs for self-actualization located at the top (Krapp, 2010).

Every person is capable and desires to move up the hierarchy toward a level of self-actualization. Unfortunately, progress is often disrupted by failure to meet lower-level needs (McLeod, 2016). Figure 21.1 exhibits what is needed according to Maslow to eventually and developmentally reach self-actualization throughout the lifespan: physiological needs to include food, water, shelter, and clothing; security and safety needs provided by family and society; love and belonging to give and receive love, appreciation, and friendship;

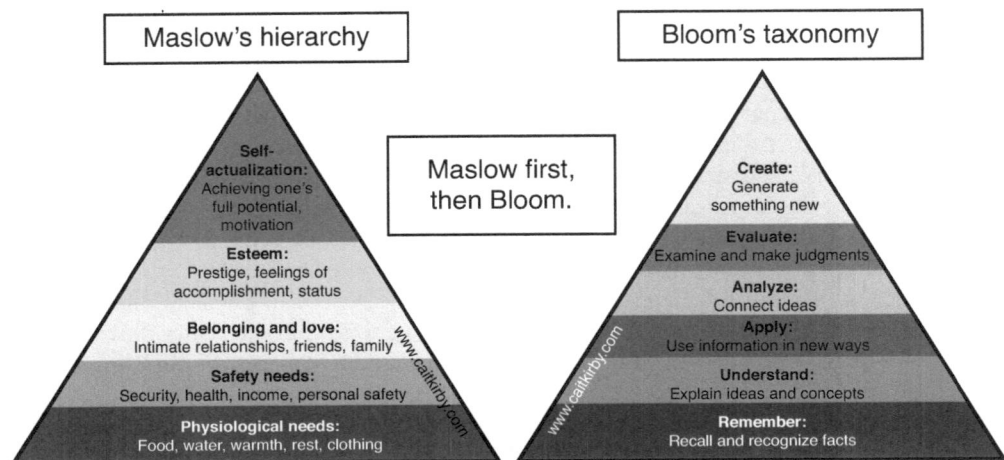

*Figure 21.1* Maslow's hierarchy of needs and Bloom's taxonomy.

This photo by unknown author is licensed under CC BY-NC-ND.

self-esteem needs, i.e., self-respect and individuality; and self-actualization, to include experiencing purpose, meaning, and realizing all inner potential.

As the importance of a stable family foundation is addressed, a crucial point is studies have shown that "children who do not get the early intervention, permanence and stability they need are more likely to act out and fail in school because they lack the skills necessary to succeed" (Children's Defense Fund, 2009a). "Bloom's taxonomy consists of six stages of teaching and learning, namely, remembering, understanding, applying, analyzing, evaluating and creating and moves from a lower degree to a higher degree" (Chandio et al., 2016). Bloom's Taxonomy divides academic learning into cognitive, affective, and psychomotor categories. The cognitive domain contains mental abilities for knowledge production; the affective domain involves continuous emotional development of mindset; and the psychomotor domain involves physical skills (Momen et al., 2022). The premise is that to successfully reach and maintain these academic goals of achievement, the cognitive, intellectual, and mental capacities represented by Bloom's framework are impacted by and aligned with Maslow's theoretical framework, "no Blooms without Maslow."

Researchers of early childhood emphasize the importance of early childhood nurturing and stimulation to help the brain grow, especially between birth and age seven, and even beyond and thus helping children thrive and be on a positive path toward successful adulthood. The importance of stimulation in the first years of life is dramatically underlined in the United States.

The Department of Education's study of 22,000 kindergartners in the kindergarten class of 1998–1999, which found that Black and Hispanic children were substantially behind when they entered kindergarten" (Children's Defense Fund, 2009b). Theoretically speaking, this information is considered crucial under the cultural analyses of the 0–7 foundational years and warrants critical attention in the completion of a thorough biopsychosocial assessment.

Stated, thousands of children in the child welfare system are already considered at risk of failing to reach self-actualization and become productive citizens of society as early as zero to seven years of age. Thousands more are not in the child welfare system but join the ranks and fail to have their basic human needs met because of the impact of poverty in their lives. Particularly with young children, their needs cannot be satisfied without a relationship with another person. The statistics paint a disturbing but accurate picture of the state of child and family welfare and its prognosis. It is no secret that many children and youth's basic needs are unmet. Thus, primary and secondary intervention methods are desperately needed for effective change. Until these ideas are embraced, child and family welfare will remain in crisis.

According to the Children's Defense Fund Report (2023a), the number of children in the United States continues to grow, reaching 74 million in 2021, and accounts for 22% of our nation's population (US Census Bureau, 2023). For the second consecutive year, children of color constituted most of all children in the United States at 50.6%. As the country grows more diverse in race, ethnicity, and other factors and increases in the number of immigrants and evolving family structures, it will be critical to consider these changing demographics when we strategize about future effective measures for meeting the needs of children, youth, and families.

Additionally, 21st-century technology is changing the dynamics of the primary agents of socialization equation via increased exposure to the multimedia sector and other caveats. Gone are the days when wandering eyes and inquiring minds were met with a rendition of the Star-Spangled Banner, the flying of Old Glory, and the static from the television network's end-of-the-day broadcasting signal. It's a new day filled with 24/7 broadcasting and exposure via the digital divide. Technology and reality television are front and center. As a result, many social critics claim today's youth face more serious and critical risks than any previous generation (Moon, 2009), and parents are convinced their children face a significant crisis.

Most experts will agree that alarming media images, deteriorating family structure, substance abuse, a culture of violence, and gang activity put youth at risk (Restore, n.d.). In recent years, attention has increasingly focused on issues such as youth crime and violence, substance abuse, gangs, school dropouts, academic performance, and other problems associated with youth who are at risk. This analysis is consistent with research regarding the primary agents of socialization and the significance of each, especially a strong family, in all our lives from birth to present (Gibson, 2019).

Interventions to which youth will respond are desperately needed! It is not about egos and self-serving motives. It is about meeting them where they are. It is about recognizing that the traditional methods of addressing child and family welfare issues have not been fully effective. Innovative and creative approaches are necessary and must be explored. Human service practitioners must work together collaboratively and with other interdisciplinary and multidisciplinary treatment professionals, advocates, and providers, including family-focused community organizations, the juvenile justice system, those responsible for effecting policies and programs, the K-12 educational system, and faith-based organizations. A micro-, mezzo-, and macro-approach that analyzes and addresses the root of the problems from cultural, practice, research, and policy-based perspectives is necessary. The following discussion provides additional insight into a select number of 21st-century problems and issues that confirm the need to "think outside the box" as responses to the child and family welfare crises are contemplated via innovative strategies, interventions, and resolutions.

### Child Maltreatment

Child maltreatment is a clear and pressing public health issue in the United States. At the federal level, the Child Abuse Prevention and Treatment Act defines child maltreatment as

> any recent act or failure to act on the part of a parent or caregiver that results in death, serious physical or emotional harm, sexual abuse, or exploitation, or an act or failure to act that presents an imminent risk of serious harm [to a child under the age of 18 years].

As such, child maltreatment includes experiences of physical, sexual, and emotional abuse and multiple forms of neglect (e.g., physical, emotional, supervisory, medical, and educational) (DePanfilis, 2006, as cited in Austin et al., 2020).

In 2018, child protective services (CPS) agencies in the United States received more than 4 million reports of suspected maltreatment involving approximately 7.8 million children (USDHHS, 2018b). Recent research indicates that, by age 18 years, more than one in three U.S. children will have had a CPS investigation for suspected maltreatment (Kim et al., 2020, as cited in Austin et al., 2020) and one in eight will have experienced confirmed (i.e., substantiated) maltreatment based on the findings of a CPS investigation (Wildeman et al., 2014, as cited in Austin et al., 2020).

As a former practitioner with over 22 years of clinical experience, being directly exposed to children and families in CPS, these problems and the following statistics mirror and represent what became a constant theme in the numerous comprehensive child and family assessments that were conducted. To witness repeated generational afflictions of poverty, neglect, helplessness, illiteracy, vocational deficits, and the inability to dream sparked a passion within me to explore innovative avenues by which to address the problems that were being faced by the child welfare system, as well as the consumers whom it serves. The revelation is that much of what is being addressed is done during the tertiary stages of prevention instead of the primary and/or secondary stages. Sometimes, there is a misdiagnosis of the actual problem because the clients' environments are often ignored. Thus, the symptoms are being addressed, and the roots of the issues are not—perhaps because of other overlooked environmental and ecological factors, including culture and diversity.

> "Child welfare services affect many families in the United States. Fully one-third of U.S. children, and one-half of Black children, will be investigated for maltreatment at some point during childhood" (Kim et al., 2017). Many of the child and family outcomes as currently defined for today's child welfare system are poor (US Department of Health and Human Services, 2018), and these outcomes are not likely to appreciably improve with current policies, organizational structures, and program strategies. In addition, because most families who are reported to CPS and investigated do not receive services, more information is needed about how to move forward with support, assistance and resolutions effectively. Parents involved with child welfare often struggle with untreated mental health and substance misuse problems, along with poverty and inadequate housing. These are some of the "root causes" of child maltreatment that must be addressed if children and youth are provided with safety and families are supported to thrive.
>
> (CWLA, 2023a)

The point is that society will pay for it now or later! Later is more costly! The implications are far-reaching and have devastating impacts across the lifespan, including the youth population who should be living their best lives and anticipating their future hopes and dreams but instead are coping with the woes of the 21st century and an unfavorable environment. The trajectory to reach Maslow's theoretical vision of self-actualization is interrupted by a marginalized life of real-world struggles. The ripple effects across the lifespan are manifesting in traumatic ways, and the common denominator in this public health crisis is child maltreatment.

Troubled teenagers who labor to cope with the stresses of life are more likely to abuse drugs and alcohol, engage in criminal activity, are sexually promiscuous, and attempt suicide. Many of these at-risk adolescents run away and eventually find themselves locked up in detention centers or living on the streets. Each year, thousands of teens who are at risk are diagnosed with clinical depression. If left untreated or ignored, it can be a devastating illness for the teen and their family. If allowed to continue, depression can lead to attempts at suicide. In high-risk teens with depression (that is, teens that have threatened or attempted suicide), four risk factors account for more than 80 percent of the risk for suicide.

(Restore, n.d.)

## Poverty and homelessness

"More than a half million children are confirmed as victims of maltreatment by the child welfare system each year. Children from unstably housed families are over-represented in child maltreatment reports, and a growing body of evidence links housing problems to maltreatment and Child Protective Services (CPS) investigations" (Marcal, 2018).

Well-established family-level risk factors for maltreatment include poverty, parental mental health and substance use disorders, and intimate partner violence. Family poverty has long been considered a significant risk factor for child maltreatment. In the child maltreatment research literature, poverty is often measured as annual household income (e.g., income below the federal poverty level), primary health insurance type (e.g., public vs. private), or participation in public benefits programs (e.g., Temporary Assistance to Needy Families) (Austin et al., 2020).

Currently, nearly 11 million, or one in seven U.S. children, live in poverty (Children's Defense Fund, 2023a; U.S. Census Bureau, 2023). By that measure, the United States is dismally compared with other wealthy countries—children under age five experience higher poverty rates than older children (Haider, 2021). Living in poverty during these critical years may impact brain development and has been shown to have significant adverse effects on the long-term well-being of children (Center for American Progress, n.d.; Sherman & Mitchell, 2017). Moreover, children of color are disproportionately represented among children in poverty, reinforcing systemic inequalities, including racial wealth gaps. The harmful effects of child poverty have enormous costs on America's society and overall economy (Hendricks & Roque, 2021) and may result in homelessness and other issues.

In what Park and colleagues (2004) call the "fishbowl effect," the heightened scrutiny that comes with homeless service use leads low-income families to become more likely to go under child welfare investigation the longer they remain in a homeless living status. Finally, children in these families may face abusive or neglectful treatment from family members; the chaotic living situations experienced by unstably housed children may expose them to many different caregivers, particularly if they experience frequent residential moves, which may heighten their risk for maltreatment. Although mothers in families struggling with housing problems may not display substantially more maltreating behaviors than similarly low-income housed families, they nonetheless likely have a myriad of other needs that contribute to overall vulnerability and capture the attention of service providers.

(Marcal, 2018)

Unfortunately, research has shown that mothers in unstably housed or homeless families are more likely than their housed counterparts to be younger, African American, unmarried, not living with a partner, unemployed, experiencing extreme financial hardship, victims of domestic violence, and suffering from depression and have more children (Curtis et al., 2013). Regrettably, the COVID-19 pandemic has only exacerbated these issues.

## COVID-19

According to the Centers for Disease Control (2024), "COVID-19 (coronavirus disease 2019) is a disease caused by the SARS-CoV-2 virus. It can be very contagious and can spread quickly. As of June 1, 2024, nearly 1.2 million people have died of COVID-19 in the United States". During the height of the pandemic, millions of parents and caretakers lost their jobs. Worsening the situation, as schools closed and switched to remote learning, many parents were forced to leave their primary occupations to provide childcare (Center for American Progress, n.d.). As a result, the share of children living with unemployed parents throughout the pandemic reached historic highs (Parolin, 2020). During the April 2020 timeframe, more than 21% of children had at least one unemployed parent. This is likely to have a disastrous impact on child poverty in the United States. Indeed, early studies have already indicated that the rate of child poverty has increased tremendously since the onset of the COVID-19 pandemic (Center for American Progress, n.d.; Haider, 2021).

In the United States, COVID-19 necessitated nationwide closures of kindergarten through 12th grade (K-12) schools and resulted in stay-at-home orders and social distancing mandates that were implemented to mitigate the spread of COVID-19 (Mayra et al., 2022). By March 25, 2020, all U.S. public school buildings were closed (Education Week, 2020). The mandated school closures are estimated to have impacted the typical school day for nearly 60 million children and adolescents enrolled in K-12 schools (Zviedrite et al., 2021). Along with increased reliance on remote learning modalities, students experienced deviations in access to meal services such as the national school breakfast and lunch programs, opportunities to engage in physical activity, and access to health services. These factors may have decreased nutrient intake and physical activity, increasing food insecurity within households (Kinsey et al., 2020).

COVID-19 has caused significant economic devastation, disconnected many from community resources and support systems, and created widespread uncertainty and panic. Such conditions may stimulate violence in families where it didn't exist before and worsen situations in homes where maltreatment, mistreatment, and violence have been a problem. Violence in the home has an overall cost to society, leading to potentially adverse physical and mental health outcomes, including a higher risk of chronic disease, substance use, depression, post-traumatic stress disorder, and risky sexual behaviors (SAMHSA, 2018).

Investigating the impacts of COVID-19 on children's mental health and ways to address them has emerged as the highest research priority, followed by studying resilience at individual and community levels; identifying and mitigating the disparate adverse effects of the pandemic on children and families of color; prioritizing community-based research partnerships; and strengthening local, state, and national measurement systems to monitor children's well-being during a national crisis (Dudovitz et al., 2021). Additionally, under-standing the full impact of COVID-19 on U.S. children, families, and communities is criti-cal to (1) document the scope of the problem, (2) identify solutions to mitigate harm, and (3) build more resilient response systems. Developing a research agenda to understand the short- and long-term mechanisms and impacts of the COVID-19 pandemic on children's healthy development, with the goal of devising and ultimately testing interventions to respond to urgent needs and prepare for future pandemics (Dudovitz et al., 2021) is crucial to moving forward and impacting change in the 21st century.

The pandemic of 2019–2020 might ultimately be remembered not just for its profound health impacts and social disruptions but as the catalyst for change and transformation, stimulating the realization of health equity and re-fashioning systems of care to sup-port optimal health development trajectories in early life and throughout the life course (Dudovitz et al., 2021). As our nation slowly regains a sense of normalcy on the other side of the COVID pandemic, another epidemic remains prevalent and unsurprisingly correlated to this unexpected crisis. The culprit is violence—it continues to decimate communities, especially communities of color (Children's Defense Fund, 2023a). Specifically, gun violence remains the number one cause of death for children ages 1–19, with the gun death rate for children at almost 5 in every 100,000 in 2020 (Pew Research Center, 2022).

According to Richardson et al. (2013), youth violence (YV) is a major public health issue that is exacerbated by contextual factors but is by no means limited to underprivileged com-munities. It is extensive, affecting all communities in one form or another at varied levels of intensity and severity. It evolves over time and is influenced by ecological factors such as societal stresses caused by ideological, economic, or public health menaces. Youth and adolescents may be victims of, witnesses to, or perpetrators of violence or a mix thereof. Additionally, violence is triggered by personal history, lack of choices and opportunities, substance use or trafficking, racism, homophobia, genderism, and other forms of discrimi-nation. One of the revelations of this comprehensive analysis is that

> the health, social, and economic impacts of COVID-19 and of the 2020 through 2021 restrictive measures aimed at bringing the pandemic under control on the incidence of youth violence and on its prevention and control initiatives have yet to be assessed at a national level,
>
> (Santaella-Tenorio and Tarantola, 2021)

substantiating the critical need for additional research, exposure, and attention to exploring 21st-century challenges via evidence-based 21st-century solutions.

### Gun Violence and Youth Violence

Per the National Center for Injury Prevention and Control, YV is the intentional use of physical force or power to threaten or harm others by young people ages 10–24. It can include incidents such as fighting, bullying, threats with weapons, and gang-related vio-lence. A young person can be involved with YV as a victim, offender, or witness. Thou-sands of people experience YV every day. It is common and negatively impacts youth in all communities: urban, suburban, rural, and tribal. Furthermore, research indicates that homicide, another form of violence, is the third leading cause of death for young people ages 10–24. It is the leading cause of death for non-Hispanic Black or African American youth (David-Ferdon et al., 2021; Sheats et al., 2018). Emergency departments treat over 800 young people for physical assault-related injuries each day (David-Ferdon et al., 2021). Welcome to the 21st century.

> Over the past few years, gun violence, notably, has risen to the forefront of public consciousness. However, much of the debate has focused on gun regulation and keeping deadly weapons out of the hands of potential killers, particularly those with mental illnesses. Unfortunately, far less attention has been dedicated to the impact of gun violence on victims. The consequences of gun violence are more pervasive and affect entire communities, families, and children. With more than 25% of children witnessing an act of violence in their homes, schools, or community over the past year, and more than 5% seeing a shooting, it becomes not just an issue of gun regulation, but also of addressing the impact on those who have been traumatized by such violence.
>
> (Finkelhor et al., 2009)

The consequences of exposure to violence on child development are real. The CWLA's National Blueprint for Excellence in Child Welfare agrees and

> serves as the foundation and framework for achieving the vision that all children will grow up safely, in loving families, with everything they need to flourish, and with connections to their culture, ethnicity, race and language. This vision for the future of child welfare requires that all children, whether they receive child welfare services, or are at risk for child abuse or neglect, will grow up safely in loving families and supportive communities.
>
> (CWLA, 2023c)

This vision points out that children and youth exposed to chronic trauma can experience inhibited brain development, producing a lasting impact on life outcomes. Exposure results in numerous skill deficits among the children and youth who live in neighborhoods that have high rates of poverty and crime.

As suggested by the research, many children experience problems with violence and aggression because they lack nonviolent conflict-resolution skills. Much of this violence and aggression is further exacerbated by emotional overload from constant exposure to violence. Children and youth exposed to violence experience significant stress and often struggle to identify and regulate their emotions because of developmental impacts from their frequent exposure to trauma. Their feelings are usually internalized and can later erupt in aggression and violence (CWLA, 2023c).

Overall, violence increases the risk for behavioral and mental health difficulties. On the microlevel, these can include future violence perpetration and victimization, smoking, substance use, obesity, high-risk sexual behavior, depression, academic difficulties, school dropout, and suicide (David-Ferdon et al., 2021). On the macrolevel, violence increases healthcare costs, decreases property value, negatively impacts school attendance, and decreases access to community support services, addressing the short- and long-term consequences of violence strains community resources. As a result, this limits the resources that states and communities can use to address other needs (David-Ferdon et al., 2016) on a primary prevention level. In 2017, the CDC reported that 3,410 children and teens were killed and 18,201 were injured with guns. In 2021, fatalities increased nearly 40% to 4,739, accounting for 13 child deaths daily related to gun violence, the highest annual number ever recorded (Children's Defense Fund, 2023b).

Babies born the year of the watershed Columbine massacre are now 24 years old. No youth today knows a world without the threat of sudden, deadly gun violence. The pandemic only exacerbated their skepticism that something like a safe space exists anywhere in their communities. Children deserve the opportunity and the right to be children. Our nation's young people deserve the chance to have a childhood free from violence and a country with leaders who ensure that they are safe in their schools, neighborhoods, and communities. Elected national, state, and local officials have enabled this violent epidemic to grow and ravage communities, specifically communities of color. It is well past time for meaningful action to ensure our children and youth can thrive and not just try to survive (Children's Defense Fund, 2023a). This is a call to action.

The Children's Defense Fund (2009b) reports that seven million youngsters—one in four adolescents—have limited potential for becoming productive adults because they are at high risk of severe problems at home, in school, or in their communities. This is one of the disturbing findings in what is known about young people aged 10 to 17 growing up in the United States today. The research referenced above has consistently shown that youth who have trouble coping with the stresses of life are more likely to abuse drugs and alcohol, engage in criminal activity and haphazard sexual behaviors, and experience emotional instability (CDF, 2009a). Many of these at-risk teens run away and eventually find themselves locked up in detention centers or homeless. "These children and adolescents are at high risk of trauma, victimization and violence. They often have unique health needs before running, including the history of physical trauma, mental illness, and substance use" (Gambon, 2020). Considering the world as it exists today, all youth are at risk. Young people globally experience these challenges to various degrees. All are exposed to ever-increasing violence, sex, drugs, and alcohol to a much larger degree than in the past through peer experiences, communities, their families, and the media, specifically social media.

## Social Media, Reality Television, Bullying, and Technology

Social media, a new study rapidly growing and gaining popularity, is ever present in modern society and has changed how people communicate with those around them. Over the past two decades, social media has expanded exponentially, now comprising a variety of websites and applications used by people of all ages around the world. Social media has been defined as web-based communication platforms with three distinct features, in which the platform (1) allows users to create unique profiles and content to share with other users, (2) creates a visible network connection between users that other users can navigate, and (3) provides users with a space to broadcast content, consume information, and interact with others in a continuous stream of information (Ellison & Boyd, 2013). Several applications (e.g., Facebook, Instagram, Snapchat) satisfy these criteria.

"Lately, studies have found that using social media platforms can harm the psychological health of its users. However, the full extent to which the use of social media impacts the public and mental health is yet to be determined" (Karim et al., 2020) but might be addictive. E-addiction is an emerging problem nowadays, and magnetic resonance imaging results reveal how addiction to social media is affecting the brain and behavior of children. Recent studies validate the reality of internet addiction disorder (Flinsi, 2018).

Further attention is warranted because young adults are the generation that most frequently uses social media; 88% of 18-to-29-year-olds indicate that they use it in some format (Smith & Anderson, 2018). Younger generations use multiple social media platforms several times a day, spending much of their time online. Thus, exploring how and why people use social media, especially young adults who use the sites most frequently, is critical. An important question is to what extent this shift to communication through social media has negatively affected the subjective well-being and mental health of younger generations (O'Day & Heimberg, 2021; Verduyn et al., 2017)?

Mental health is defined as a state of well-being in which people understand their abilities, solve everyday life problems, work well, and significantly contribute to their communities' lives (WHO, 2004). There is a debate presently going on regarding the benefits and negative impacts of social media on mental health (Berryman et al., 2018). Yet, social networking is a crucial element in protecting our mental health. Both the quantity and quality of social relationships affect mental health, health behavior, physical health, and mortality risk (Umberson & Montez, 2010).

The Displaced Behavior Theory may help explain why social media shows a connection with mental health. According to the theory, people who spend more time in sedentary behaviors such as social media use have less time for face-to-face social interaction, both of which have been proven to be protective against mental disorders (Karim et al., 2020). However, social theories found that social media use affects mental health by influencing how people view, maintain, and interact with their social network (Khalaf et al., 2023). From the studies that have been conducted on the impacts of social media, it has been discovered that the prolonged use of social media platforms such as Facebook may be related to negative signs and symptoms of depression, anxiety, and stress (O'Reilly et al., 2018). Furthermore, social media can create a lot of pressure to make the stereotype that others want to see and be as popular as others (Karim et al., 2020), which leads to another real-world public health problem. A form of bullying identified as cyberbullying is connected to this pastime.

The Centers for Disease Control (CDC) defines bullying as any

> unwanted aggressive behavior(s) by another youth or group of youths, who are not siblings or current dating partners, that involves an observed or perceived power imbalance and is repeated multiple times or is highly likely to be repeated. Bullying may inflict harm or distress on the targeted youth including physical, psychological, social, or educational harm.

Bullying can also occur through technology, which is called electronic bullying or cyberbullying (Gladden et al., 2013). A young person can be a perpetrator, a victim, or both (also known as "bully/victim"). Bullying is a frequent discipline problem reported by nearly 14% of public schools as a daily or at least once a week occurrence. Reports of bullying are highest in middle schools (28%), followed by high schools (16%), combined schools (12%), and primary schools (9%). Reports of cyberbullying are highest in middle schools (33%), followed by high schools (30%), combined schools (20%), and primary schools (5%) (Diliberti et al., 2019; Farrington & Baldry, 2010; Hoehe & Thibaut, 2020).

The digital revolution has changed, and continues to change, our world and our being. Significant aspects of our lives have moved online due to the coronavirus pandemic, and social distancing has necessitated virtual togetherness. There is ample evidence that the use of digital technology may influence human brains and behavior in both negative and positive ways. As Richard Hodson in the Nature Outlook on "Digital Revolution," 2018, concluded, "An explosion in information technology is remaking the world, leaving few aspects of society untouched. In the space of 50 years, the digital world has grown to become crucial to the functioning of society" (Hodson, 2018). Intertwined with this digital transformation is reality television.

The last decade has seen an explosion in both the popularity of reality television programming and the use of social networking sites. Murray and Ouellette (2009) argued that reality television (TV) has become one of the most popular forms of entertainment in the United States due to its inexpensive production costs and the ability of editors to highlight natural and manufactured drama and comedy easily. However, reality television is a matter of great concern, and reality shows have deviated from what they intended to be. Reality shows have become a paradox; the reality aspect is gradually vanishing. The structure of the programs is no longer spontaneous. The focus is more on portraying the show as reality rather than letting the program happen as an interaction between participants. Reality shows have become a mixed genre of television programs. Reality programs differ from cinema and other forms of content due to the aura of realism and spontaneity they invoke (Calvert, 2004, p. 56).

This has been a popular trend over the past decade with the advent of many television shows solely on creating drama through a scripted sequence, ensuring the audience is intrigued enough not to wonder about its authenticity. A significant debate arises about the ethical nature of such an interaction. Some say that it is a part of how the entertainment industry has grown, defending its use of techniques to toy with the audience, which includes our youth. Others mention that such a method employed in television programs reflects a sad reality of our society. According to the critics' opinion, such shows play with viewers' emotions, using inappropriate techniques that will have a harmful effect on society and the lives of viewers (Arulchelvan, 2019), our most impressionable young viewers.

Ferrucci et al. (2015) utilized previous literature to investigate the intriguing link between the reality television programming that college students watch and how they behave on Facebook. Specifically, they examined whether individuals who watch reality programming "model" some of the mediated "real" behavior they see on television and then enact those behaviors on their Facebook and social media accounts, possibly a connection to cyberbullying and the exposure of internet trolls.

Consider the lessons children and young adults are learning from reality programs and their content. Humans typically do things to get pleasure or avoid pain. For most of us, hurting others causes us to feel pain. And we don't like this feeling. This suggests two reasons people may harm the harmless—either they don't feel the others' pain, or they enjoy feeling the others' paiin (McCarthy-Jones, 2020). Being unkind to others isn't just "whipping" them up. It is a form of mental cruelty. Welcome to reality television that appears to be here to stay, and parents need to be aware that these short television series are promoted heavily and often tailor-made for young viewers. However, they are rarely appropriate for impressionable young minds (Arphan, 2001). The consequences and the implications for our families, future generations, and our communities are far-reaching and serious.

Additionally, the influence of media on society has expanded exponentially and into ever-diversified forms.

Reality TV allows Americans to fantasize about gaining status through automatic fame. Ordinary people can watch the shows, see people like themselves, and imagine that they could become celebrities by being on television. It does not matter as much that the contestants are often shown in an unfavorable light; the fact that millions of Americans, including our children and youth, are paying attention means the contestants are important (USEDmedia, n.d.). In all their various forms, media today are shaping our world in more ways than ever. Gone are the days when the television networks discontinued broadcasting at midnight, and viewers were greeted with the Star-Spangled Banner as the stations sounded off until the following day. Presently, beyond what children may see at home, they are continuously surrounded by messages and images in community institutions, advertisements, TV shows, songs, and other spheres that reinforce negative habits that often correlate with abusive behavior. Technology and social media have both a positive and a negative impact on children. It seems important to comprehend the benefits and adverse effects of technology and media to utilize them effectively for the optimal growth and development of the future generation (Flinsi, 2018).

Different types of violence are connected and often share root causes. A prime example is bullying, which is a form of YV and an adverse childhood experience (ACE) that is linked to other forms of violence through shared risk and protective factors, including child maltreatment. Thus, addressing and preventing one form of violence may have an impact on preventing different forms of violence (Farrington & Baldry, 2010). Therefore, effectively addressing 21st-century woes must originate from further research and collecting and assessing a plethora of data from the micro, mezzo, and macro-environmental influences.

## A Culturally Focused 21st-Century Response

The primary mission of the social work profession is to enhance human well-being and help meet the basic and complex needs of all people (Butler et al., 2021), focusing on those who are vulnerable, oppressed, or living in poverty. The previously discussed public health caveats are 21st-century issues that require a different approach and strategy to mitigate and/ or eliminate the havoc being wreaked on children and families. The Social Work response differs from other professions because practitioners focus on the person and the environment as a part of the solution. Social workers deal with the external factors that impact a person's situation and outlook and create opportunities for assessment and intervention to help clients and communities cope effectively with their reality and change that reality when necessary. Social workers help clients deal with how they feel about a situation and what they can do about it (NASW, n.d.). Competent Social workers are equipped with the skill set to be practitioners who view problems holistically and are prepared to plan interventions aimed at multiple levels of systems related to client concerns. Including culture and diversity in developing effective interventions is mandated and not optional.

A holistic approach considers multiple dimensions of human functioning, such as biological, social, and psychological factors. Client goals and needs specifically suggest culturally appropriate interventions rather than letting interventions inspire the selection of compatible client goals. In other words, competent social workers base their interventions on findings from the assessment rather than fitting clients into intervention models regardless of identified problems and goals (Zastrow & Kirst-Ashman, 2015). In short, we avoid the cookie-cutter approach and treat each case uniquely. We strategically remain cognizant that client problems are also influenced by micro-, mezzo-, and macro-systems, including individual relationships, relationships with organizations and groups, and social norms or more extensive policies that affect clients' everyday lives.

Theoretically, the strengths perspective and social justice frameworks are enduring elements in social work practice (Saleebey, 1996). The focus of the intervention includes understanding the interaction between the biological, psychological, social, cultural, and spiritual aspects of human development and the impact on human functioning across the lifespan, including an understanding of the helping and change process. Our professional comprehension and strategic interventions are strongly aligned with theories. The growing use and support of these evidence-based best practices suggest that scientific results, including quantitative and qualitative designs, must inform social work practices. Findings from social work practice are used to inform research through organizational or government reports and publications of scholarly work, such as this manuscript.

"Due to the complexity of factors that create the need for culturally focused child welfare services, interdisciplinary responses are important." Future research, solutions, and interventions should address how to use team-based care in building 21st-century child welfare service systems, using the best of what works well in healthcare and other interdisciplinary/ multidisciplinary settings. Research has found that relationships between parents and caregivers and youth that are warm, open, and communicative, include appropriate limits, and provide reasoning for rules for behavior are associated with higher self-esteem, better performance in school, and fewer adverse outcomes such as depression or drug use in children and teenagers. Thus, in addition to a focus on culturally appropriate micro- and macro-interventions, resolutions should include cross-cultural differences in parenting that are strongly related to the attitudes, beliefs, traditions, and values of the culture or ethnic group within which the family belongs (mezzo). These parenting practices are also related to the social and economic context in which these families are situated (APA, 2009).

In addition to reducing risk factors and developing protective factors and resiliency among youth and families currently suffering from mental health and other problems, human service professionals agree that communities must help children and youth who are at risk to develop protective factors to shield them from the opposing challenges that frequently result from exposure to traumatic life events. Preventing childhood exposure to maltreatment, violence, and other traumas and mitigating the impact of constant exposure is too large a job for any one group or organization. Child welfare, prevention, and mental health agencies cannot tackle this problem alone. Agencies must embrace the message of CWLA's National Blueprint (CWLA, 2023c) and encourage communities to take responsibility for the well-being of children and youth on the primary prevention level. Combating the negative impact of violence on children and youth requires the collaboration of teachers, principals, social workers, counselors, police officers, doctors, nurses, parents, friends, and more. Each person has a role to play on the micro-, mezzo-, and macrolevels of intervention, be it screening for exposure to ACEs, mitigating the impact of violence through emotional support, or preventing violence through community activism and policy initiatives. Only when all facets of society recognize the actual adverse effects that exposure to these traumatic child and family welfare factors has on the well-being of children, youth, families, and communities and actively work to address these problems will substantive change take place.

The reality is that fighting a community's culture is an uphill battle, presently netting few positive results. However, when communities, families, children, and youth are empowered to work together and challenge negative values and dynamics, they can begin to change the culture of violence and reduce community-wide fear. While change may not be an overnight process, it is essential to encourage communities to take ownership of the safety and well-being of all children, youth, and families. Consistent with the standards in CWLA's National Blueprint resource document (CWLA, 2023b), recommendations for intervention include working one-on-one with families, children, and youth to help them build their protective factors, developing resiliency, regulating their emotions, strengthening coping strategies, and transforming negative life views into ones of hope for a better future. It is also important to teach parents how to model nonviolent and constructive behaviors for children and educate them on positive methods of discouraging violent alternatives (CWLA, 2023a).

Addressing the social, emotional, and physical well-being and mental health needs of children and youth exposed to gun violence is a complex process that requires proper identification and assessment of those exposed. It also requires sufficiently trained providers and advocates in age-appropriate, evidence-based, and trauma-informed treatment settings to understand all environmental concerns concurrently. In addition, it requires our society to find ways to reduce the actual number of children and youth who are initially exposed to gun violence. This is no easy task, given the many settings in our world that contain violent situations or imagery: schools, homes, communities, the media, and social media (CWLA, 2023b). While it will take collaboration between various agencies and specific communities for a significant drop in child and youth exposure to violence to occur, many professionals are already committed to the cause (CWLA, 2023a), acknowledging that practice doesn't always match policy.

Nevertheless, preventing YV requires understanding and addressing the factors that put people at risk or protect them from tumultuous environments. Long-standing systemic health and social inequities have put many people from racial and ethnic minority groups at increased risk. It is essential for prevention efforts to consider societal conditions disproportionately experienced by Black or African American youth and young adults. This includes conditions like concentrated poverty and residential segregation. It also includes other forms of racism and disparities that limit opportunities to grow up in healthy, violence-free environments. Effectively addressing the root causes of violence and the critical public health status of child and family welfare is essential to reducing the high rates of violence in communities of color (Sheats et al., 2018). The implications are far-reaching.

Projecting the future, calculated responses should include research about interventions that must continue to focus on risk and protective factors at the macro or community and societal levels to strengthen the evidence base for population-wide primary prevention strategies. Such approaches can potentially create contextual environments in which families and children thrive (Austin et al., 2020). Crucial to 21st-century interventions include the development of culturally focused strategies that support children and their families through policy, program, and practice methods and avenues. While we call out the need for more excellent housing, income, mental health, and substance abuse treatment supports for families, these are areas where other systems beyond child welfare need to do more to help families and to do so in a more coordinated and collaborative manner (CWLA, 2023b). The 21st Century Call for Action is imminent: The children and youth, our future generations, can't wait for tomorrow; the time is now.

## Questions for Reflection

1 What post-COVID changes and challenges have you identified in the population that you serve? What was your response to addressing the issues?
2 Discuss some of the personal and professional challenges that you have encountered with 21st-century digital technology and cyberbullying. How have you effectively addressed the problems?
3 How can human service practitioners who work with CPS prepare for and cope with compassion fatigue and secondary trauma? What advice would you give new/beginning child welfare social workers and human service practitioners?

# References

American Psychological Association. [APA]. (2009). *Parents and caregivers are essential to children's healthy development.* Author.

Arphan, A. (2001). Examining the influence and significance of reality tv on contemporary popular culture. Common Good Ventures. https://www.commongoodventures.org/posts/the-impact-of-reality-tv-on-popular-culture-a-deep-dive-into-its-influence-and-significance/

Arulchelvan, S. (2019). Understanding reality television: A study of tamil television reality shows the impact on the audience. *Anthropological Research and Studies, 9*(1), 79–86. https://doi.org/10.26758/9.1.8

Austin, A. E., Lesak, A. M., & Shanahan, M. E. (2020). Risk and protective factors for child maltreatment: A review. *Current Epidemiology Report, 7*(4), 334–342. https://doi.org/10.1007/s40471-020-00252-3

Barkan, S. (2012). Agents of socialization. In *Sociology: Comprehensive Edition* (v. 1.0). https://2012books.lardbucket.org/books/sociology-comprehensive-edition/s07-03-agents-of-socialization.html

Berryman, C., Ferguson, C., & Negy, C. (2018). Social media use and mental health among young adults. *Psychiatric Quarterly, 89*, 307–314. https://doi.org/10.1007/s11126-017-9535-6

Bitsko, R. H., Holbrook, J. R., & Robinson, L. R. (2016). Health care, family, and community factors associated with mental, behavioral, and developmental disorders in early childhood states, 2011–2012. *Morbidity and Mortality Weekly Report, 65*, 221–226. https://doi.org/10.15585/mmwr.mm6509a1initiative/search/tag/437451662899965125

Butler, L., Arya, V., Nonyel, N., & Moore, T. (2021). The rx-heart framework to address health equity and racism within pharmacy education. *American Journal of Pharmaceutical Education, 85*(9), 984–992.

Calvert, C. (2004). *Voyeur nation: Media, privacy, and peering in modern culture.* Critical Studies in Communication and in Cultural Industries. Westview Press.

Center for American Progress. (n.d.). *An expanded child tax credit would lift millions of children out of poverty.* https://www.americanprogress.org/article/expanded-child-tax-credit-lift-millions-children-poverty/.

Centers for Disease Control and Prevention (n.d.). *Violence prevention.* https://www.cdc.gov/violence-prevention/index.html.

Centers for Disease Control. (2024). *COVID-19.* https://www.cdc.gov/covid/index.html

Chandio, M. T., Pandhiani, S. M., & Iqbal, R. (2016). Bloom's taxonomy: Improving assessment and teaching-learning process. *Journal of Education and Educational Development, 3*(2), 203–221.

Children's Defense Fund. [CDF]. (2009a). *Promising models for reforming juvenile justice systems.* https://staging.childrensdefense.org/child-watch-columns/health/2009/promising-models-for-reforming-juvenile-justice-systems/

Children's Defense Fund. [CDF]. (2009b). *Cradle to Prison Pipeline® Fact Sheet.* https://staging.childrensdefense.org/wp-content/uploads/2018/08/cradle-to-prison-pipeline-overview-fact-sheet-2009.pdf

Children's Defense Fund [CDF]. (2023a). *Child population.* 2023 State of America's Children® Report. https://www.childrensdefense.org/tools-and-resources/the-state-of-americas-children/soac-child-population/.

Children's Defense Fund. [CDF]. (2023b). *Gun violence.* 2023 State of America's Children® Report. https://www.childrensdefense.org/tools-and-resources/the-state-of-americas-children/soac-gun-violence/.

Child Welfare League of America. [CWLA]. (2023a). *National research agenda project for a 21ˢᵗ Century child and family well-being system.* Executive Summary. Annie E. Casey Foundation, Casey Family Programs, William T. Grant Foundation. https://nationalresearchagenda.org/. https://framerusercontent.com/assets/ZbUu92H764UDhxqTvLRQqyV5OQQ.pdf.

Child Welfare League of America. [CWLA]. (2023b). *Building a 21st century research agenda: Using evidence to promote better outcomes for families.* Executive Summary. Annie E. Casey Foundation, Casey Family Programs, William T. Grant Foundation. https://framerusercontent.com/assets/ZbUu92H764UDhxqTvLRQqyV5OQQ.pdf.

Child Welfare League of America. [CWLA]. (2023c). *Family and community support.* https://www. cwla.org/our-work/practice-excellence-center/family-community-support/

Curtis, M. A., Corman, H., Noonan, K., & Reichman, N. E. (2013). Life shocks and homelessness. *Demography, 50,* 2227–2253. https://doi.org/10.1007/s13524-013-0230-4

David-Ferdon, C., Vivolo-Kantor, A. M., Dahlberg, L. L., Marshall, K. J., Rainford, N., & Hall, J. E. (2016). *Youth violence prevention resource for action: A compilation of the best available evidence.* National Center for Injury Prevention and Control, Centers for Disease Control and Prevention.

David-Ferdon, C., Clayton, H. B., & Dahlberg, L. L. (2021). Vital signs: Prevalence of multiple forms of violence and increased health risk behaviors and conditions among youths—United States, 2019. *Morbidity and Mortality Weekly Report, 70,* 167–173. https://doi.org/10.15585/mmwr.mm7005a4

DePanfilis, D. (2006). *Child neglect: A guide for prevention, assessment, and intervention.* Child Abuse and Neglect User Manual Series. U.S. Department of Health and Human Services, Administration for Children and Families, Administration on Children, Youth and Families, Children's Bureau Office on Child Abuse and Neglect. file:///C:/Users/irma_/Downloads/neglect.pdf. https:// www.researchgate.net/publication/242514380.

Diliberti, M., Jackson, M., Correa, S., & Padgett, Z. (2019). Crime, violence, discipline, and safety in U.S. public schools: Findings from the school survey on crime and safety: 2017–18 (NCES 2019–061). U.S. Department of Education. National Center for Education Statistics. https://nces.ed.gov/pubsearch

Driscoll, A., & Nagel, N. G. (2008). *Early childhood education: Birth-8. The world of children, families, and educators* (pp. 175–176). Pearson Education Inc.

Dudovitz, R. N., Russ, S., Berghaus, M., Iruka, I. U., DiBari, J., Foney, D. M., Kogan, M., & Halfon, N. (2021). COVID-19 and children's well-being: A rapid research agenda. *Journal of Maternal Child Health, 25*(11), 1655–1669. https://doi.org/10.1007/s10995-021-03207-2

Education Week. (2020). *The coronavirus spring: The historic closing of U.S. schools (a timeline).* https://www.edweek.org/leadership/the-coronavirus-spring-the-historic-closing-of-u-s-schools-a-timeline/2020/07

E-learning Support Initiative. [ELSI]. (2016). *Sociology: Understanding and changing the social world.* University of Minnesota Libraries Publishing. https://doi.org/10.24926/8668.2401

Ellison, N. B., & Boyd, D. (2013). Sociality through social network sites. In W. H. Dutton (Ed.), *The Oxford handbook of internet studies* (pp. 151–172). Oxford University Press. https://doi. org/10.1093/oxfordhb/9780199589074.013.0008

Farrington, D., & Baldry, A. (2010). Individual risk factors for school bullying. *Journal of Aggression, Conflict and Peace Research, 2*(1), 4–16. https://doi.org/10.5042/jacpr.2010.0001

Ferrucci, P., Tandoc, E., & Duffy, M. (2015). Modeling Reality: The connection between behavior on reality tv and facebook. *Bulletin of Science Technology and Society, 34,* 99–107. https://doi. org/10.1177/0270467614564153.

Finkelhor, D., Turner, H., Ormrod, R., Hamby, S., & Kracke, K. (2009). Children's exposure to violence: A comprehensive national survey. *Juvenile Justice Bulletin.* https://www.ncjrs.gov/pdffiles1/ojjdp/227744.pdf

Flinsi, M. (2018). *Impact of technology and social media on children. International Journal of Pediatric Nursing.* 4(1).

Gambon, T. B. (2020). *Helping runaway youths: Report outlines risk factors, interventions.* American Academy of Pediatrics. AAP Publications.

Gibson, I. J. (2019). *The 21st century crisis of intimate partner violence among African american male victims: Up close and personal with an unnoticed population (a social work response).* Mountain Arbor Press.

Gladden, R. M., Vivolo-Kantor, A. M., Hamburger, M. E., & Lumpkin, C. D. (2013). *Bullying surveillance among youths: Uniform definitions for public health and recommended data elements* (Version 1.0). National Center for Injury Prevention and Control.

Grusec, J. E. (2011). Socialization processes in the family: Social and emotional development. *Annual Review of Psychology, 62*(1), 243–269. https://doi.org/10.1146/annurev.psych.121208.131650

Haider, A. (2021). *The basic facts about children in poverty.* Center for American Progress. https://www.americanprogress.org/issues/poverty/reports/2021/01/12/494506/basic-facts-children-poverty/

Hendricks, G., & Roque, L. (2021). *An expanded child tax credit would lift millions of children out of poverty.* Center for American Progress. https://www.americanprogress.org/article/expanded-child-tax-credit-lift-millions-children- poverty/

Hodson, R. (2018). Digital revolution. *Nature, 563*(7733). p. 1. https://doi.org/10.1038/d41586-018-07500-z

Hoehe, M. R., & Thibaut, F. (2020). Going digital: How technology use may influence human brains and behavior. *Dialogues in Clinical Neuroscience, 22*(2), 93–97. https://doi.org/10.31887/DCNS.2020.22.2/mhoehe

Honeycutt, H. (2019). Nature and nurture as an enduring tension in the history of psychology. Oxford Research Encyclopedia of Psychology. Oxford University Press. Retrieved 14 Jul. 2025. https://oxfordre.com/psychology/view/10.1093/acrefore/9780190236557.001.0001/acrefore-9780190236557-e-518

Karim, F., Oyewande, A. A., Abdalla, L. F., Chaudhry-Ehsanullah, R., & Khan, S. (2020). Social media use and its connection to mental health: A systematic review. *Cureus, 12*(6). https://doi.org/10.7759/cureus.8627

Khalaf, A. M., Alubied, A. A., & Rifaey, A. A. (2023). The impact of social media on the mental health of adolescents and young adults: A systematic review. *Cureus, 15*(8). https://doi.org/10.7759/cureus.42990. PMID: 37671234; PMCID: PMC10476631.

Kim, H., Wildeman, C., Jonson-Reid, M., & Drake, B. (2017). Lifetime prevalence of investigating child maltreatment among US children. *American Journal of Public Health, 107*(2), 274–280. https://doi.org/10.2105/ajph.2016.3035

Kinsey, E. W., Hecht, A. A., Dunn, C. G., Levi, R., Read, M. A., Smith, C., Niesen, P., Seligman, H. K., & Hager, E. R. (2020). School closures during COVID-19: Opportunities for innovation in meal service. *American Journal of Public Health, 110*(11), 1635–1643.

Krapp, E. K. (2010). *Gale encyclopedia of nursing and allied health 3: 1500–1503.* Gale Virtual Reference Library.

Kuna, J. (2014). An overview of bronfenbrenner's ecological systems theory, with practical applications. *Self-Improvement.* https://www.slideshare.net/John_Kuna_PsyD/bronfenbrenner-34175734

Lum, D. (2010). *Culturally competent practice: A framework for understanding* (4th ed.). Brooks/Cole: Cengage Learning.

Lumen Learning. (n. d.). Agents of socialization. Module 4: socialization. Introduction to Sociology. https://courses.lumenlearning.com/wm-introductiontosociology/chapter/agents_of_socialization/

Macionis, J. J. (2009). *Society: The basics* (10th ed.). Pearson Education.

Manouchakian, M. (2018). *The debate of nature versus nurture.* Lebanese University. Faculty of Letters and Human Sciences—Dekwaneh Branch. English Literature and Language Department. https://www.researchgate.net/publication/348191103_The_Debate_of_Nature_Versus_Nurture

Marcal K. E. (2018). The impact of housing instability on child maltreatment: A causal investigation. *Journal of Family Social Work, 21*(4–5), 331–347. https://doi.org/10.1080/10522158.2018.1469563

Mayra, S. T., Kandiah, J., & McIntosh, C. E. (2022). COVID-19 and health in children and adolescents in the US: A narrative systematic review. *Psychology School, 29*, 10.1002/pits.22723. https://doi.org/10.1002/pits.22723

McCarthy-Jones, S. (2020). Why some people are cruel to others. BBC. https://www.bbc.com/future/article/20201016-why-some-people-are-cruel-to-others

McLeod, S. A. (2016). *Maslow's Hierarchy of Needs.* https://www.simplypsychology.org/maslow.html

Momen, A., Ebrahimi, M., & Hassan, A. (2022). Importance and implications of theory of bloom's taxonomy in different fields of education. In *Proceedings of the 2nd International Conference on Emerging Technologies and Intelligent Systems* (pp. 515–525). https://doi.org/10.1007/978-3-031-20429-6_47

Moon, J. S. (2009). *Youth ministry: It starts sooner than you think! A youth ministry case study report.* https://core.ac.uk/download/479618799.pdf

Murray, S., & Ouellette, L. (2009). *Reality TV: Remaking television culture* (2nd ed.). New York University Press.

National Association of Social Work (NASW). (n.d.). *Why choose the social work profession?* https://www.socialworkers.org/Careers/Career-Center/Explore-SocialWork/Choose-the-Social-Work-Profession

National Youth-at-Risk Conference, S. (NYARCP). (2011). *Successful programs for empowering youth: Overcoming poverty, violence and failure.* NYAR Savannah Program 2011. https://digitalcommons.georgiasouthern.edu/cgi/viewcontent.cgi?article=1327&context=nyar_savannah

O'Day, E. B., & Heimberg, R. B. (2021). Social media use, social anxiety, and loneliness: A systematic review. *Computers in Human Behavior Reports, 3,* 100070. ISSN 2451- 9588. https://doi.org/10.1016/j.chbr.2021.100070

O'Reilly, M., Dogra, N., Whiteman, N., Hughes, J., Eruyar, S., & Reilly, P. (2018). Is social media bad for mental health and wellbeing? Exploring the perspectives of adolescents. *Clinical Child Psychology and Psychiatry, 23,* 601–613.

Park, J. M., Metraux, S., Brodbar, G., & Culhane, D. P. (2004). Child welfare involvement among children in homeless families. *Child Welfare, 83*(5), 423–436.

Parolin, Z. (2020). Unemployment and child health during COVID-19 in the USA. *The Lancet, 5,* e521–e522, https://www.thelancet.com/action/showPdf?pii=S2468- 2667%2820%2930207-3

Payne, M. (2014). *Modern social work theory* (4th ed.). Palgrave Macmillan.

Perez-Felkner, L. (Forthcoming). Socialization in childhood and adolescence. In J. DeLamater, & A. Ward (Eds.), *Handbook of social psychology* (2nd ed.). Springer Publishing.

Peterson, C., Parker, E. M., D'Inverno, A. S., & Haileyesus, T. (2023). Economic burden on us youth violence injuries. *Journal of the American Medical Association Pediatrics.* 177(11), 1232–1234. https://doi.org/10.1001/jamapediatrics.2023.3235

Pew Research Center. (2022). *What the data says about gun deaths in the U.S.* https://www.pewresearch.org/fact-tank/2022/02/03/what-the-data-says-about-gun-deaths-in-the-u-s/

Restore. (n.d.). *At-risk-youth treatment programs.* https://www.restoretroubledteens.com/At-Risk-Youth-Treatment-Programs/

Rettew, D. (2017). Nature versus nurture: Where we are in 2017. *Psychology Today.* https://www.psychologytoday.com/ie/blog/abcs-child-psychiatry/201710/nature-versus-nurture-where-we-are-now?msockid=1d913953f61651f10bb05b73eb764de

Richardson, J. B. Jr., Brown, J., & Van Brakle, M. (2013). Pathways to early violent death: The voices of serious violent youth offenders. *American Journal of Public Health, 103*(7), e5–16. https://doi.org/10.2105/AJPH.2012.301160

Rothschild, T. (n.d.). *Rothschild's introduction to sociology.* Simple Book Publishing.

Saleebey, D. (1996). The strengths perspective in social work practice: Extensions and cautions. *Social Work, 41*(3), 296–305.

Santaella-Tenorio, J., & Tarantola, D. (2021). Youth violence: Prevention and control. *American Journal of Public Health, 111*(S1), S8–S9. https://doi.org/10.2105/AJPH.2021.306320

Šaras, E. & Perez-Felkner, L. (2018). Sociological perspectives on socialization. Oxford Bibliography. 10.1093/obo/9780199756384-0155.

Sheats, K. J., Irving, S. M., Mercy, J. A., Simon, T. R., Crosby, A. E., Ford, D. C., Merrick, M. T., Annor, F. B., & Morgan, R. E. (2018). Violence-related disparities experienced by Black youth and young adults: Opportunities for prevention. *American Journal of Preventive Medicine, 55*(4), 462–469. https://doi.org/10.1016/j.amepre.2018.05.017

Sherman, A., & Mitchell, T. (2017). *Many studies find that economic security programs help low-income children succeed over the long term.* Center on Budget and Policy Priorities. https://www.cbpp.org/research/poverty-and-inequality/economic-security-programs-help-low-income-children-succeed-over

Smith, A., & Anderson, M. (2018). *Social media use in 2018.* Pew Research Center. https://pewresearch.org/internet

Substance Abuse and Mental Health Services Administration (SAMHSA). (2018). Trauma and violence. https://www.samhsa.gov/mental-health/trauma-violence.

Swelindawo, M. P. (2019). An investigation into repeated admission of abused women with mental illness in a psychiatric institution: A case study of selected outpatients in Port Elizabeth. https://core.ac.uk/download/492499083.pdf

Traver, A. (2021). *Introduction to sociology.* https://core.ac.uk/download/425647060.pdf

Umberson, D., & Montez, J. K. (2010). Social relationships and health: A flashpoint for health policy. *Journal of Health and Social Behavior, 51,* 54–66. https://doi.org/10.1177/0022146510383501

US Census Bureau. (2023). *Accessed via quick facts.* https://www.census.gov/quickfacts/fact/table/US/PST045222#PST045222

U.S. Department of Education, National Center for Education Statistics. (2004). *Average length of school year and average length of school day, by selected characteristics: United States, 2003–04.* Private School Universe Survey (PSS). https://nces.ed.gov/surveys/pss/tables/table_2004_06.asp.

U.S. Department of Health & Human Services (USDHHS). (2018b). *Child maltreatment.* Annual Report. Administration for Children and Families, (ACF) Children's Bureau (CB). https://acf.gov/sites/default/files/documents/cb/cm2018.pdf

USEDmedia.org. (n.d.). *YouTube drama bringing in the views.* https://usedmedia.org/2018/08/05/youtube-drama-bringing-in-the-views/

Verduyn, P., Ybarra, O., M. Résibois, M., J. Jonides, J., & Kross, E. (2017). Do social network sites enhance or undermine subjective well-being? A critical review. *Social Issues and Policy Review, 11,* 274–302. https://doi.org/10.1111/sipr.12033

Wildeman, C., Emanuel, N., Leventhal, J. M., Putnam-Hornstein, E., Waldfogel J., & Lee, H. (2014). The prevalence of confirmed maltreatment among U.S. children, 2004 to 2011. *Journal of the American Medical Association Pediatrics, 168*(8), 706–713.

World Health Organization. (2004). *The World health report: 2004: Changing history.* https://www.who.int/whr/2004/en/

Zastrow, C., & Kirst-Ashman, K. (2015). *Empowerment series: Understanding human behavior and the social environment* (10th ed.). Thomson.

Zviedrite, N., Hodis, J. D., Jahan, F., Gao, H., & Uzicanin, A. (2021). COVID-19-associated school closures and related efforts to sustain education and subsidized meal programs, United States, February 18–June 30, 2020. *PLoS One, 16*(9), e0248925.

# 22 Being Still ... Reflections about Professionalism, Friendship, and Internalized White Supremacy in Human Services

*Jasalynne Northcross*

Reflecting on my career, I cannot ignore the impact of the Great Recession in the late 2000s and the COVID-19 pandemic on my personal and professional development. I earned a bachelor's degree in psychology in 2010. It took about six months to land a full-time job at an adult day care center. I entered into human services ready to take on the challenge because it was important to me to have a career that involved working with people and helping them accomplish their goals. At my interview, the supervisor said that most people do not last long at the agency. The salary was low, and the work was physically demanding. This job exposed me to social workers, and I quickly became interested in the profession and saw it as a way to positively impact my community. Most social workers I know were called to the human services profession for similar reasons. As I considered graduate school, one of my major priorities was to choose a profession that aligned with my values and was secure enough to endure a global financial crisis. Social work seemed like it could accomplish both goals. I believed that I could do what I loved, while earning enough money to support myself.

It is important to note which of my identities are most relevant for this chapter. I am the oldest daughter of the oldest daughter, which means I was raised to be responsible and self-sufficient. I am a dark-skinned, cisgender, queer woman, which means that, even in Black spaces, I often feel "othered." These intersecting identities add a layer of social stress that impacts how I navigate my personal and professional identity (Harris, 2014; Robinson-Wood et al., 2015). I am keenly aware that my intersecting identities pose challenges for me that others may not experience or be aware of.

I graduated from the Howard University School of Social Work in 2017. The first years of my social work career were challenging financially and emotionally. I worked at a couple of non-profit organizations, a hospital, and for the local government. Life as a novice social worker presented several challenges. My first employer lost their government contract which meant that dozens of recently hired employees, mostly new graduates, were laid off within weeks of starting the job. I worked for supervisors who expected staff to be available around the clock, completed home visits that ended as late as 8:00 pm, used outdated and inefficient case management systems, transported clients in my personal vehicle, and completed massive amounts of paperwork.

I felt like I was finally hitting my stride when I was offered a position with the federal government in 2022. I was excited because I thought I was going to experience the dream that was promised to me years prior by a friend, who is in a related profession, and warned me that it would take a few years after graduate school before life would feel stable financially. I had finally reached what I thought was the pinnacle of success. At a young age, my family encouraged me to consider government work because it is stable and secure. In fact,

DOI: 10.4324/9781003531258-26

prior to earning an MSW degree, I researched federal jobs to ensure that I was choosing a profession that would permit me to obtain a federal job.

I wanted to make an impact on my new team and was eager to take my career to the next level. Initially, I felt supported by leadership. I received high scores on evaluations and positive feedback from my local and regional leadership. The director of the office was transparent about her difficulty with staff retention, something that she attributed to the pandemic. I was surrounded by social workers, either my friends or office buddies, who were experiencing burnout and compassion fatigue. It seems so obvious now, but at the time, I did not see how that environment was impacting me physically, spiritually, and emotionally. The fatigue was normalized in that environment.

My job was three positions rolled into one. It was clear that there was no way to do my job in 40 hours. In fact, everyone was behind, but the work never stopped or slowed down. Chronic work stress and the nature of the work I was doing caused physical and emotional exhaustion that caused me to experience burnout (Newell, 2020). I wanted to advance my career and thought myopically that progress was tied to what my employer would allow.

The director in my office expressed their intention to get support for our team but lacked time, resources, or interest in supporting the vision of the clinical staff. I was interested in transitioning to a leadership position because I believed that I could be a change agent and turn the culture of the office around. I believed in the mission of the organization and had a vision of how it could improve service delivery and staff morale, and retention. Despite a history of high-performance evaluations and community service leadership positions, I faced barriers as I tried to transition into leadership.

Toxic office politics, staffing shortages, vicarious trauma, deplorable office facilities, and inefficient technology, I found myself feeling stressed, burned out, and beginning to question my place in this profession. The issues I was confronted with at this job were no different from what I had experienced previously at the adult day program, as a child welfare social worker, hospital social worker, and the other human services positions I held previously.

Six years into my career as a licensed social worker, I woke up most mornings wondering where I went wrong. How did I end up in a job that felt like a dead end after completing two degrees and earning advanced licensure? It felt like I was living a nightmare. At a low point, I questioned my skill set. My mentors, colleagues, family, and friends saw me as more talented than I saw myself. What I felt more than doubt was deep and long-lasting hopelessness. As a mental health professional with training in suicide prevention, I knew that it was not safe for me or my clients to have these feelings; something had to change.

In reflection, I realize that I had internalized one of the three pillars of white supremacy (capitalism/slavery), financial stability seduced me into offering myself as a commodity for the machine (Smith, 2016). I signed up for more training at my job, partnered with my colleagues to complete special projects, and tried to come to work eager to take on the day's challenges. I watched colleagues get opportunities that were not offered to me and felt powerless. The way the office operated kept the people at the bottom at the mercy of the employer, who was more concerned with the costs and results than employee welfare or client outcomes (Del-Villar, 2021). Several offices I worked in operated in a similar fashion, and I believe that this structure pits employees against each other because they are fighting for scarce resources.

One night I was at dinner with a friend who works in the finance industry. She is a Black woman who immigrated to America when she was in elementary school. As I listened to her talk about her experiences with racism in her office, I sat in awe at how similar we felt. I was stunned by how similar our experiences were. We felt stuck, unprotected, and upset. We have four degrees between the two of us and a mountain of student loan debt, but we found ourselves going to work daily in systems that were not designed for us and/or interested in our protection. In this conversation, we identified and named our experiences, which was pivotal in my resistance to the oppressive nature of my former employer (Robinson-Wood et al., 2015).

I started a journey of self-discovery during the period of the COVID-19 pandemic that positively impacted my sense of self-worth. I lived alone in a studio apartment and quarantined myself. I felt blessed and privileged to work from home but isolated. I spent a lot of time thinking about areas of my life that I had neglected and began to realize that, until that point, I had not thought about my sexuality outside the context of a relationship or the desire to be in one. A forever student, I started attending virtual webinars offered by Afrosexology, a sexual health organization that focuses on Black liberation, pleasure, healing, and community.

As I thought about my dissatisfaction with social work, I began to imagine what liberation would feel like in my professional life. Ultimately, I decided that for the sake of my overall wellness, it was best to walk away from a career in the federal government and create a new path for myself. Standing on a solid foundation of courage, faith, and ancestral protection, I decided to apply my skills toward something personally enriching. I left government work to become a full-time therapist with a specialty in sex. I have more flexibility and control over my schedule now, which allows me to be creative with my professional endeavors; I am pursuing dreams that I once thought were out of reach. I never could have imagined the doors that have opened since I made this change.

## Questions for Reflection

1  Share your experiences navigating office politics and burnout.
2  Which of your identities are most relevant to your role? How do your identities inform how you show up at school or work?
3  What is your life's mission, and what do you need to know or do to maintain your focus on it?

## Bibliography

Cooke, C. D., & Hastings, J. F. (2024). Black women social workers: Workplace stress experiences. *Qualitative Social Work: Research and Practice, 23*(3), 499–514. https://doi.org/10.1177/14733250231151954

Del-Villar, Z. (2021). Confronting historical White supremacy in social work education and practice: A way forward. *Advances in Social Work, 21*(2/3), 636–653. https://doi.org/10.18060/24168

Harris, L. N. (2014). Black, queer, and looking for a job: An exploratory study of career decision making among self-identified sexual minorities at an urban historically black college/university. *Journal of Homosexuality, 61*(10), 1393–1419. https://doi.org/10.1080/00918369.2014.928170

Newell, J. M. (2020). An ecological systems framework for professional resilience in socialwork practice. *Social Work, 65*(1), 65–73. https://doi.org/10.1093/sw/swz044

Robinson-Wood, T., Balogun-Mwangi, O., Boadi, N., Fernandes, C., Matsumoto, A., Popat-Jain, A., & Zhang, X. (2015). Worse than blatant racism: A phenomenological investigation of microaggressions among Black women. *Journal of Ethnographic and Qualitative Research, 9*(3), 221–236.

Smith, A. (2016). Heteropatriarchy and the three pillars of white supremacy: Rethinking women of color organizing. In INCITE! Women of Color Against Violence (Ed.), *Color of Violence: The INCITE! Anthology* (pp. 66–73). Duke University Press. https://doi.org/10.2307/j.ctv1220mvs.9

# 23 Access to Artificial Intelligence (AI) Art

## Healing Trauma and Transforming Children and Youth in Marginalized Communities— Leading Human Service Conversations: Cultural Considerations and Social Justice

*Treva Gray Jones*

### Introduction

The use of artificial intelligence (AI) art has the potential to assist children and youth in healing from the disastrous mental health crisis in the United States. Five out of ten children and teens are dealing with trauma stories (Kooij et al., 2022). Approximately 5.0 million teenagers aged 12–17 in the United States experienced at least one major depressive episode; adolescent females had a higher rate of major depressive episodes, 29.2%, than boys, 11.5% (National Institute of Mental Health, n.d.). One in five children does not get the appropriate level of care needed to relieve their symptoms (CDC, 2020). Thirteen percent of youth struggle with functionality because of serious thoughts of suicide (Hink et al., 2022). Twenty percent of young people reported at least one episode of major depressive disorder; three million youth were not able to obtain the treatment they needed, and 8.5% of youth have private insurance that does not cover mental health services (MHA, 2024). African American children and youth from disadvantaged and marginalized communities bring trauma to school; it is carried at home and is a part of their daily lives (SAMHSA, 2016). In this section on AI and the use of AI art, the chapter considers the suffering of underserved children and youth in marginalized communities and how virtual healing can be offered.

Innovative trauma-informed mental health practices that use intermodal expressive arts through the use of AI art are novel and innovative. In this chapter, there are demonstrations and case examples of how to engage children and youth and provide sample prompts regardless of which AI art tool is used. The demonstration includes pages for personalized books and coloring pages that can be converted into a collection of coloring pages that may be used as helpful tools to encourage adolescents to regulate their nervous system in a way that helps them process information. This new idea may help children and youth from disadvantaged areas feel better about their mental health, make them stronger, help them heal, and change their lives.

### The Importance of Bridging Trauma-Informed Care with AI Art

#### What Is Trauma-Informed Care?

The trauma-informed approach is a term used in social services and healthcare facilities that involves understanding and responding to the effects of all traumas and recognizing their impacts or potential impacts. It also places a high emphasis on the psychological, physical, and emotional safety of survivors and providers to create opportunities to rebuild the sense of empowerment and control and once everyday life experience. The key principles include

DOI: 10.4324/9781003531258-27

safety, trustworthiness, transparency, peer support, collaboration and mutuality, empowerment, voice, choice, cultural-historical, and gender issues (SAMSHA, 2016).

Trauma can stem from various sources, including natural disasters, abuse, and violence. The aftermath of Hurricane Katrina in 2005, for instance, left an indelible mark on thousands of children and youth. They experienced displacement, loss of loved ones, and significant disruptions to their lives. Studies indicate that the trauma from such events can have long-lasting effects on mental health, leading to conditions like PTSD, anxiety, and depression (Kessler et al., 2008).

In an Afrocentric world, for this writer, it has been more effective to start with culture first when treating survivors of trauma. This helps to build rapport and establish safe connections with the individuals who receive treatment. In this research, the writer discovered the power of culture first when engaging with adolescent survivors of Hurricane Katrina and COVID-19. The work is to better understand the person's history and where they come from and figure out how it has driven their beliefs today.

### AI Art (What Is It)

AI-generated art encompasses digital images created through the use of a large language model of machine learning augmented by AI algorithms (Elgammal et al., 2017). It can include images that show promise and work to create, with the assistance of AI, to increase and leverage machine learning for everyone (Smith, 2021). It also equalizes the playing field so that everyone can have access to AI. AI art is a form of AI that is increasingly used and can be accessed 24/7.

Children can be creative outside of the gaming world. Access to other tools, such as AI art, may help to provide a way for them to create avatars to help them relax, relate, and cope with what may be happening in their experience, as well as give voice to it when humans are not accessible or available. They can then relate the information to the provider or adult caregiver when they engage with them. AI decreases the disparity between those who have and those who do not have economic disparities and financial limitations in all domains, including art. Art includes a variety of forms, such as sculpture, music, poetry, and digital painting (Malchiodi, 2012). Recently, these innovative artistic experiences have been used to integrate AI art to reduce stress among adolescents at a mental health practice in Stone Mountain, Georgia.

### Integrating AI Art with Maslow's Hierarchy of Needs

In this chapter, there are case examples of how to engage children and youth and provide sample prompts regardless of which AI tool is used. The demonstration includes pages for personalized books and coloring pages that can be used as helpful tools to encourage adolescents to regulate their nervous system in a way that helps them process information. This new idea can help kids and teens from disadvantaged areas feel better about their mental health, make them stronger, help them heal, and change their lives.

### Reflection and History

During the evacuation of Hurricane Katrina, Facebook emerged as a crucial platform that allowed evacuees to mark themselves safe and connect with family, high school classmates, and friends. Today, Facebook may be used to connect communities based on shared interests in numerous ways. Before Katrina, Myspace was a popular social media tool. Today, children and youth have access to and can create many additional trauma-informed tools that will give more insight into what is happening within their minds. According to Ford et al. (2015), access remains a challenge for African American children and youth in marginalized communities due to limited access to health services that offer access to activities that teach the regulation of emotional circuits. It may also include limited access to distrust for providers who do not look like them (Asante, 2003). Racial inequality and Eurocentric models are not designed with African Americans in mind (Benjamin, 2019). Further systematic barriers and economic disparities, skin color, racial background, discrimination, transportation, educational disparities, living conditions, and more pressing necessities may contribute to reduced access in marginalized communities (Ali et al., 2021).

Children and youth can further enhance their ability to create avatars similar to gaming tools to tell many stories that heal trauma in effective and meaningful ways. Once the stories are created using AI art and digital animation, the color can be removed, creating individualized coloring books. These coloring books can offer soothing and supportive inner healing so that they can normalize their expectations, hopes, and experiences for better future outcomes. They can also create themselves as superheroes who will grow up to make the world a better place. They envision themselves as leaders who will bring hope and innovation into their own communities. The coloring books with themselves as the leading hero will create lasting reminders of their commitment to not giving up on themselves, their loved ones, and their communities.

## Hurricane Katrina

Natural disasters that cause negative mental health consequences for children and adolescents are becoming more common and catastrophic, but the restorative resources are limited (Meltzer et al., 2021). As America comes upon the yearly anniversary of Hurricane Katrina, many New Orleanians reflect on the daily trauma narratives that the Katrina babies continue to live with post-evacuation. Although it appears that the rest of the country was able to resume their normal lives, the children and youth of New Orleans continue to remember Hurricane Katrina every August. When the levees were breached, the children and youth who are now late teens and emerging adults experienced overwhelming distress. They had to relocate to cities across the United States, never to return to what they knew to be home. As providers see these children in offices around the country, many may not link child symptoms to Katrina because the children may not tie the evacuation to their current symptoms. Providers may not realize that the children and adolescents who are now late teens or young adults may be suffering from depression, trauma, grief, and loss, but it is not understood to be tied to the sudden uncertainty of a mass evacuation. Many returned to New Orleans and could not attend school for months. Many never returned as residents. Who checks on those children and youth who have grown up? Americans may never recover the entire story tied to them. Some may receive assistance in New Orleans, but many children and youth throughout the United States may not.

As families continue to visit and have Zoom and Facebook live parties, bridal showers, gender reveal, holidays, and other celebrations and funerals, the city of New Orleans, all these years later, is still not the same. Technology and AI art can be taught to African American children by someone who looks like them to feel a sense of secure attachment in mental health and emotional wellness group settings during the school day (enrichment hours) and in after-school settings (Ali et al., 2021). It can also be taught by trained trauma-informed providers in local communities and in online group settings. It can be used to offer daily opportunities for grounding with their roots in New Orleans. They do not have to wait for celebrations, birthday parties, or family celebrations to relax. They can implement these skills regularly to manage emotional circuits (APA, n.d.). It would not impact parents being forced to take time off from work. Children and youth demonstrate high levels of resilience post-Katrina. If there were AI art platforms, they could have connected sooner and not have felt the long duration of idleness while waiting extensively to start new schools. More opportunities to effectively continue education would have made a major difference in the lives of children. Many children and adolescents were left behind socially, emotionally, and academically because of inadequate resources and lack of access (Madrid & Grant, 2008).

## COVID-19

Children and youth across the world experienced something equally traumatic with separation due to COVID-19. As a country, we cannot ignore the painful post-traumatic reactions of the pandemic. Children are still suffering from the inability to connect (Ali et al., 2021; Ford et al., 2015; SAMHSA, 2016). They are living in a social media age where it is easy to build "pseudo-connections," making it even harder to connect with humans and build secure attachments (Ali et al., 2021); although the pandemic period of isolation has passed, the children and youth's nervous system may still see social media connection as safe because it was the safest access to use during COVID-19 (Bozzola et al., 2022). It is easier to connect to social media than to access human connection (Otte, 2020). They may also experience social anxiety, fear, humiliation, teasing, rejection, bullying, and ridicule (SAMHSA, 2016). Children need secure attachments more than they ever have before. Therapists and mental health providers are seeking ways to help adolescents have a secure attachment within themselves through efforts such as trauma-informed care, mindfulness practices, self-awareness, and emotional regulation efforts (Weare, 2013). Art and AI-generated art have been game changers that have assisted with these efforts. AI is a technology that allows computers to perform tasks that typically require human intelligence. In the context of art therapy, AI can generate images or provide tools that aid in the therapeutic process. Human capacity is limited because adult caregivers, parents, and teachers have other responsibilities that tend to need their attention (work, other children, and other social determinants). AI art is not put in place to replace parent–teacher and caregiver involvement. It is there to supplement their participation when parents, teachers, and caregivers cannot be present.

AI art therapy can help specifically African American children and youth regulate their nervous system through expressive arts. If they feel they have skills with drawing, they get to use their own ability; however, if they do not feel they have the skills to draw, we enter props that provide images to help them visualize and manifest the things that are happening within their imagination. Adolescents are then encouraged to seek to create imagery like the avatars they use when playing their favorite video game. Afterward, they imagine themselves traveling through the challenges of life and coming out victorious, similar to their engagement with video games.

This innovation has offered a new level of activity and engagement. The results are that they can move from not seeing themselves in a positive light in magazines, books, and social media outlets to seeing themselves in a positive light. For example, we turn adolescents into superheroes or positive images. There is a lack of highlighting African American representation of strong leadership abilities. Children should be taught African American history daily, as well as those who are making history every day (Asante, 2003). Children see extraordinary African American leaders in their daily lives and oftentimes in proximity, such as community organizers, small business owners, first responders, military personnel, teachers, barbers, hair stylists, athletes, technology developers, innovators, doctors, attorneys, and local government officials. Other positions of influence may only be seen on media outlets: musicians, entertainers, and high-ranking government officials, such as the president or vice president of the United States. While some leaders are closer than others, African American children and youth need to see as many positions of African American influence in their daily lives as possible so they can have access to role models who may make a difference through the art of influence. Although we have come a long way thus far, children still struggle with seeing reflective images of African American leaders of daily influence in everyday advertisements such as magazines, book covers, television shows, and other social media platforms. To bring imagery and possibility closer to African American children and youth, AI art can be used as an immediate access point to manifest pictures and other innovative ideas of Large Language Model artistry.

## The Role of AI Art for Adolescents in Marginalized Communities

Creating AI art using AI can make it immediately possible in real time for everyday children in African American communities to be able to access resources like books, puzzles, and games where the highlighted characters look like them. Children can thrive and build communities using technology platforms that allow them to engage in their artistic abilities while offering them connections now more than at any other time in history.

Art has a rich history in the African American community, dating back to the Harlem Renaissance and even further back to Africa (Patton, 1998; Pawłowska, 2014). Art's impact on the brain's limbic system, particularly in regulating emotions and stress responses, underscores its therapeutic value (Malhotra et al., 2024). AI-generated art therapy taps into this by providing personalized experiences that stimulate positive neurochemical reactions, such as cortisol reduction, dopamine release, and activation of mirror neurons. Expressive arts, a person-centered modality founded by Natalie Rogers, help children and adolescents learn concepts of unconditional positive regard, congruence, and empathy, increasing play among children (Jones, 2024).

## Discovery of AI Art to Assist Adolescents

There are many ways to engage adolescents with art. However, they have interests that are specific to their memories. For the people of New Orleans, the culture is unlike other states. For example, there are cultural customs and places like Canal Street (where streetcars are used as public transportation), the French Quarter, Treme, St. Charles Avenue, uptown, Ninth Ward, Mardi Gras, parades, Jazz, Brass Bands, Zulu, hand-painted coconuts, and the annual Zulu Ball. There is a rich culture of the New Orleans second lines, Super Sundays, the New Orleans Jazz Festivals, and 30 years of the Essence Festival, which has been held in New Orleans since its "party with a purpose" inception in 1995. There is the creation of handmade Indian costumes, Super Sunday celebrations, and a host of other culturally relevant histories that should be remembered in the hearts of the children who evacuated from New Orleans. In the wake of Katrina, all the reminders of its rich culture are stagnated as it continues to hold its title as the disaster of the century (Horowitz, 2020). Ray Nagin, the mayor at that time, and the rest of its citizens felt abandoned (Nagin, 2007). Children needed help to connect with others according to the Children's Defense Fund (n.d.). Using AI art, paintings, and images can allow adolescents to reclaim their connections by recreating images of their unique culture and connection.

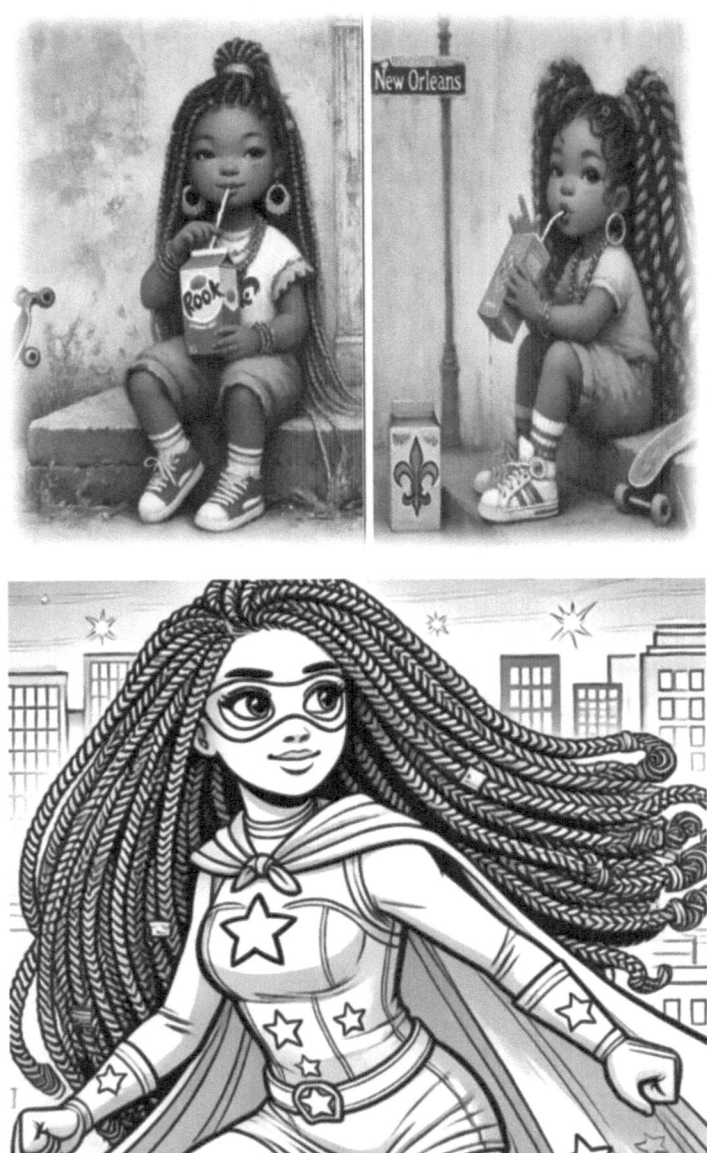

The above images are of adolescent girls proud to be from the 9th Ward of New Orleans, Louisiana. She celebrates her unique style and heritage. They want to remain grounded in rich culture, although they relocated to a new state after Hurricane Katrina. Images like these can be created using AI prompts and can be mounted to a wall or area of their choosing as a reminder of what is true and feels authentic to who they are as individuals. They can share memories and reflections on what they have survived, how they made it to where they are now, and what they would like to achieve in their future. They can create Afrocentric art to help them create a path specific to them.

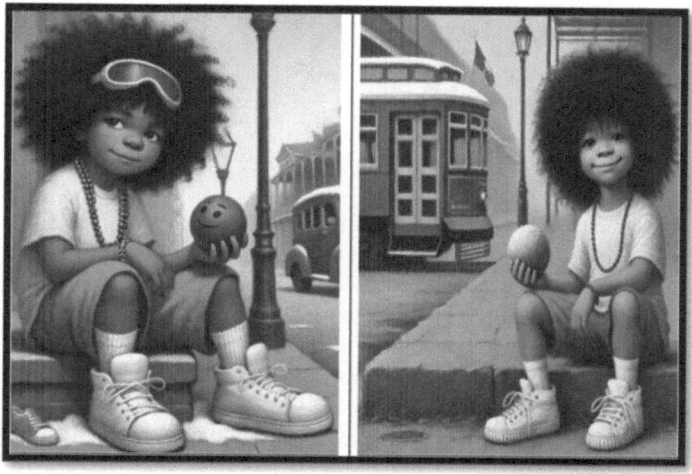

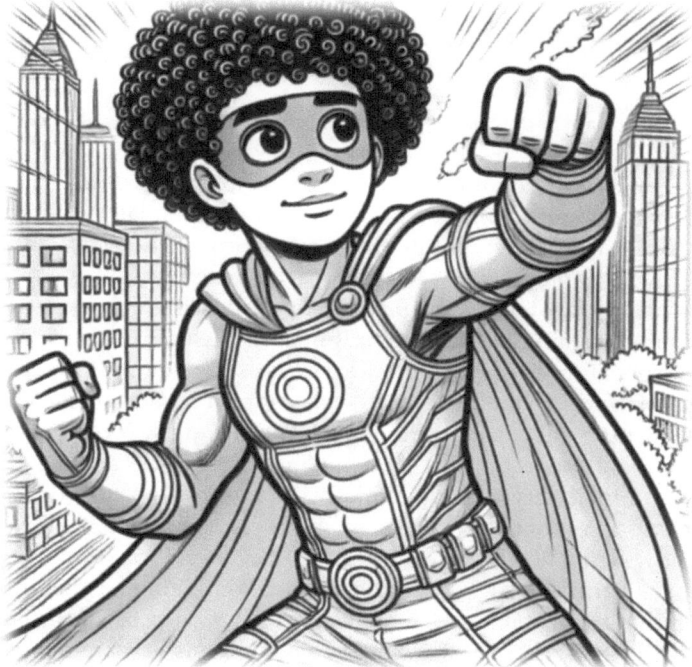

This image can remind the adolescent male of a positive memory of living in the 7th Ward in New Orleans before Katrina hit. It can also be used as an image to foster resilience and remind the adolescent of a time of feeling positive. Conversations about opportunities, hope, and future planning may emerge as a result of AI art.

Although this demonstration was specific to youth from New Orleans, it can be modi-fied to specifics related to whatever demographic is described by the adolescent in the session. For example, when identifying a calm and peaceful place in the child's and youth's memory, the adolescent will have a specific memory. The therapist or provider will type in the memory and ask the AI tool to recreate an image. The AI art image is verified to ensure the image is appropriate and then shared with the adolescent. The therapist then asks the person what they are noticing during the activity. The dialogue and conversation continue.

## Innovative Community Building

### Mental Health Professionals

Therapists and other healthcare providers can be trained to provide this useful interaction to children to add a higher level of engagement to the therapy sessions. Other non-therapeutic platforms may also be able to strengthen resilience in adolescents in marginalized communities. AI-generated art can support mental health interventions by building on foundational theories such as cognitive development by Piaget, EMDR by Shapiro (2018), trauma-informed principles (SAMHSA, 2016), and the neurobiology of chronic stress (McEwen, 2017). Incorporating AI-generated art into adolescent treatment can be a significant advancement in trauma-informed care in marginalized communities (SAMHSA, 2016). It can be integrated into online platforms to expand access and can develop useful coping techniques, promote trust in relationships, and strengthen coping skills such as visualization, relaxation, deep breathing, and comfort (Haque & Rubya, 2023).

### Black Developers

We need African American developers to create low-cost or free-access content suitable for children, adolescents, and teens. By engaging Black developers, AI art will include an Afrocentric perspective through a cultural lens. They can also speak to the AI system in culturally relevant, inclusive, and affirming language, which is the foundation for America's African American youth. They will also incorporate African American values, cultural expressions, and knowledge to effectively communicate with the target audience. It will foster positive outcomes by incorporating content that reflects the Black lifestyle. It will use Afrocentric resources as a foundation for improving culturally centered self-imagery (Asante, 2003; Benjamin, 2019).

The AI artwork content is still new—clear images with appropriate fingers, arms, and facial features would be extremely helpful. Currently, time is spent requesting the image to try again for clearer images. It may still consume time and require a quick review to verify the image. Collaborating with grant programs that offer funding to providers seeking to offer these services to adolescents in underserved communities would make a positive difference. Establishing partnerships with non-profits to provide AI Art tools would better prepare communities to operate efficiently. Simplifying interfaces that would offer adolescents easy access would reduce the time spent learning how to engage in the modality. Training cultural sensitivity and educational integration to mental health therapists on the proper use of their tools and all the amenities would better assist them in working with adolescents in marginalized communities.

### Community Partnerships

Establishing partnerships within local community organizations and cultural institutions can promote access to the use of AI art in marginalized communities. Providing a QR code that leads to web-based resources for adolescents would be an effective starting point. Offering mentorship opportunities that connect adolescents with AI art, similar to online boys' and girls' clubs, would be ideal for healing. It may remove barriers to transportation and provide human-assisted engagement and connection. Teaching youth to use the images and providing them with events to share their images would build engagement and connection.

## Awareness and Outreach

It is important to use marketing, outreach, community involvement, and campaigns to increase awareness of AI art tools available for adolescents. By identifying and involving local community members in these awareness campaigns, support and participation can be enhanced. These awareness campaign efforts will celebrate creativity through AI art; engage adolescents, their loved ones, and communities; and help expand online platforms. Additionally, they will create social media materials to attract more adolescents and involve adolescent-based partners who serve underrepresented groups. Online awareness resources will be allocated to provide adolescents with website tutorials and help build the necessary skills to use these tools effectively.

### Access to Funding

Funding is essential to provide a supportive infrastructure, which includes technical support such as online assistance, help desks, regular updates, and notifications of new features. This funding would also ensure the creation of a safe online environment that offers live interactions and a self-guided platform for users. A platform similar to IXL.com, which helps users grasp basic concepts through interactive learning, would be particularly beneficial. This infrastructure will ensure that users have the necessary support and resources to engage with the materials effectively.

## Conclusion

The integration of AI-generated art using trauma-informed care principles can significantly impact the lives of African American children and youth in marginalized communities. This transformative approach leverages technological innovation and personalization, facilitating engagement while preserving rich history and memories. It offers healing and is culturally relevant for adolescents to express themselves as never before. AI art platforms empower adolescents to visualize and narrate positive experiences, create avatars, instill hope, and build resilience. To fully realize these benefits, it is essential to ensure equitable funding and access, especially for African American children and youth in marginalized communities. Collaborative efforts can create an inclusive environment that meets immediate mental health needs while establishing a foundation for long-term emotional wellness and strength. This innovative approach allows adolescents to have fun through quality engagement during their development stages while continuing to honor the legacy of African American art, keeping their stories alive for many years to come. Intentional and coordinated measures should be taken to respond to this call to action and secure access for African American children, the forgotten under-resourced community who needs it most.

## Questions for Reflection

1 Why is it important for children and youth to have a sense of safety through a trauma-informed lens?
2 How can AI art aid in the recovery from trauma for African American children and youth?
3 What is necessary for children and youth to have access to funding resources that will reach them in their local community?

## References

Ali, E., Letourneau, N., & Benzies, K. (2021). Parent-child attachment: A principle-based concept analysis. *SAGE Open Nursing, 7*, 1–18. https://doi.org/10.1177/23779608211009000

American Psychological Association. (n.d.). *Emotion regulation: Helping children manage their emotions.* https://www.apa.org/topics/parenting/emotion-regulation

Asante, M. K. (2003). *Afrocentricity: The theory of social change* (Rev. ed.). African American Images.

Benjamin, R. (2019). *Race after technology: Abolitionist tools for the new Jim Code.* Polity Press.

Bozzola, E. et al. (2022). The use of social media in children and adolescents: Scoping review on the potential risks. *International Journal of Environmental Research and Public Health, 19*(16), 9960. https://doi.org/10.3390/ijerph19169960

Centers for Disease Control and Prevention. (2020). Mental health surveillance among children—United States, 2013–2019. *MMWR Supplements, 69*(4), 1–28. https://www.cdc.gov/mmwr/volumes/71/su/su7102a1.htm

Children's Defense Fund. (n.d.). *Katrina's children—Still struggling.* Children's Defense Fund. https://www.childrensdefense.org/

Elgammal, A., Liu, B., Elhoseiny, M., & Mazzone, M. (2017). CAN: Creative adversarial networks, generating "art" by learning about styles and deviating from style norms. *arXiv preprint arXiv:1706.07068.* Available at arXiv.

Ford, J. D. et al. (2015). Social, cultural, and other diversity issues in the traumatic stress field. *Posttraumatic Stress Disorder,* 503–546. https://doi.org/10.1016/B978-0-12-801288-8.00011-X

Haque, M. R., & Rubya, S. (2023). An overview of chatbot-based mobile mental health apps: Insights from app description and user reviews. *JMIR mHealth and uHealth, 11*(1), e44838. https://doi.org/10.2196/44838

Hink, A. B., Midi, C. M., & Larios, C. M. (2022). Adolescent suicide—Understanding unique risks and opportunities for trauma centers to recognize, intervene, and prevent a leading cause of death. *Current Trauma Reports, 8*(2), 41–53. https://doi.org/10.1007/s40719-022-00223-7

Horowitz, A. (2020). *Katrina: A history, 1915–2015.* Harvard University Press.

Jones, T. (2024, August). *A trauma-informed practice: Integration of eye movement desensitization and reprocessing (EMDR) and AI art for African American youth* (Capstone project). Unpublished manuscript.

Kessler, R. C., Galea, S., Jones, R. T., & Parker, H. A. (2008). Mental illness and suicidality after Hurricane Katrina. *Bulletin of the World Health Organization, 86*(10), 745–823. https://doi.org/10.2471/BLT.08.060442

Kooij, L. H., O'Brien, K. P., Myrick, A. C., & van Harmelen, A. L. (2022). Common elements of evidence-based trauma therapy for children and adolescents. *European Journal of Psychotraumatology, 13*(1), 2079845. https://doi.org/10.1080/20008198.2022.2079845

Madrid, P. A., & Grant, R. (2008). Meeting mental health needs following a natural disaster: Lessons from Hurricane Katrina. *Professional Psychology: Research and Practice, 39*(1), 86. https://psycnet.apa.org/doi/10.1037/0735-7028.39.1.86

Malchiodi, C. A. (2012). *Handbook of art therapy.* Guilford Press.

Malhotra, B., Jones, L. C., Spooner, H., Levy, C., Kaimal, G., & Williamson, J. B. (2024). A conceptual framework for a neurophysiological basis of art therapy for PTSD. *Frontiers in Human Neuroscience, 18*, 1351757. https://doi.org/10.3389/fnhum.2024.1351757

McEwen, B. S. (2017). Neurobiological and systemic effects of chronic stress. *Chronic Stress, 1*, 2470547017692328. https://doi.org/10.1177/2470547017692328

Meltzer, G. Y., Rende, R., & Esposito-Smythers, C. (2021). The effects of cumulative natural disaster exposure on adolescent psychological distress. *The Journal of Applied Research on Children: Informing Policy for Children at Risk, 12*(1), 6.

Mental Health America. (2024). Youth data 2024. *MHA.* https://mhanational.org/news/mha-releases-2024-state-of-mental-health-in-america-report/#:~:text=The%20nation's%20youth%20continue%20to,had%20serious%20thoughts%20of%20suicide.

Nagin, R. (2007). *Newsmakers 2007 cumulation*. Encyclopedia.com. https://www.encyclopedia.com/journals/culture-magazines/nagin-ray

National Institute of Mental Health. (n.d.). Major depression. *NIMH*. https://www.nimh.nih.gov/health/statistics/major-depression#:~:text=An%20estimated%205.0%20million%20adolescents,compared%20to%20males%20(11.5%25)

Patton, S. F. (1998). *African American art*. Oxford University Press.

Pawłowska, A. (2014). *The ambivalence of African-American culture: The New Negro Art in the interwar period*. Department of Art History, University of Łódź.

Shapiro, F. (2018). *Eye movement desensitization and reprocessing (EMDR) therapy* (3rd ed.). Guilford Press.

Smith, J. (2021). ArtMind: AI-driven therapeutic art platform shows promise. *Journal of Innovative Mental Health, 10*(3), 45–59. https://doi.org/10.1037/imho0000123

Substance Abuse and Mental Health Services Administration. (2016). Trauma-informed care in behavioral health services. *SAMHSA*.

Weare, K. (2013). Developing mindfulness in children and young people: A review of the evidence and policy context. *Journal of Children's Services, 8*(2), 141–153. https://doi.org/10.1108/JCS-12-2012-0014

# 24 Creating a Beloved Community
## A Radical Approach to Unlearning Racism

*Tracy Robinson Whitaker*

### Creating a Beloved Community: A Radical Approach to Unlearning Racism

Human service organizations are special places. They fulfill a very important role in society. These agencies take on the huge challenge of filling the gaps faced by those who experience disparity, injustice, and inequality. These organizations work with people living in poverty and with its collateral consequences, which include poor health outcomes, food insecurity, incarceration, poor education, and shortened lifespans. These organizations are also aware of the impact of racism, oppression, and injustice on these same communities. The varied missions of these organizations have one collective goal—that all people have access to a quality of life that will allow them to pursue their own goals and dreams. This overarching mission is closely related to the Reverend Dr. Martin Luther King, Jr.'s vision of the Beloved Community (King Center, n.d.). According to the King Center, the Beloved Community is one in which

> poverty, hunger and homelessness will not be tolerated because international standards of human decency will not allow it. Racism and all forms of discrimination, bigotry and prejudice will be replaced by an all-inclusive spirit of sisterhood and brotherhood.
>
> (King Center, n.d.)

The Beloved Community does not evolve from a series of legislative or government mandates but rather from "the manifestation of individual persons engaging in acts of loving self-sacrifice" (Patterson, 2018, p. 124). Habitat for Humanity CEO Jonathan Reckford stated, "This will never be a world of equality, of fairness, of human decency that leave no room for poverty or prejudice or violence, unless we build it" (*PR Newswire*, 2018).

Creating a Beloved Community is an idea that can be applied not only to the greater community (*PR Newswire*, 2019) but also to the workplace (Jones et al., 2008). In 2018, Habitat for Humanity launched a national initiative to honor Dr. King's legacy and make the concept of a Beloved Community a reality by "strengthening its commitment to build a world where everyone has a decent place to live and the opportunity for a better future" (*PR Newswire*, 2018). Similarly, Jones et al. (2008) describe how "businesses might incorporate Dr. Martin Luther King Jr.'s social justice of themes of belongingness and connectedness in way beneficial to desirable organizational outcomes" (p. 457).

Human service organizations are perfectly suited to provide the foundation for the Beloved Community. These organizations demonstrate a fierce commitment to justice. There is boldness to human service work that can be harnessed to strengthen communication between colleagues. There is a sense of purpose in this work that can deepen connections to co-workers and community members.

DOI: 10.4324/9781003531258-28

If the ideal of a Beloved Community can be achieved, the human service workforce is likely to be the group to do it. The tenacity, strength, and perseverance of this workforce should not be underestimated. This workforce believes in the impossible. These workers provide services and support to those neglected by other systems. They close gaps of despair and open doors of opportunity. They are a force to be respected, admired, and sometimes feared. With the serious goals these workers have embraced, the human service workplace is no place for fence-sitters or for those who are comfortable with systemic inequities and disparities. This workforce believes in the concept of an equal society. There is an unspoken mandate that the human service workplace reflects the integrity, ferocity, and commitment to justice embodied by their mission statements and their staff.

Addressing racism in the human service workforce should be a natural outgrowth of the work of these organizations, yet these workplaces are increasingly charged to confront inequities and to prioritize anti-racism, diversity, and inclusion within their environments (Abramovitz & Zelnick, 2022). Although the gains of the civil rights, LGBT, and disability rights movements resulted in more people with diverse backgrounds in the workplace, less attention has been paid to ensuring that all workers feel included, welcomed, and protected from racist and derogatory interactions while at work. The dual pandemics of COVID-19 and racism that erupted in 2020 fueled an interest in making workplaces less racist and more inclusive. Much of the attention was on the corporate sector, with many people assuming that the human service workplace was already diverse, anti-racist, and inclusive. These assumptions about the human service workplace were often shared by the workers themselves. However, many human service workers were surprised to find that racism was as much a part of their work environment as it was for their colleagues in the private sector (O'Connor & Netting, 2009).

> Paradoxically, while belonging to professions dedicated to upholding ethics and values that are inconsistent with racism, human service professionals are part of a society structured by racism, serving clients who are either beneficiaries or targets of racism, working in agencies that reflect society's institutional racism and that employ practitioners who experience conscious, unconscious and internalized racism when providing services.
>
> (Miller & Garran, 2017, p. xviii)

It is difficult for people to model what they have not experienced or affirm what they do not believe. How do human service professionals provide hope to their clients when they feel marginalized and devalued at work? How do they model empowerment when they are ostracized or punished for using their voices for self-advocacy?

Most people are familiar with the concept of racism and how it manifests in policies and actions that conspire to create a society marked and marred by inequality, division, and disparity. However, the racial reckoning of 2020 amplified how people *experience* racism's unequal and unfair interactions in their lives.

For white people, racism is a phenomenon that can be observed but may not be experienced. White people enjoy white privilege, which is "unearned benefits afforded to White individuals because of their race-based group membership" (Deamer et al., 2024, p. 2). White privilege allows white people to avoid acknowledging or interacting with racism unless they choose to do so. They are "exempt from things that are 'racial'" (Nolan, 2022). Regardless of their individual intentions, white people exist within structures that reward them for their whiteness and oppress others who are not white (Dull et al., 2024). They are also complicit in maintaining a racial system of oppression because of their inextricable link to the benefits of this system (Dull et al., 2024).

Even as some people acknowledge their white privilege, others reject the idea that they have unfairly benefited from a racialized system. Their denial of their white privilege is often correlated with the idea of meritocracy or earned rewards (Deamer et al., 2024). Despite myriad data to the contrary, the belief in equal opportunities for success persists as a strongly held idea. This unyielding belief in the myth of meritocracy is correlated with higher levels of denial of white privilege and less support for race-based social policies such as affirmative action (Deamer et al., 2024).

The Black Lives Matter movement arose from the collective sense of fear, despair, and anger among African Americans that there were no consequences for murdering Black people, even children. There were no consequences when police killed 12-year-old Tamir Rice for holding a toy gun; for shooting unarmed 18-year-old Michael Brown in the street; and for the self-appointed vigilante who murdered 17-year-old Trayvon Martin. In addition, the ever-ready smart phone has captured how racism interrupts the lives of regular people doing regular things such as having a cookout in the park (Lipsky, 2018); bird-watching in Central Park (Ransom, 2020); going for a swim in their neighborhood pool (Proto, 2018); or jogging in the middle of the day (Vera, 2020). These events showed the world that not only would law enforcement intervene recklessly and wantonly in their lives but that any white person could interfere in the lives of people of color with impunity. As the last tragic moments of George Floyd's life were witnessed, first by bystanders and then by the world, it became abundantly clear that the actions of the police were not tempered by concerns of repercussion. For African Americans and other people of color, racism is not an abstract concept but a powerful, destructive force that seeks to limit not only the quality of their lives but the longevity of their lives as well. For people who must live with its effects, racism is much more than an idea.

Racism is violent, destructive, mean, and vicious (Coates, 2015). It punishes and rewards unequally. Racism is stupid and drives simplistic thoughts and reactions. It explains societal inequities through a lens of personal failures and character flaws. Racism promotes and embraces mediocrity because it is based on false pretenses and the insane proclamations of white supremacy (Whitaker et al., 2021).

In the workplace, racism hinders careers and opportunities. Racism shuts down innovation and creativity. Workplaces with diversity have been shown to be more productive (Helfrich, 2021) but only when people are included enough to contribute. People cannot freely contribute to places that doubt their criteria for belonging. People who feel devalued will not offer their best creative solutions and ideas.

In the human service workplace, racism affects the type and quality of services that clients receive. Racism creates boxes from which clients cannot escape. It hinders potential and drives self-fulfilling negative prophecies. It fuels one-size-fits-all solutions. Racism creates artificial divides between what is good for *us* and good enough for *them*.

In the workplace, people know how to respond to threats to their safety and those around them. If someone noticed smoke rising from a trash can at work, they would be desperate to extinguish it and alert their colleagues. If that smoke turned into a fire and professional intervention were necessary, there would be no hesitation to call on experts to prevent the fire from ravaging the workplace. People would likely warn each other and help their colleagues escape the danger. No one would be expected to work while the fire was raging. Only when the fire is fully extinguished and the smoke has cleared, would it be considered safe for employees to return.

Yet, many people go to jobs with smoldering racism in the air. Racism at work is worse than a fire. It is its own special disaster. Its embers burn slowly all the time, waiting for the next eruption into full-blown flames. It sanctions dangerous and harmful interactions and creates unsafe working environments. And, in general, people who start the fires are not punished or removed from the workplace, leaving others to breathe the toxic fumes.

Many people, including those who work in human service organizations, understand the damage that racism causes in the workplace and in society. Attuned and sensitive to disparities and discrimination, these people have tried valiantly to extinguish racism where they work. They have engaged in "difficult dialogues," "critical conversations," and "racial reckonings." They have hired consultants, participated in trainings, and taken steps forward or backward in diversity walks. They have participated in countless conversations about intersectionality, privilege, and oppression. They have attempted to broaden their perspectives and walk in another's shoes. These efforts have been earnest attempts to eradicate racism, bias, and harm from their work environments. Yet, despite good intentions and myriad trainings, conversations about diversity and inclusion can lead to increased isolation, confusion, and resentment among colleagues (Moran, 2018).

One of the challenges in addressing diversity and anti-racism in the workplace is the continuing centering of whiteness as the norm. The concept of diversity has meant adding color to previously white environments, such as higher education, neighborhoods, and workplaces. However, this framework reinforces whiteness as the constant variable, influenced by the intermittent, limited, and controlled presence of people of color. A second challenge is based on undoing racism as an appeal to the intellect. Diversity trainings may focus on providing historical background and sharing personal experiences as mechanisms to build understanding and empathy and to promote self-reflection (Malcome & Holmberg, 2023). This approach, "when people know better, they will do better," is based loosely on the Maya Angelou quote, "Do the best you can until you know better. Then when you know better, do better." However, changes in behavior do not necessarily follow increases in knowledge. This is true for individuals and for building inclusive work environments (Kaledaiscope Group, n.d.). In fact, diversity training can inadvertently reinforce notions of the power and responsibility of white people for correcting racism. If the takeaway from a diversity training is that one group is responsible for "rescuing" another group, existing ideas about power and superiority may be strengthened.

It is unreasonable to think that because people have chosen a particular career, they have somehow immunized themselves from the influences of the larger society. Media images of different groups, political statements about desirable and dangerous people, and segregated communities and institutions reinforce ideas about the difference between people. This near-steady diet of bias has fueled even deeper divisions between people.

Becoming anti-racist is a process that involves courage and vulnerability. If a person believes that they are already anti-racist and that their words and actions and unimpeachable, that person poses the biggest threat to a vulnerable community. If they cannot understand their co-workers' differences, how will they understand a community with whom they are likely to have many more differences? If their language is casually careless, how will they know when they are the reason the client rejects services? People who work with vulnerable populations owe it to those populations to be in a constant state of learning, listening, and appreciating.

To be anti-racist is to first acknowledge that racism is our default place of familiarity. Coates (2014) describes white supremacy as a "force so fundamental to America that it is difficult to imagine the country without it." As a result of these strong cultural underpinnings around inequality, racism has become America's default first language. Bergman (2019) states that "our language, like our national society, has racism built in and it is so extensive and subtle (especially to White people) that we often do not notice it" (p. 412). Studies have found that even children as young as three years can express racial biases (Winkler, 2009). According to Dull et al. (2024), "all youth in the United States are social-ized into a society that is marked by white supremacy, anti-Blackness, and anti-Indigeneity" (p. 52). As a result, the American populace is fluent in speaking about racism, bias, and stereotypes.

When phrases such as "you people," "those people," or other denouncements of division are thrown around, there is no question about who is identified with the good and who is included with the bad. People of color learn to code-switch—changing voices and language styles, to appear less black or brown and more white (Kramer & Atkins, 2023). In-group conversations often describe the frustrations caused by those bearing other demographic characteristics. Conversations with friends of diverse backgrounds are engaged in carefully and often laden with invisible land mines. Too often, even these conversations take a nega-tive turn when one party discovers that their friend sees and experiences the world in a way that is very different from their own.

How do people who have a cultivated language steeped in racism learn the language of anti-racism? Anti-racism is a different language (Bergman, 2019; Corneau & Stergiopou-los, 2012). Anti-racist language involves examining default racialized terms and avoiding language that reinforces oppression (Bergman, 2019; Corneau & Stergiopoulos, 2012). Anti-racist language is also devoid of stereotypes about groups and generalizations that stigmatize people of color. It requires intentionality and focus. When people learn a new language, they are usually timid in the beginning. They know they are learning and are often hesitant to practice the new language in front of others. They anticipate that they will mispronounce words, that their accents will not be quite right, and that they will be corrected. However, they usually do not conflate correction with an inherent flaw within themselves. They are in a learning process, and mistakes are a part of the process.

Learning the language of anti-racism is similar. The difference is that most people believe they are already fluent in the language of anti-racism and are not prepared to make mistakes. When they say something that offends someone, those who are serious about anti-racism usually take it to heart and feel terrible. In human service organizations, this does not have to be the path. Everyone can learn the language of anti-racism together. The larger society is so segregated that many people do not know that their in-group references might be offensive to some outside their group. People experience membership in multiple groups simultaneously. The common phrases they may use with one community may differ from the phrases they use with another group of friends. Therefore, just as learning a new lan-guage can be exciting, so too can learning the language of anti-racism.

This is where the concept of the Beloved Community has application. The goal of anti-racism is a healthy and thriving community, not protecting the fragile feelings of our colleagues. Anti-racism is not just an appeal to the mind and the ego; it requires an engage-ment of the heart. How do human service professionals love their clients and their col-leagues enough to protect them not only from the political and socioeconomic mayhem of racism, but also enough to correct them as they learn the language of anti-racism together? How might services be impacted by workers whose ethos was a fierce commitment to com-munity well-being?

The workplace is one of the most diverse environments that people encounter, making it the ideal place to learn and practice anti-racism.

Heretofore, the anti-racism, diversity, equity, and inclusion movement or moment was centered on bringing attention to microaggressive words and actions. This "calling out" of racism created its own backlash because of the assumptions that accompanied it. The callers-out were angry and hostile; the called-out were misjudged and embarrassed (Whitaker, 2023). Even in diversity trainings, people talked about how they were treated when they identified racist behaviors among their co-workers (Malcome & Holmberg, 2023). Yet, there is another scenario that can be imagined. Everyone on the team should be a "caller-out." They should call out not to embarrass but out of a deep love to see their colleagues move more gently, more consciously, and more intentionally in the workplace. They should call out to make sure that clients are not unintended victims of misspoken words. This level of connection is not always comfortable. It is the same discomfort that we feel when a friend has spinach in their teeth, a splash of lunch on their face, or toilet paper on their shoe. We really don't want to say anything. It is uncomfortable, and we know that the friend will feel a moment of embarrassment and perhaps shame. But we speak up, not to exert superiority, but to shield our friend from further embarrassment. We know their moment of embarrassment will be temporary and that they will be more grateful than embarrassed that we intervened. It is likely that these call-out moments will be challenging in the beginning and will likely require courage, humility, vulnerability, and, fundamentally, goodwill. The leadership in these organizations can model both calling out and being called out with an attitude that welcomes correction and exhibits trust.

This is the opportunity that human service organizations have. They already have inherent strengths in the organizations that will facilitate the building of a Beloved Community. They already have a workforce that is committed to doing well. This workforce is there because of a compatibility with the organization's mission and a desire to be a part of a positive change in the world. The workforce is likely to be more diverse than other work environments, giving the staff a broad arena within which to practice their new skills with a variety of different people. Third, an improved human service work environment will translate into improved services. Workers who respect each other and, more importantly, like each other, bring a more positive energy into the lives of clients than co-workers who merely tolerate each other. The demonstration of respect and collegiality between co-workers speaks louder and more clearly than any mission statement.

When there is trust and goodwill between colleagues, misstatements that would have led to hurt feelings can instead become powerful teaching moments where humor and vulnerability can replace hubris and superiority. I recall a time when a colleague of the Muslim faith asked me to take a poster tube on an airplane for him. He said that he was sure to be targeted by TSA if he showed up with the long tube. I took the tube from him and opened it, saying, "You can't be too sure," and smiled. This response caught him off guard, but we both ended up laughing. However, there was a hint of pain beneath our laughter. It was painful that my dear colleague needed to spend any time thinking about how to avoid being targeted. It was painful that he needed to ask someone else to do a minor task to sidestep the racial profiling of Muslim men on airplanes. However, there was so much goodwill between us, I felt comfortable pretending that I, too, was complicit in Muslim stereotyping. As an African American woman, I felt the pain of racial profiling as it loomed large over the heads of my brother, husband, and son. This moment of vulnerability and solidarity deepened our connection. Racism causes pain, and becoming fluent in anti-racism both exposes and heals that pain. When a co-worker understands how something affects someone they now care deeply about, the pain is spread, and there is a shared commitment to its eradication.

Discussions about becoming anti-racist do not have to be painful confrontations about privilege and oppression. They can be exciting opportunities in which people learn about each other and become more intentional, authentic, and present in their conversations. Human service organizations already have the right people, the right mission, and the right motivation. Because their work is with vulnerable communities, these organizations should want to protect these communities as much as they want to advocate on their behalf. By consciously unlearning racism, human service organizations can cultivate cultures of courage, empathy, and deep caring. Building on Dr. King's vision of the Beloved Community, human service organizations have the power to create workplace cultures that are genuine, dynamic, and fiercely committed to community well-being.

## Questions for Reflection

1  Dr. King believed that, through love, we could transform our communities and society. Why don't we talk about love more in human service work?
2  How do we build cultures of trust and goodwill in the workplace that can lead to authentically pursuing anti-racism?
3  Why do human service organizations sometimes protect people who bring racist and toxic energy into the workspace? What makes them so valuable?

## References

Abramovitz, M., & Zelnick, J. R. (2022). Structural racism, managerialism, and the future of the human services: Rewriting the rules. *Social Work, 67*(1), 8–16, https://doi.org.proxyhu.wrlc. org/10.1093/sw/swab051

Bergman, M. E. (2019). Civility, anti-racism, and inclusion. *Industrial and Organizational Psychology, 12*, 412–418. https://doi.org/10.1017/iop.2019.80

Coates, T. (2015). *Between the world and me*. Spiegel and Grau.

Coates, T. (2014, June). The case for reparations. *The Atlantic.* https://www.theatlantic.com/magazine/archive/2014/06/the-case-for-reparations/361631/

Corneau, S., & Stergiopoulos, V. (2012). More than being against it: Anti-racism and anti-oppression in mental health services. *Transcultural Psychiatry, 49*(2), 261–282.

Deamer, S. K., Sonnentag, T. L., & Wadian, T. W. (2024). The effects of morally reframed messages on white individuals' attitudes toward white privilege. *Psychological Reports,* 23:332941241265316, 1–27.

Dull, B. L., Rogers, L. O., & Charlson, E. (2024). "I don't think there is much racism left": A critical analysis of white adolescents' (un)awareness of white privilege. *Qualitative Psychology, 11*(1), 52–74, https://doi.org/10.1037/qup0000283

*PR Newswire.* (2018, January 15). Habitat for Humanity unveils nationwide 'Beloved Community' initiative to bring Dr. Martin Luther King Jr.'s vision of access,). equality and opportunity for all into action.".

Helfrich, T. (2021, April 2). How diversity can help with business growth. *Forbes.* https://www.forbes.com/sites/forbestechcouncil/2021/11/12/how-diversity-can-help-with-business-growth/

Jones, J. R., Wilson, D. C., & Jones, P. (2008). Toward achieving the "Beloved Community" in the workplace: Lessons for applied business research and practice from the teachings of Martin Luther King, Jr. *Business & Society, 37*(4), 457–483.

Kaleidescope Group. (n.d.). *Knowledge is insufficient to change behavior.* https://kgdiversity.com/news-thinking/knowledge-is-insufficient-to-change-behavior/#:~:text=Knowledge%20is%20important%20but%20insufficient,knowledge%20will%20not%20do%20that

King Center (n.d.). *The Beloved Community*. The King Center. https://thekingcenter.org/about-tkc/the-king-philosophy/

Kramer, P. S., & Atkins, A. (February 7, 2023). What is Black fatigue and code-switching, and why do they matter to organizations? *National Institutes of Health, Office of Equity, Diversity and Inclusion.* https://www.edi.nih.gov/blog/opinion/what-black-fatigue-and-code-switching-and-why-do-they-matter-organizations

Lipsky, J. (2018, May 14). White woman who called cops on a Black bbq in Oakland is now a meme. *Newsweek.* https://www.newsweek.com/white-woman-who-called-cops-black-bbq-oakland-now-meme-925341

Malcome, M. L., & Holmberg, B. (2023). Becoming antiracist social workers. In L. S. Abrams, S. E. Crewe, A. J. Dettlaff, & J. H. Williams, (Eds.), *Social work, White supremacy, and racial justice.* Oxford University Press. https://doi.org/10.1093/oso/9780197641422.003.0014

Miller, J. L., & Garran, A. (2017). *Racism in the United States: Implications for the helping professions.* Springer.

Moran. B. (2018, July 30). Diversity is difficult. The Brink. https://www.bu.edu/articles/2018/diversity-is-difficult/

Nolan, S. (February 7, 2022). It's time for white people to have tough conversations with their white friends and relatives. *Time.* https://time.com/6145211/white-people-tough-conversations-race/

O'Connor, M. K., & Netting, F. E. (2009). *Organization practice: A guide to understanding human services* (2nd ed.). Wiley & Sons.

Patterson, J. M. (2018). A covenant of the heart: Martin Luther king Jr., Civil Disobedience, and the Beloved Community. *American Political Thought: A Journal of Ideas, Institutions, and Culture,* 7(1), 124–151.

PR Newswire. (2018). Habit for Humanity unveils nationwide "Beloved Community" initiative to bring Dr. Martin Luther King Jr.'s vision of access, equality and opportunity for all into action. https://www.prnewswire.com/news-releases/habitat-for-humanity-unveils-nationwide-beloved-community-initiative-to-bring-dr-martin-luther-king-jrs-vision-of-access-equality-and-opportunity-for-all-into-action-300582041.html

Proto, D. (2018, July 6). Woman was racially profiled when she tired to use her neighborhood pool. *ABC News.* https://abcnews.go.com/US/woman-claims-racially-profiled-neighborhood-pool/story?id=56406803

Ransom, J. (2020, July 6). Amy Cooper faces charges after calling police on black bird watcher. *New York Times.* https://www.nytimes.com/2020/07/06/nyregion/amy-cooper-false-report-charge.html

Vera, A. (2020, May 4). A Georgia man was chased and killed while jogging, his mother says. *CNN US.* https://www.cnn.com/2020/05/04/us/ahmaud-arbery-jogging-georgia-shooting

Whitaker, T. (2023). Calling out racism in social work: Why we should and why we don't. In L. S. Abrams, S. E. Crewe, A. J. Dettlaff, & J. H. Williams (Eds.), *Social work, White supremacy, and racial justice* (pp. 231–242). Oxford University Press. https://doi.org/10.1093/oso/9780197641422.003.0014

Whitaker, T., Alfrey, L., Gates, A., & Gooding, A. R. (2021). White supremacy. In D. Bailey, & T. Mizrahi (Eds.), *Encyclopedia of macro social work* (pp. 2652–2667). Oxford University Press. https://doi-org.proxyhu.wrlc.org/10.1093/acrefore/9780199975839.013.1586

Winkler, E. N., (2009). Children are not colorblind: How young children learn about race. *PACE: Practical Approaches for Continuing Education, 3*(3), 1–8.

# 25 Multiculturalism in Human Services
## Challenges and Solutions

*Beverly Edwards*

In recent years it has become increasingly evident that human services agencies must become more multicultural to appropriately serve diverse and disenfranchised people. This need is apparent given the increases in populations of color, people who are elderly, and people with disabilities; the widening income gap; and the dismantling of the public welfare sector (Bocage, Homonoff, & Riley, 1995; Ferguson, 1996; Gutiérrez & Nagda, 1996; Hasenfeld, 1996, as cited in Hyde, 2004). Human services managers must also contend with greater gender, race, and age diversity in the service workforce (Asamoah, 1995; Brody, 1993; Iglehart, 2000; Shin & McClomb, 1998, as cited in Hyde, 2004). Under the auspices of multicultural development, activities have been undertaken in response to these trends—awareness training, hiring and retention plans, and improved outreach and service delivery systems (Ferguson, 1996; Fong & Gibbs, 1995; Hyde, 1998; Iglehart; Iglehart & Becerra, 1995, as cited in Hyde, 2004). Given the current times in which we live, it is apparent that human services agencies need to become more multicultural to adequately address the needs of diverse and marginalized people. Yet, comprehensive multicultural development often remains elusive.

Research has shown that there are indications that human service organizations need to be more accessible when underrepresented groups either seek or are in the pipeline of providers. To facilitate outcomes for all populations, Wilson et al. (2019) assert that the Multicultural Counseling Competencies (MCC) model, which deals with awareness, knowledge, and skills, should emphasize the application concept more. Furthermore, the population of the United States is increasing with more diversity, and this diversity is on pace to make the U.S. demography browner in complexion than ever before. With this gradual change in demography, racial and ethnic populations, women, people who are part of the LGBT community, and people with disabilities are among those underrepresented groups that encounter access barriers to behavioral health and other services. Given this backdrop, the MCC was created to address the counterproductive outcomes of many underrepresented groups. The creators of the MCC also understood that the competencies could be applied to groups that might not be considered underrepresented as well. As human service organizations will encounter increased numbers of people seeking services from underrepresented groups, it is becoming increasingly important to acknowledge that the application principle might not be as evident as other concepts in the MCC. As underrepresented groups increase in numbers, human service providers understand that applying the MCC is important to move the needle with more productive outcomes with all who seek human and other kinds of services in our society (Wilson et al., 2019, p. 242).

DOI: 10.4324/9781003531258-29

## Literature Review

Moreover, in the social work discipline, social workers should understand culture and its function in human behavior and society, recognizing the strengths that exist in all cultures, particularly when they work with individuals in human service or social service organizations. According to the National Association of Social Workers (NASW) Code of Ethics, social workers should have a knowledge base of their clients' cultures and be able to demonstrate competence in the provision of services that are sensitive to clients' cultures and to differences among people and cultural groups. Social workers should obtain education about and seek to understand the nature of social diversity and oppression with respect to race, ethnicity, national origin, color, sex, sexual orientation, gender identity or expression, age, marital status, political belief, religion, immigration status, and mental or physical ability. Consequently, social workers who provide electronic social work services should be aware of cultural and socioeconomic differences among clients and how they may use electronic technology. Lastly, social workers should assess cultural, environmental, economic, mental or physical ability, linguistic, and other issues that may affect the delivery or use of these services (NASW, 2021).

Given the challenges of rising immigration by people from a variety of social and cultural backgrounds to societies with mature welfare systems, human services organizations have had to adapt their activities to significant demographic change. In Hajighasemi's article (2023), where he writes about this challenge, he speaks to the relevance of this demographic change in countries such as Sweden where immigration has occurred rapidly, and as such urban areas have become increasingly inhabited by marginalized groups as a result (Hajighasemi, 2005; Kings, 2011, as cited in Hajighasemi, 2023, p. 247). The number of impoverished neighborhoods characterized as marginalized across Sweden increased from 7 in 1998 to more than 70 in 2008 (SCB, 2017, as cited in Hajighasemi, 2023). Management of the effects of the rapid exclusion has become a considerable challenge to the welfare institutions. Similarly, because of performance issues raised in nursing homes and home care for the elderly during the COVID-19 pandemic, it recognized the ability to revise service provision to changes in care recipients' needs and preferences as of great importance. At the same time, the large number of service users and service providers in these organizations who are of ethnic origin and the issues of multicultural competences and cultural sensitivity in human services organizations are now receiving wider attention (Rambaree & Nässén, 2020, as cited in Hajighasemi, 2023, p. 247).

Even though the pandemic might be considered an extraordinary event, in social work research, however, the importance of social and cultural differences in the work of human services organizations has become increasingly obvious in recent decades (Fong & Furuto, 2001; Green-Hernandez, 2006; Harrison & Turner, 2011; Lum, 2007; Lusk et al., 2017, as cited in Hajighasemi, 2023, p. 248). Previous research (Ahmadi, 2008; Hajighasemi, 2019; Kamali, 2002, p. 51) has identified the need for the social services sector to adapt to the demands of a pluralistic and multi-ethnic society. The working conditions for social workers have steadily deteriorated in recent years to the extent that social work is considered one of the occupations most exposed to stress-related illnesses (Barck-Holst, 2020, as cited in Hajighasemi, 2023). One of the main reasons for the deteriorating working environment is the extensive cuts made to the welfare sector (Hajighasemi, 2004). The discrepancy between the reduction in funding for social services and a growing need to provide social support to vulnerable groups has placed welfare service providers in the difficult position of mediating

(Hasenfeld, 2010, as cited in Hajighasemi, 2023) between users with high expectations and the authorities that allocate fewer resources to service organizations.

### Cultural Competence Models

Since multicultural environments are constantly changing, the organization, and its managerial and operational staff, should also be expected to constantly renew their cultural competences in an ongoing and fluid process. From this perspective, the contextual, experiential, and developmental processes of learning strengthen the ability of operational staff to understand and meet the needs of clients (Balcazar et al., 2010, as cited in Hajighasemi, 2023, p. 251). Most of the models that suggest a process of enhancing cultural competence highlight the need for, and willingness of, organizations to be open to adapting their services to the changing and new needs of their client groups. Less emphasized, however, is the importance of the degree of diversity among employees or the impact of multi-ethnic staffing on the diversity-related activities and development plans of these organizations. To meet this shortcoming, Hyde and Hopkins (2004, as cited in Hajighasemi, 2023, p. 251) suggest two criteria that can be used in evaluating the performance of organizations in developing strategies for pursuing diversity goals: (1) the degree of diversity among employees relative to their clients, and (2) the existence of diversity-related activities and development plans. A significant underrepresentation of employees from ethnic backgrounds in relation to the clients may indicate a deviation from diversity goals (Hyde & Hopkins, 2004, as cited in Hajighasemi, 2023, p. 252). One consequence of this deficiency is that the organization might lose natural access to the cultural competence that ethnically diverse staffing provides. This shortcoming could limit the existence of diversity-related activities in the organization, as well as the quality of diversity planning, which is the second important criterion in examining diversity development in an organization. The existence of such a plan can be used to assess the measures and initiatives that aim to make diversity part of the organizational culture. In cases where an organization offers only individual preventive measures against discrimination or competence-enhancing diversity initiatives, it is arguable that the diversity climate is weak or moderate. A robust diversity climate requires a significantly stronger commitment and a long-term diversity strategy (Cox, 2001; Hyde & Hopkins, 2004).

Accordingly, cultural competence is a multifaceted ability that requires a long learning process. Recruiting ethnic staff who already possess such competence is often a more rapid, affordable, and convenient way of handling the cultural challenges that human services organizations face. Having a knowledge of the social and cultural characteristics of multicultural environments and their effects on social relations is a prerequisite for creating a culturally sensitive service strategy (Hajighasemi, 2023, p. 251). Despite that, in recent years, the focus has been on the growing need for ethnic sensitivity as a professional skill in social work (Valtonen, 2008). The need was identified primarily to explain the difficulties that arise in communications between social workers and ethnic minority clients. The issue became prevalent following extensive refugee immigration in the late 1990s, when service organizations experienced a growing deficiency in the management of ethnic minority clients (Kamali, 2002, as cited in Hajighasemi, 2023, p. 251). The new paradigm emphasized the need for a shift from labeling clients as the cause of the problems to drawing attention to the structural shortcomings of welfare organizations and their strategies for advocating the assimilation of migrants into the majority culture.

Subsequently, Hajighasemi's research found that the recruitment of social workers from migrant backgrounds has become part of a broader social policy strategy to make social services more culturally sensitive. A multicultural workforce would possess more of the crucial skills of social work, such as information gathering, an understanding of migrant clients' social problems, and the ability to manage their specific needs. Adoption of this strategy has had positive effects but also reduced the complexities associated with ethnic clients to purely cultural aspects. Hajighasemi also found that a change of perspective was needed that emphasized the significance of cultural differences. Instead of considering immigrants' lack of knowledge of the norms and values of service organizations as a shortcoming, attention turned to the low degree of cultural sensitivity in these organizations as the reason for their inefficiency (Skytte & Montesino, 2006, as cited in Hajighasemi, 2023, p. 250).

Diversity topics are more likely than not to remain critical to human services and social work education. Therefore, diversity frameworks clearly need to remain at the core of pedagogy from a first-year course of study to ensure practice is respectful and sensitive. The exploration of topics linked to diversity, often the source of tensions within and outside a university (Arieli et al., 2012; Laurs et al., 2013, as cited in Lenette, 2014, p. 120), can yield discussions rich in the exchange of personal viewpoints and narratives when facilitated in a supportive way. Similarly, institutional commitment can challenge perceptions of how cultural diversity issues should be taught in university settings and understood in practice contexts. Therefore, students should be exposed to a range of courses on diversity and be immersed in a culturally safe environment to ensure their learning in an introductory course is reinforced by appropriately integrated content in the broader curriculum over time (de Anda, 2007, as cited in Lenette, 2014, p. 121).

The overall aim of teaching about multiculturalism or cultural diversity is to encourage students to "continuously examine, challenge, question, and expand their cultural assumptions" (Lee & Greene, 2004, p. 24, as cited in Lenette, 2014, p. 121). This process is particularly relevant for first-year students from culturally homogeneous (usually white, middle-class) backgrounds with limited exposure to ethnically and culturally (and otherwise) diverse communities (Saleh et al., 2011, as cited in Lenette, 2014). Thus, courses on cultural diversity should not only value students' lived experiences and biographies but also create an atmosphere where students explore how their own cultural frameworks and biases affect their ways of seeing the world and relating to others (de Anda, 2007, as cited in Lenette, 2014) as this can assist the students with dealing with the many challenges of a multicultural society. It is with the expectation that courses on multiculturalism will provoke human services and social work educators to consider how teaching diversity in a critical manner, particularly to first-year students, can be enriched by the core tenets of cultural safety.

## Solutions or Strategies

To achieve and/or provide social support to vulnerable groups, ethnically sensitive strategies are required that enable human service organizations to create and constantly develop new programs and working methods that keep services compatible with the cultures, needs, and integration processes of new social groups. Ethnic sensitivity means awareness among staff members of their own and their clients' ethnic affiliations and expectations and that they must meet and treat people from other cultural backgrounds in a conscious and sensitive way (Green-Hernandez, 2006, as cited in Hajighasemi, 2023, p. 248).

Furthermore, Hajighasemi's (2023) research, which was designed to survey the preparedness of four Swedish human services organizations to enhance their cultural sensitivity when providing cultural congruent care and services to culturally diverse client groups, found that a lack of cultural sensitivity is particularly evident in smaller units with specialized work functions and with sensitive missions. Additionally, staff diversity creates opportunities for innovative working environments, which enables the exchange of knowledge and experience and thus the integration of a culturally sensitive approach into welfare services (Hafford-Letchfield et al., 2014).

By providing culturally sensitive care staff from the same communities as the patients with the greatest communication difficulties, most of the problems linked to cultural diversity were prevented or resolved. Access to ethnic minority staff has been an investment with a double return. This proactive attitude in employing ethnic staff can be compared with the school sector's lack of ambition to take advantage of the cultural capital that teachers from ethnic backgrounds possess. This weak enthusiasm can be explained by a lack of interest from the school system in immersing itself in or caring about cultural differences in the home environments of its pupils (Sernhede, 2011, as cited in Hajighasemi, 2023, p. 258). Ethnic minority pupils are perceived to have sufficient ability to absorb the prevailing norms and values of society and follow the curricula set out by the National Agency for Education. This strategy is in line with the main task of the school system, which is to actively influence and stimulate students regardless of background to embrace the common values of society (Skolverket, 2009, p. 8, as cited in Hajighasemi, 2023, p. 258). The prevalent opinion in the school system seems to be that these goals can best be achieved if students, regardless of cultural or ethnic background, are included in a common culture based on the dominant democratic norms and values of society (Avery, 2016).

Lastly, social services organizations with a diverse staff and board membership provide a dynamic platform for regular and continuous dialogue on everyday activities and are more receptive to valuing and implementing culturally sensitive approaches. Human services organizations with representative staff and management boards have a greater capacity or ability to design sustainable plans for the development of a diversity strategy (Allen & Montgomery, 2001, as cited in Hajighasemi, 2023). A comparison of the plans of the human services organizations surveyed in Hajighasemi's (2023) study to increase cultural competence revealed that the most pronounced measure was the recruitment of staff from an ethnic minority background. Such staff, and those with special cultural competence more generally, are considered the most effective, long-term, and sustainable investment in increasing cultural competence. Moreover, for many schools of social work, educating and training environments that are welcoming of multicultural perspectives are a goal.

## Questions for Reflection

1 What can we do to address the multicultural society we are becoming to provide services to those who are different?
2 How can human service organizations deliver services to those who are different, given that their staff may not be trained in cultural competence?

## References

Avery, H. (2016). *Moving together: Conditions for intercultural development at a highly diverse Swedish school.* Jönköping University, School of Education and Communication.

Cox, T. (2001). *Creating the multicultural organization.* Jossey-Bass.

Eagan, J. L. (2024, January 19). Multiculturalism. In *Encyclopedia Britannica.* https://www.britannica.com/topic/multiculturalism

Hafford-Letchfield, T., Lambley, S., Spolander, G., & Cocker, C. (2014). *Inclusive leadership: Managing to make a difference in social work and social care.* Policy Press.

Hajighasemi, A. (2023) Enhancing diversity climates in human services organizations. *Journal of Ethnic & Cultural Diversity in Social Work, 32*(5), 247–260. https://doi.org/10.1080/15313204.2021.1984357

Hyde, C. A. (2004). Multicultural development in human services agencies: Challenges and solutions. *Social Work, 49*(1), 7–16. https://doi.org/10.1093/sw/49.1.7

Hyde, C. A., & Hopkins, K. (2004). Diversity climates in human service agencies. *Journal of Ethnic & Cultural Diversity in Social Work, 13*(2), 25–34. https://doi.org/10.1300/J051v13n02_02

Lenette, C. (2014). Teaching cultural diversity in first year human services and social work: The impetus for embedding a cultural safety framework. A practice report. *The International Journal of the First Year in Higher Education, 5*(1), 117–123. https://doi.org/10.5204/intjfyhe.v5i1.196

National Association of Social Workers. (2021). *Code of ethics.*

Valtonen, K. (2008). *Social work and migration: Immigrant and refugee settlement and integration.* Ashgate.

Wilson, K. B., Pitt, J., Acklin, C., Gines, J., Chao, S.-Y., & Stewart, J. (2019). Facilitating application of the multicultural counseling competencies. *Rehabilitation Research, Policy, and Education, 33*(4), 234–244. https://dx.doi.org/10.1891/2168-6653.33.4.234

# Section IV

# Leading Conversations about Human Services and Education

# 26 Creative Means to Address Mental Health in the African American Community

## Arts, Advocacy, and Awareness

*Denise F. Brown*

## Mental Health

The concept of mental health is determined by an individual's emotional, social, and psychological well-being (SAMHSA, 2020). Mental illness and/or mental disorders fall under the umbrella of mental health; however, mental health has a much broader scope. Mental health focuses on well-being and how to sustain emotional, psychological, and social stability (SAMHSA, 2020). There is a difference between mental illness and mental health, and it is possible to struggle with mental illness and develop coping strategies to improve mental health (Benton, 2018). It is also possible to not actively suffer from mental illness but still have mental health issues or problems that interfere with daily living. For example, being in a dysfunctional relationship can cause stress and anxiety but not mental illness (Benton, 2018).

## Mental Illness

Mental illnesses are diagnosable mental disorders involving health conditions that cause changes in emotion and behavior and overall distress in functioning socially as well as in family and work life (American Psychiatric Association [APA], 2021a). African Americans make up 13.4% of the United States population, and, of them, approximately 16% (4.8 million) have reported having a mental illness (Mental Health America [MHA], 2020). Accordingly, African Americans are more likely than white people to report feelings of emotional distress, sadness, and feelings of hopelessness due to the stigma around mental illness and/or lack of access to treatment (National Alliance on Mental Illness [NAMI], 2022). Although mental illness and psychological distress are present in the African American community, African Americans are less likely than white people to seek traditional treatment, such as seeing a therapist or taking medication (NAMI, 2022). Seeking traditional mental health treatment has consequently been seen as a sign of weakness within the Black community (NAMI, 2022). Approximately 63% of African Americans tend to view mental illness as a sign of weakness, meaning more than half of African Americans may have this perception of mental illness (NAMI, 2022). This may result in a reluctance to seek professional help due to misunderstanding and mistrust in the healthcare system, along with a sense of discrimination and unfair treatment (NAMI, 2022). In addition, many African Americans report negative perceptions and attitudes about mental illness (NAMI, 2022; MHA, 2020). This may mean they are less likely to report or identify as having psychological disorders and/or seek help (MHA, 2020). A current report from MHA highlights the complications associated with African Americans not wanting to ascribe to having psychological disorders

DOI: 10.4324/9781003531258-31

(MHA, 2020). However, exposure to learning about mental illness could help to reduce negative beliefs about mental illness among African Americans (MHA, 2020).

## Defining Mental Illness, Stigma, and African American Perceptions

It is important to understand how mental illness is perceived in the African American community. Furthermore, it is essential for undergraduate students in the course to evaluate the definition of mental illness and what it means according to the APA. The APA source defining mental illness is assessed to identify stigma within the African American community when mental illness is housed in a Westernized framework. Mental illnesses, as explained by the APA, are diagnosable mental disorders (APA, 2021a, b). The term "diagnosable disorders" is further explained in class to clarify that mental illness is a disorder, just like medical disorders, and requires medical treatment. Challenges in mental functions are chronic and biological in nature (APA, 2021a, b). Negative perceptions of mental illness within the African American community stem from Westernized misinterpretations of African Americans' mental health (Umeh, 2019). Comparing people of African descent with animals without the capacity to have human emotions is long-standing brainwashing within American culture (Umeh, 2019). Over time, it has been necessary to debunk the concept of mental illness being a "White person's issue" (Umeh, 2019). Mental illness, health, and well-being are human conditions not confined to just white people (Umeh, 2019). However, treatment should not be dictated by white people's standards since it contributes to African Americans' distrust in Westernized mental healthcare. The challenge of seeking help continues to be prevalent in the African American community, as the perception of mental illness is also rooted in the idea that having a mental illness is a weakness (Umeh, 2019). In summary, two concepts are covered in this special topic course: (1) learning about what mental illness is and how it is interpreted in the African American community, and (2) the relationship between mental illness and mental health.

In the context of this study, "stigma" can be defined as negative and discriminatory attitudes about mental illness (Caddell, 2020). Understanding what stigma is regarding mental illness allows students to put in perspective how to define behaviors that could be identified as stigmatizing mental illness. The stigma around mental illness and mental health contributes to the challenge of properly identifying mental illness for the purpose of seeking treatment (Caddell, 2020). Mental health is a productive method to address advocacy in the African American community. Emphasizing mental healthcare to focus on emotional, psychological, and social well-being is a holistic approach to reducing stigma around mental illness.

## Becoming a Mental Health Advocate

Students can begin to deconstruct the role of an advocate as a representative and voice of those who may not have visibility, under-resourced, or are unsure about how to engage in self-advocacy. (Fuller, 2020). More specifically, a mental health advocate, as Fuller (2020) explains, can shatter stereotypes and stigmas associated with mental illness. Advocacy can also provide a mechanism to understand that it is important to be aware of mental health overall. Fuller describes different actions that can be taken to present mental illness as a challenge that can be overcome, rather than an obstacle that is negatively viewed or consistently ignored due to shame and ignorance (Fuller, 2020). Because stigma around mental illness in the African American community is such an expansive issue, utilizing varied avenues to help reduce those stigmas can enhance the professionalism of any mental health advocate. Advocating "artistically" is open for interpretation and, as mentioned in this study, has a range of outlets, such as literary art, performance art, and the visual arts. Advocates can use existing knowledge and passions to help bring awareness. Advocacy using the arts to increase knowledge of mental health can occur through experience, information, and access to resources. Advocates can use their personal stories as well as creative resources to help promote the idea of the overall process of mental health and well-being.

## Arts, Advocacy, and Awareness

According to the NAMI (2022), while the experience of being Black in America varies tremendously, there are shared cultural factors that play a role in helping to define mental health and supporting well-being, resiliency, and healing. Part of this shared cultural experience, family connections, values, expression through spirituality or music, reliance on community, and religious networks—are enriching and can be great sources of strength and support. The cultural experiences shared through specific examples, such as music, religion, community, and spirituality, are documented as historical coping mechanisms for promoting well-being (Hollow, 2019; Morin, 2020; NAMI, 2022). Thus, although such cultural practices can be creative and helpful means of support for mental health and well-being, negative attitudes around mental illness can be considered counterproductive.

This study examines creative means to address mental health and its stigma in the African American community through arts, advocacy, and awareness. Considering this view, the role of the arts (literary, visual, and performance) as they relate to social causes may be expanded to include art as an advocacy and awareness tool in helping to address social issues. In addition, art can be used to promote awareness of psychological disorders within the African American community to reduce associated negative ideas and attitudes.

African American artistic expression to promote awareness about social issues, such as police brutality and discrimination, has been useful in raising community awareness (Haque, 2020). Likewise, using art to increase awareness about the stigma associated with mental illness and mental health is apparent in many organizations. The mission of some organizations has been to address misinformation and stereotypes about mental illness through art and music (Johnson & Johnson, 2021). The Champions of Science organization suggests that using art to reduce the stigma around mental illness helps all people, not just students, to understand mental illness from different perspectives while promoting empathy (Johnson & Johnson, 2021). This special topic course aims to demonstrate an avenue of utilizing what is already apparent in the African American community, and that is artistic expression—the art of bringing awareness to the unique struggles of African Americans.

## Course Goals

In the course, students learn to differentiate mental health from mental illness. Students also learn creative means to address mental health, mental illness, and stigma as an essential part of the course. Students are made aware that the cultural practices of African Americans could lead to non-traditional means of coping and gaining a sense of well-being. Students recognize the arts as an effective source of creative means to promote awareness. Advocacy is presented to students on how to shed light on perceptions around mental illness, as it differs and is interrelated to mental health. Finally, students present their own creative means without prior artistic training to demonstrate an awareness of mental health. Ultimately, expressions such as music and visual arts provide a different perspective on advocating the concepts of mental health and well-being (Hollow, 2019).

## Qualitative Inquiry

This qualitative inquiry aims to gain insight into the experiences of students participating in the special topics course for the spring of 2024 as it relates to the course student learner outcomes (CSLOs), also known in this study as the course objectives.

These CSLOs provide a lens for students' perception of the class in terms of what knowledge and experience they obtained from learning about African American mental health, well-being, and artistic advocacy. Bloom's Taxonomy provides a lens for the course objectives as students will be assessing two levels of learning, analyzing artistic expression for advocacy, and applying the learning experience with a performance (Nurmatova, & Altun, 2023). The research questions (RQ-1 and RQ-2) were developed to guide the content for the questionnaires, and the questions were designed to reflect students' experiences with taking the class relative to the CSLOs. The research questions are listed in the next section.

## Research Questions

For this qualitative inquiry, two research questions were derived from the course objectives.

**RQ 1:** Is analyzing the terminologies related to this course helpful in bringing awareness around African American mental health and well-being and mental illness?

1. Do you have a better assessment of African American mental health and well-being and the difference between the two?
2. How would you explain the historical framework of African American mental health?
3. How would you explain mental health and well-being?
4. How would you describe advocacy for African American mental health/well-being in terms of bringing awareness to other communities?
5. How has learning about advocacy for African American mental health helped you in identifying your own advocacy tools?
6. Has learning about artistic advocacy as a tool for bringing awareness helped you create your own artistic advocacy?

**RQ 2:** Can creative means through artistic expression be utilized in advocating the awareness of mental health and well-being regardless of artistic ability?

1. Do you have a better understanding of bringing awareness about mental health and well-being through cultural and artistic expressions?
2. Can you identify how the arts can be an effective tool to advocate for mental health and well-being? If so, in what ways?
3. What was your experience of utilizing creative means through artistic expression to advocate for African American mental health and well-being?
4. Do you feel most people, regardless of artistic ability, could use artistic expression to bring awareness about mental health and well-being?
5. Would you suggest that those who choose to go into the helping profession use creative means/artistic expression to increase awareness of mental health and well-being?

6 Did you have a specific artistic (literary, performance, or visual) ability or experience prior to this special topic course?

## Data Plan

This special topics course was taught in the spring semester of 2024 at a historically Black college/university. The spring semester special topics course began on January 8, 2024, and ended on April 22, 2024. Students received instructions according to the course material, as displayed on the syllabus. Each student was allowed to choose an artistic expression (literary, visual, or performance), as an advocacy tool in bringing awareness around African American mental health issues and well-being. The mental health issues addressed included, but were not limited to, mental illnesses, stigmas around mental illnesses, and the importance of psychological well-being. The artistic advocacy presentations were presented during the spring semester. The presentations consisted of students creating their own artistic expression through visual art, literature, or performance (dance, singing) to bring awareness about the mental health and well-being of Black people. Examples of the presentations included spoken words about depression, mental health stigma, poverty, a song about colorism, and a dance that represented discrimination and oppression.

After the presentations were completed on April 17, the following week, students were provided with a questionnaire, and those who completed the questionnaire earned five extra credit points. The students' earned grades were not affected if the questionnaire was not completed. This was to ensure that students would not feel pressured to complete the questionnaire for their final grade. The artistic advocacy presentations accounted for a 45% portion of their final grade, with classroom participation and weekly assignments accounting for the other 55%.

Since there was no perceived risk to recruiting student participants, on April 15, 2024, consent forms were given to each student, and the instructor reviewed the consent forms during regular class time, at noon in room 296 of Dickey Hall. The students were provided with an explanation of the consent form in addition to an explanation of the questionnaire as it related to the CSLOs. Students were given an opportunity to ask questions about the research and consent forms. After the consent forms were reviewed, each student was given time to review them again before making a final decision to participate in completing the questionnaire. On April 17, students were invited to participate in completing the questionnaire once the consent forms were signed and given back to the instructor. The questionnaire was given to each student who signed a consent form. The instructor explained the questionnaire in addition to informing the students that its completion was voluntary and for extra credit. The students were instructed not to include their names for the protection of privacy. Once each student completed the questionnaire, the questionnaire forms were transcribed by the instructor.

### Data Analysis

This qualitative inquiry evaluated student experiences by using artistic expression as an advocacy tool. The researcher's main goal was to assess whether there were any themes surrounding the learning experiences of participants in this course based on the objectives. Participants' personal experiences provided deeper insight into the interpretation of course objectives. In addition, thematic coding revealed the proficiency achieved related to course objectives among students who were not professional artists. Developing an artistic, expressive performance for the final presentation was mandatory; however, having previous artistic experience or ability was not a requirement.

Out of the 27 students who were registered for the class, 16 completed the questionnaire. The questions were then transcribed by the researcher, and feedback was captured in charts and a table to illustrate the thematic coding, which was used to break down the data into themes and codes based on the CSLOs (Naeem et al., 2023). Each question for which participants provided feedback was color-coded to identify phrases that were similar and/or repetitive, as they related to the course objectives. All color-coded phrases were then grouped into codes, and each code was formed from themes discovered in the phrases. The phrases that were identified as having themes were counted to calculate the number of responses. For example, question number one under RQ-1 had 14 responses that were classified as having a theme. The number of responses was entered into a table to provide an overview. The charts and table in the following sections provide the complete data for all of the questions.

### Course Student Learner Outcomes

- Define course terminologies, including mental health and mental illness/stigma
- Interpret and analyze historical references as well as current events relating to African Americans and mental health/illnesses
- Describe advocacy initiatives within the African American community
- Develop and present advocacy projects utilizing creative means i.e., literary, visual, and/ or performing arts

The chart below displays the thematic coding for questions 1–6 under RQ-1, "Is understanding the terminologies related to this course helpful in bringing awareness around African American mental health and well-being and mental illness?" Each question from the questionnaire reflects one of the CSLOs from the syllabus, which is also included in the chart. The CSLOs were developed based on the measurable concepts of defining, interpreting, describing, and developing. Students were asked to provide feedback based on their level of knowledge regarding advocacy in the action of bringing awareness around African American mental health and well-being. The first question asked students to provide feedback on their assessment of mental health and well-being. Below is a breakdown of participant responses.P-3 Yes.

P-4 Yes.

P-6 Yes, I do.

P-7 Yes, I do have a better assessment of African American Mental Health.

P-10 Yes, this class has distinguished a difference between the two.

P-11 Yes, I do.

P-12 *This course did in fact enhance my knowledge about the difference between mental health and African American* well-being.

The themes for question suggested "yes I do have a better assessment of mental health and well-being." The number of responses, 12 out of 16, demonstrated a theme, with two other participants' feedback not directly answering the question. The second question asked participants to explain the historical framework of African Americans and mental health. Participants' responses were examined for descriptions of the history of mental health related to African Americans. The 12 responses for question 2 had very similar phrases related to stigma, slavery, and discrimination as it related to Blacks' mental health; the similar responses most likely reflected answers students retrieved from class notes. Below are some examples.

P-1 The historical framework of African American mental health is deeply intertwined with the legacy of slavery, racial oppression, and systemic discrimination.

P-2 American mental health is deeply rooted in systemic oppression, starting from slavery through segregation and ongoing discrimination.

P-3 A lot of African American mental health is a result of the deep traumatic history of slavery, which is rooted in the DNA of America.

P-4 Mental health has not been appreciated in the African American communities based on the stigmas placed in the African American communities. Most of the stigmas are embedded in racism and slavery.

P-5 Historically, African Americans have been wrongfully diagnosed with mental illnesses in various medical fields. In the psychology mental health field, there are not as many African Americans in the field, which can be uncomfortable for clients who may not be able to open up as much to people they see may be different than them.

P-6 African American community is unique in that mental health wasn't addressed for a long time. There was/still is a stigma toward mental health within the African American community. Over time people within the community have shed more light on it. Black people have used the arts to express mental health/social problems.

P-7 The historical framework of African American mental health is deeply intertwined with centuries of systemic oppression, including slavery, segregation, and ongoing racial discrimination.

P-8 Slavery, discrimination, and social status have all had an impact on African Americans' mental health history. For example, slave owners and white racists have spread myths that enslaved Black Americans are immune to mental disease.

P-9 The history of dealing with the traumatic experiences was addressed by expressing themselves creatively as early as the 1800s, when slaves brought awareness to one another about their feelings and/or how they wanted to carry out their freedom from captivity.

For question 3, two themes were developed to highlight the pattern of responses explaining mental health and well-being. For mental health, the theme emerged as emotional and psychological stability, and for well-being, the themes of satisfaction, fulfillment, and coping emerged. The following are a couple of responses.

P-1 Mental health refers to a person's overall psychological and emotional well-being. Well-being is the concept that encompasses many aspects such as satisfaction and happiness.

P-2 Mental health refers to a person's emotional, psychological, and social well-being. Well-being, on the contrary, encompasses more than just the absence of mental illness; it includes factors like life satisfaction, fulfillment, and the ability to cope with life's challenges in a positive and productive way.

The participants seemed to identify mental health and well-being as a state of being stable. Participant responses did not shed light on distinguishing between mental health and mental illness and well-being. The researcher noted the need for a clearer breakdown of the terminology during class lectures to equip students with more clarity around distinguishing between mental health (which includes mental illness) and well-being.

The graph below shows questions 4, 5, and 6. These questions relate to how the participants explained artistic advocacy as a tool for bringing awareness. The purpose was to assess whether participants could interpret art as a tool for outreach in the community by identifying and creating artistic advocacy for themselves. The themes based on participant responses provided insight into participants' acknowledgment of advocacy in terms of community engagement as it relates to diversity and culture and mental health access. Participants' themes for creating individual artistic advocacy were interpreted as using the voice for messaging to outer communities; thus, the pattern of responses was attached to a general theme of vocal expression.

## Graph of Themes for RQ-1 Questions 1–6

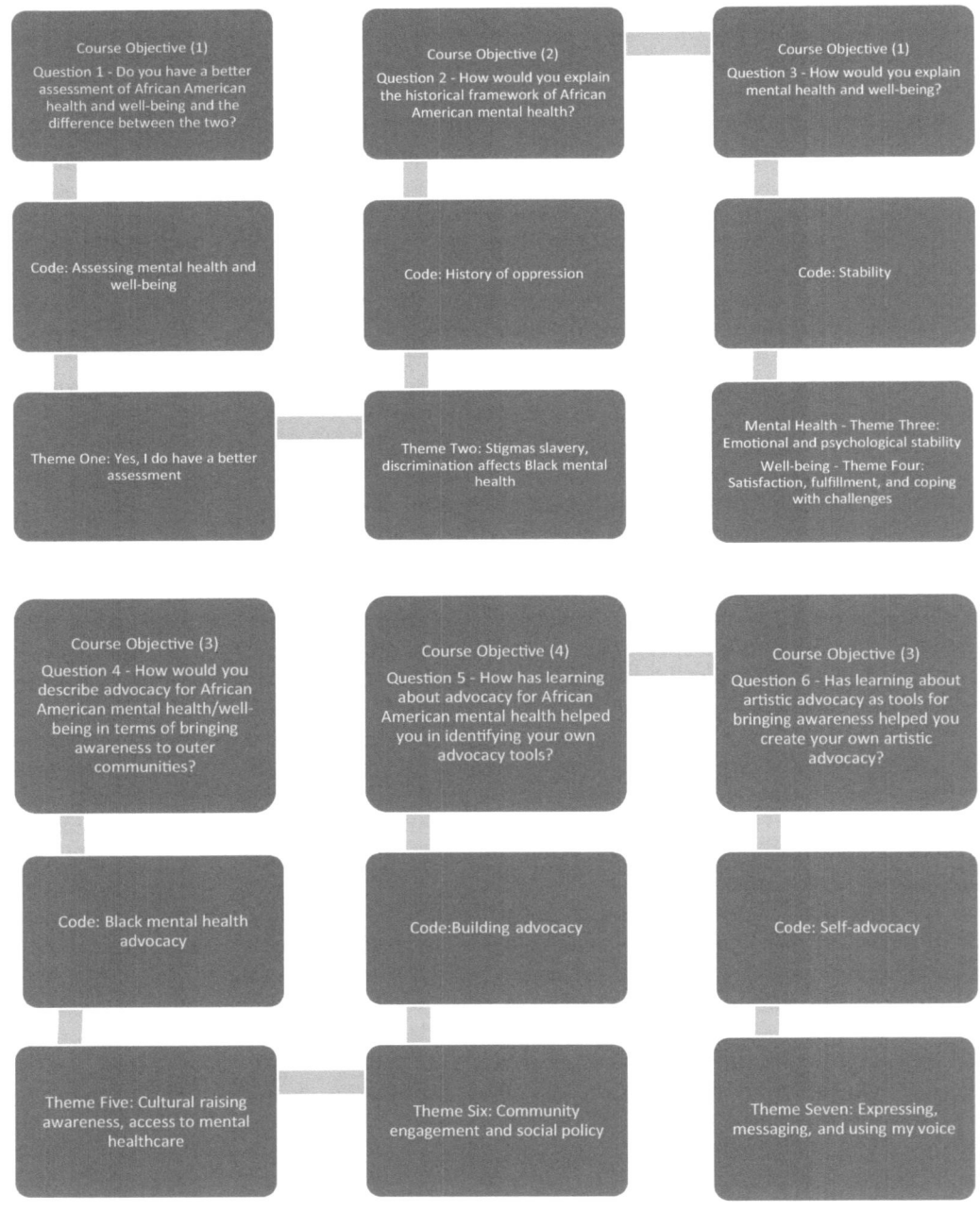

The graphs in the following section represent questions 1–6 for RQ-2, "Can creative means through artistic expression be utilized in advocating the awareness of mental health and well-being regardless of artistic ability?" The first question asked the participants to explain their understanding of bringing awareness through cultural expressiveness, specifically related to mental health and well-being. Examples of responses include as follows:

P-1 Yes

P-2 Yes, absolutely. Cultural artistic expressions offer a unique and powerful avenue for raising awareness about mental health and well-being

P-3 Yes, I wouldn't say that I was never aware, but I never actually thought about how acceptable artistic expression really is to people, and Black people are very gifted with that.

P-4 Yes, to my understanding, culture brings a huge role in mental health advocacy. It needs to be understandable and relatable for people can appreciate the benefits of mental well-being.

The second question elaborates on questions about artistic advocacy and its effectiveness, and the third question relates to participants' experiences utilizing creative means via artistic expression to advocate for African American mental health and well-being. Topics included mental health and well-being, African American mental health and well-being, and using creative expressions related to literary, performance, and the visual arts. Participants' responses showed 14 out of 16 with themes for the first two questions. The themes resulted in "Yes, I do have a better understanding of bringing awareness through cultural artistic expression about mental health and well-being" and "Yes, the arts are an effective tool to bring awareness to mental health and well-being and reduce the stigma in the African American community." The third question consisted of two themes related to experiences utilizing creative means: "Yes, it was a great experience," and "Utilizing the arts was a challenging experience."

Questions 4, 5, and 6 under RQ-2 point to artistic advocacy outside of the classroom. These last set of questions are geared toward assessing participants' perception of artistic advocacy as a universal concept that anyone can use as a tool, particularly in the helping profession. Participants were asked a final question about their personal artistic abilities; this question was to assess if participants had artistic abilities before taking the course. Out of 13 participants who directly answered the question, 8 answered that they had no prior artistic (literary, performance, or visual) ability or experience, and 5 responded that they did have prior experience. Three of the participants did not answer the question directly. Participants also provided feedback that represented support for artistic advocacy being utilized in the helping profession.

## Graph of Themes for RQ-2 Questions 1–6

| RQ-1 Responses | RWT Q-1 | RWT Q-2 | RWT Q-3 | RWT Q-4 | RWT Q-5 | RWT Q-6 |
| --- | --- | --- | --- | --- | --- | --- |
| 16 | 12 | 12 | 13 | 10 | 11 | 9 |
| RQ-2 Responses | RWT Q-1 | RWT Q-2 | RWTQ-3 | RWT Q-4 | RWT Q-5 | RWTQ-6 |
| 16 | 14 | 14 | 9 | 12 | 11 | 13 |

## Table of Responses with Themes (RWT) to RQ-1 and RQ-2: Total of 12 Questions

The table above shows the sequence of responses to each question. This table provides an overview of the patterns of responses. Themes were frequent for most of the questions. The responses demonstrated how often students were able to provide feedback. There were a

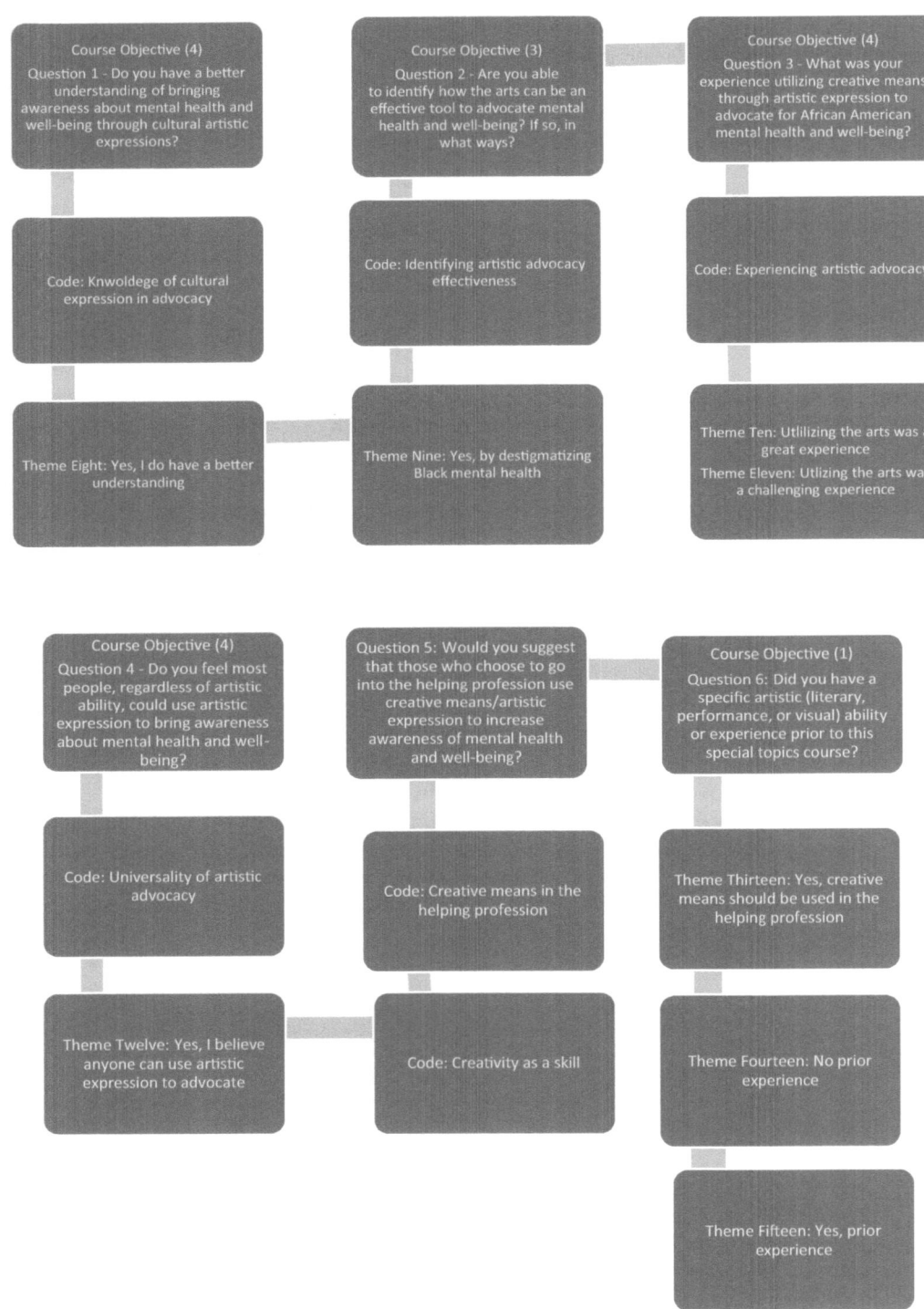

total of 15 themes, based on 12 questions. The themes were broken down for each question. The purpose of having a theme for each question was to specify how the responses more clearly represented the CSLOs and to provide an overview of what students gained from the class experience.

## Course Student Learner Outcomes

The questions were aligned with the CSLOs to better evaluate how the participants interpreted their learning experiences in the classroom (Nurmatova, & Altun, 2023). The purpose of the CSLOs was for the students to define course terms, interpret the history of mental health and well-being within African American communities, describe artistic advocacy, and, finally, develop their own artistic presentation. The alignment of CSLOs with the research questions was necessary to better capture whether the course objectives were met through students' responses and recall of the course content. The feedback from the participants revealed that, although students were able to grasp a significant portion of the course content, modifications can be made to better address CSLOs in the future. Examples of course modifications include changes in course instruction, lectures, and explanations of course terminology. The next section summarizes the main themes around the CSLOs.

## Conclusion

This qualitative inquiry was written to analyze the feedback from students and develop thematic coding around student responses as they related to the CSLOs. Thematic coding was utilized to provide a final assessment of students' experiences in artistic expression as an advocacy tool for the final performance presentation. The results were documented to further provide insight into the impact of this special topics course as it related to course learner outcomes as documented on the syllabus. Based on student feedback, 15 themes were developed, and those themes can be summarized within the CSLOs: (1) defining mental health and well-being and the differences between the two, (2) interpreting the history of African Americans and mental health and well-being, (3) describing what artistic advocacy is and how it is used, and (4) developing an artistic advocacy presentation. Based on the researcher's assessment, course learner outcomes were moderately achieved. Participants declared an adequate understanding of the development of artistic advocacy to demonstrate a performance presentation. Participants were able to moderately elaborate on the challenges of utilizing artistic advocacy to bring awareness to others, such as in front of peers, faculty, and widespread university audiences. According to the themes, participants reported a productive learning experience on the benefits of artistic advocacy. This special topic course, "Creative Means to Address Mental Health in the African American Community: Arts, Advocacy, and Awareness," will continue to be taught in the spring semesters, and further data analyses will be conducted to assess how students gain insight into the "arts" as an advocacy tool within the African American community.

## Reflective Questions for Consideration

1  If this special topic course were taught as a required course, what would be the justification?
2  What changes could be made to make this course more applicable to students going into the helping profession?
3  Could this course be taught as a cross-listed course for other disciplines in the social sciences?

## References

American Psychiatric Association. (2021a). *What is mental illness?* https://www.psychiatry.org/patients-families/what-is-mental-illness

American Psychiatric Association. (2021b). *Stigma, prejudice and discrimination against people with mental illness.* https://www.psychiatry.org/patients-families/stigma-and-discrimination

Benton, S. (2018, April 12). *The difference between mental health and mental illness.* https://www.psychologytoday.com/us/blog/reaching-across-the-divide/201804/the-difference-between-mental-health-and-mental-illness

Caddell, J. (2020, July 3). *What is stigma?* https://www.verywellmind.com/mental-illness-and-stigma-2337677

Fuller, K. (2020, June 24). *What does it mean to be a mental health advocate?* https://www.nami.org/Blogs/NAMI-Blog/June-2020/What-Does-It-Mean-to-Be-a-Mental-Health-Advocate

Haque, D. (2020, October 5). *Art can be used as a tool for advocacy and social justice.* https://thetempest.co/2020/10/05/news/social-justice/art-as-advocacy/

Hollow, M. (2019, January 29). Fighting the stigma of mental illness through music. *The New York Times.* https://www.nytimes.com/2019/01/29/well/mind/fighting-the-stigma-of-mental-illness-through-music.html

Johnson and Johnson. (2021). *Champions of science: The art of ending stigma project launches to combat stigma about mental illnesses through education and artistic creation.* Johnson & Johnson jnj.com/media-center/press-releases/champions-of-science-the-art-of-ending-stigma-project-launches-to-combat-stigma-about-mental-illnesses-through-education-and-artistic-creation.

Mental Health America. (2020). *Mental Health America's Advocacy Network is a powerful voice for change.* https://mhanational.org/issues/advocacy-network

Morin, A. (2020, October 26). *Exploring the mental health stigma in African American communities.* verywellmind.com/exploring-the-mental-health-stigma-in-black-communities-5078964

Naeem, M., Ozuem, W., Howell, K., & Ranfagni, S. (2023). A step-by-step process of thematic analysis to develop a conceptual model in qualitative research. *International Journal of Qualitative Methods, 22,* 1-18. https://doi.org/10.1177/16094069231205789

National Alliance on Mental Illness [NAMI]. (2022, April 8). *Erasing mental health stigma in the Black community.* https://www.nami.org/african-american/erasing-mental-health-stigma-in-the-black-community/

National Council for Mental Wellbeing. (2019). *Stigma regarding mental illness among people of color BH365.* https://engage.thenationalcouncil.org/communities/community-home/digestviewer/viewthread?GroupId=55&MessageKey=c348ee0f-4858-4a55-b16b-77f99aa52486&CommunityKey=9f102bb3-8160-4927-bb13-d05b672b532d

Nurmatova, S. & Altun, M. (2023). A comprehensive review of bloom's taxonomy integration to enhancing novice EFL educators' pedagogical impact. *Arab World English Journal (AWEJ), 14*(3), 380-388. https:// doi.org/10.24093/awej/

Substance Abuse and Mental Health Services Administration [SAMHSA]. (2020). *What is mental health?* https://www.samhsa.gov/data/data-we-collect/nsduh-national-survey-drug-use-and-health/national-releases/2020

Umeh, U. (2019). *Mental illness in the Black community, 1700-2019: A short history.* https://www.blackpast.org/african-american-history/mental-illness-in-black-community-1700-2019-a-short-history/

# 27 Addressing Empathy Deficits in College-Age Students Utilizing Social Work Pedagogy amid Social Shifts

*Sandra R. Williamson-Ashe*

## The Current Landscape

For years, there has been a notable decline in the empathy levels of college students. Data from the University of Michigan empathy study of 2009 was compared with data from the 1979 study (Swanbrow, 2010). The 14,000 participants show a decline of 30% in empathy levels (Swanbrow, 2010). This decline is supported and increased by the rapid advances of mediated communications and the regeneration of saturated traumas. The instantaneous breaking news, the uncertainties of the pandemic, and the visible wars of racial injustices and inequalities, experienced in intense people isolation, promote stress, emotional turmoil, bewilderment, and overthinking, contributing to apathy and a lack of empathy.

Americans are exposed to three times more media-type information than they were three decades ago (Swanbrow, 2010). This media familiarity is not limited to the explosion of social media but also to the health crisis of the nation and the combative racial climate. The health crisis that not only affected the United States but also international nations held no levels of predictability with individuals, leaving them in a tremendous state of uncertainty. The Institute of Health Metrics and Evaluation indicates that COVID-19-related deaths totaled 1,046,845 in the fall of 2022 (COVID-19 Projections, 2022). During the COVID-19 lockdown, daily levels of risk saturated the televised airways and social media, tethering individuals and families to their devices for status reports. And although Black Americans are cognizant of their skin color and the responses it brings on a daily and situational basis, during the COVID-19 lockdown, the overwhelmingly violent demonstrations of rejection and hatred based on race were played out on every avenue possible. From podcasts, television news, and talk shows, to social media posts, comment responses, and blogs, each communication route was contaminated with its own macroaggressions while the world pivoted with microaggressions.

The intricacies that have penetrated the lives and cultures of individuals in this media-pandemic-racial reckoning are significant. This pandemic-centered collision includes the overabundance of news that saturates any and all communication devices. It is noted that, in the domination of information, too much news leads to increased worry, making it difficult to concentrate, adding high levels of anxiety that over time negatively affect one's mood and lead to depression (Campbell, 2022).

The United Way of the National Capital Area surveyed respondents pre- and post-pandemic to reveal that 37% of Americans report a decline in their empathetic levels by up to 20% (United Way NCA, 2022). Because the University of Michigan's empathy comparison studies are pre-pandemic college student surveys, it may be reasonable to consider that the decline in current students' empathetic level may now be more substantial. The student

DOI: 10.4324/9781003531258-32

empathy levels were previously better; now the United Way survey reports that the empathy levels of general Americans (which could include students) have declined; certainly, toxicity from the recent challenging happenings would heighten the probability of empathetic decline.

According to Erik Erickson's stage 6 of the theory of psychosocial development, adults between the ages of 18 and 40 are centered on forming intimate, loving relationships while pursuing long-term commitments (McLeod, 2018). Important to note with the unprecedented non-socialization practices of the pandemic is that, according to Erickson, the avoidance of commitment and intimacy could lead to isolation and result in depression (McLeod, 2018). This is the formula that the contagiousness of the pandemic required individuals, particularly students, to operate (McLeod, 2018). Regrettably, as young adult college students were in intimacy versus isolation stages, the world was supporting isolation out of safety and inviting hatred and division instead of the ultimate goal of stage 6, love.

Young collegiate adults experience the greatest amount of relationship discord and call into question their purpose in life (Kellam & Degges-White, 2017) without any consideration for modern-day climate changes. If students' psychosocial development during the collision of heightened acts of the media-pandemic-race conflicts was not enough to derail young adult development, consider that the mission of collegiate institutions is not only intellectual development but also emotional and social development (Kellam & Degges-White, 2017). The institutions that young college adults merge and structure their lives around for academic, social-emotional development are severed in the pandemic isolation safety protocols.

The elevated complexities for traditional-aged college students' psychosocial development and growth may be more pronounced in consideration of their developmental momentum alongside the collision of current-day events. Erickson's theory of psychosocial development is not the only theoretical perspective that provides vision to the positioning of young adults in this current-day climate. Arthur Chickering's seven vectors for identity also provide a psychosocial student development model that continues to deliver clarity for students while in college. This model continues the social and emotional and adds the physical and intellectual factors in the formation of the student's identity development in college. Chickering's 1969 model was revised with Reisser in 1993. The seven vectors include developing competence, managing emotions, moving through autonomy toward interdependence, developing mature interpersonal relationships, establishing identity, developing purpose, and developing integrity (Robinson, n.d.). As mentioned, students question their purpose at this developmental time; it stands to reason that they are seeking to develop positive relationships (developing purpose) in vision of their values (developing integrity), and affirming their values only adds in the process of a healthy self-concept (establishing identity) (Robinson, n.d.).

In conjunction with already waning college students' loss of empathy, the addition of their developmental cycles, alongside the racial aggressions, the pandemic, and the tensions of news bombarding all communication devices, will generate an intensity among young adults in the coming years. This intensity would presumably be magnified for social work students as a result of their already harbored troublesome circumstances that formulated their desired entry into the social work program. Social work students have reported that their selection of the discipline is the result of life struggles, and these traumas have resulted in empathy decay (Williamson-Ashe, 2019). With lowered levels of empathy, students will have difficulty controlling their emotions, maintaining relationships, and understanding the feelings of others (Robbins, 2021). Empathy can lead to greater happiness, improved communication skills, reduced negativity, and transcendent relationships (Robbins, 2021).

To develop mature interpersonal relationships, students will foster their ability to accept others, appreciate commonalities, and respect differences (Robinson, n.d.). During a climate that questions the value of life for marginalized populations, 50% of young adults aged 18–34 supported the U.S. protests for police wrongdoing after the death of George Floyd (Statista Research Department, 2020). This population made up the greatest number of protest supporters. Deductively, there could be theoretical support for the college-aged young adults accepting others and showing an appreciation for the common humanity.

Managing emotions encompasses college students managing their reactions to events—this supports the choice to engage in protests. In competence, college students are intellectually reasoning with critical thinking to make decisions, while interpersonal competence promotes college students communicating and working well with others (Robinson, n.d.), which would explain the coordinated efforts of protesting behaviors. Earnestly, protesting behaviors exceed the physical street marches; they include policy review and dissection, integrity in candidacy and voting, and the relentless process of challenging the seemingly comfortable and mediocre. This transition into more cognitive and intangible protests has been comported as a result of the previous two decades of intrusive mediation communication. The receipt of massive bundles of information with an unlimited trajectory inundates the narratives people are required to filter, interpret, and resolve, creating the need for variation in protests.

Historically, college-aged students have been a tremendous force for social justice changes. The movement reinforced through the neighboring deaths of two unarmed Black people, George Floyd and Breonna Taylor, catapulted college campuses to lifelong changes with the previously advanced Black Lives Matter. Student activism has encouraged police reform, dismantling systemic barriers that disproportionately affect Black students, student organizations evolving an amplified Black voice, Black art recognizing Black Lives Matter, the renaming of buildings, the deconstruction of confederate monuments, student athletes flattering activism, campus mascots challenged to be culturally appropriate, and diversity initiatives being introduced at alarming rates (Thompson, 2021); some institutions have hired diversity, equity, inclusion officers at the senior administrative levels.

These equalizing efforts benefit all individuals, despite their life circumstances, and are inclusive of everyone. The collegiate forces for justice accepted the commonalities of people and appreciated their differences, reflecting how young adults develop interpersonal relationships. Reverend Dr. Martin Luther King, Jr. stated, "Injustice anywhere is a threat to justice everywhere" (King, 1963/2004). At the moment that college students use their vocal energies to stimulate progress by challenging inequalities, differences are recognized and respected. And, as Dr. King wisely noted, any lack of humanity limits the humanity for others; interdependence from autonomy is one of Chickering's vectors in college student development.

## The Challenge, The Growth

As a nation, the blame for what is incorrect and the accolades for what is correct may be seemingly shared across and among all the members. This would ring true if there were equal contributions from everyone. But even with the desire to be an equal and regular contributor, the opportunities are different for different people. Unfortunately, differences here also mean inequality, discriminatory practices, and the marginalization of races through power imbalances. Being a member of society exposes all persons to the same societal norms; both the person oppressed and the oppressor have been taught the same societal expectations and are exposed to the governance of the majority and the power preferences.

With the social construct of race, there is an intentional societal categorization into in-groups and out-groups, referred to as social identity theory. Group membership is powerful; this type of categorization leads to favoritism or discrimination toward members of other groups (Janse, 2020). Social identity theory has three mental processes involved in identifying in-groups versus out-groups or us versus them: social categorization, social identity, and social comparison (Janse, 2020).

As a way for individuals to organize themselves into categories, according to social categorization, they seek to understand the social world around them based on their group. Group members emphasize the similarities between themselves and other in-group members and the differences between themselves and other out-group members (Janse, 2020). In social identity, behavior is important. Group members behave as they believe members of their group should (Janse, 2020). And the final stage, social comparison, where group members begin to compare their group with other groups, using social status and prestige (Janse, 2020).

Social identity theory explains that knowing your identified group aids people in learning more about their category and environment, and individuals are not isolated to one category; multiple associations are possible: race, religion, social class, gender, and politics, to name a few. Stereotyping behaviors are a part of the formula used to put people into social groups and exacerbate society's explained cognitive process of us (in-group) against them (out-group), competitiveness and comparison. Group membership carries emotionality within the connectivity; therefore, the stereotype-prejudice-racism, rivalry, and social competition for resources and the protection and elevation of one's self-esteem are theoretically explained in the social identity theory (McLeod, 2019).

The college student stage of life has a complex positioning that is only increased in complexity when married to the underpinnings of social identity theory. As explained in the theory, there is competition between the in-group and out-group that is seemingly normalized through the theoretical explanations of how competitiveness is associated with a vie for resources and what is interpreted as a process related to pride. The in-group considers their associated category as being better than the out-group, intentionally seeking or decisively creating negative characteristics to make their category more prominent. This means that the differences seen by members of the in-group are embellished and can result in the non-courageous stereotypes and prejudiced behaviors in opposition to members of the out-group. The outcome of this societal division is racism. In the collegiate realm, members of the underrepresented groups—the out-group—may tend to take fewer college credits per semester; they are perceived by the in-group to lack academic rigor and interest or be incapable of executing learning strides equal to those of in-group members. These embellishments, as external assumptions, have shared threads with racial socialization practices, making it an effortless transition to prejudiced behaviors. Fewer credits authentically resemble a need by the out-group to work externally to finance the expenses of college and living. This leaves restricted hours available for class enrollment hours and restricted time to seek academic study groups and advisement.

Having been an enforced social norm in behaviors and institutional operations, the permanency of racism in society shows limited signs of departure, but there are indications of efforts to reduce the macroaggressions of racism. A clear tug-of-war befalls the racial reckoning, as diligently as the oppressed group challenges their minimized status and current state of affairs, the group desiring to maintain the power differential and hierarchy clinches their current position with reverence. In the tug-of-war, society will continue to harbor and maintain the racial divide. The extensive history of stereotypes and prejudiced behaviors is woven into social structures and policies effortlessly; this will remain an area of contention. The intertwined roots of racism are multilayered and bottomless, growing both toward the light and deeper beneath the surface. The continuation of racism in the future will likely develop the creativity of microaggressions into new layers, but the same combat remains.

The derogatory messages directed at members of the out-group masked as harmless exchanges result in microaggressions that, over time, contribute to increased depression and anxiety, making racism a mental health crisis (Reed, 2022). There are three forms of racial microaggressions: microassaults, microinvalidations, and microinsults (Reed, 2022). Microassaults are meant to hurt, verbal or non-verbal; they are direct and deliberate racist attacks (Reed, 2022). Microinvalidations, also verbal or non-verbal, invalidate people's feelings and life experiences (Reed, 2022). Microinsults are belittling, insulting, subtle comments, sometimes unconscious, but racially charged (Reed, 2022).

> One study examined the racial climate and microaggressions at college campuses and found that African American students experienced more depression, self-doubt, frustration, and isolation that impacted their education as a result. The experience of having to question whether something happened to you because of your race or constantly being on edge because your environment is hostile can often leave people feeling invisible, silenced, angry.
>
> (Reed, 2022)

The impact of intense community endemic disease can result in things such as fear of the workplace or gathering spaces that feel threatening to individuals, causing them to change their behavior (Madhav et al., 2017). Trauma is considered a global health problem, and the public health model that would identify causes is most concerned with preventive health (Magruder et al., 2017). As the years progressed, the approach to the unprecedented pandemics would have a behavioral component based on a multilevel social-ecological approach that included society, community, relationships, and the individual (Magruder et al., 2017). This public health approach to trauma provides strategies and opportunities for intervention (Magruder et al., 2017). The prevention framework, considered a classic, has three levels. The first level prevents disease occurrence, the second level is early intervention for a cure, and the third level is prevention of the disability that accompanies the disease (Magruder et al., 2017). As a systems-level model, this approach considers the interactions between the person and their environment important and contributory to one's health and behavior.

For future occurrences, following the social-ecological model as a framework for the prevention of the associated traumas that accompany a public health crisis could be advantageous. This means that, in the future, how society responds to possible and actual endemic diseases may look different as a behavioral approach intentionally accompanies intervention. The social-ecological model outlines that an individual's health is affected through the interactions they have with the community and the physical and social environments. The social-ecological approach was known prior to the onset of the COVID-19 pandemic, but prior to this, as a society, complacency left individuals vulnerable to the nation's successful survival and health, well-being precedents. With the harsh realities of the recent pandemic, tomorrow's public health threats will have fewer traumatizing accompaniments.

Social work students trained at the onset and during the learning curve of the COVID-19 pandemic, while also in their relational development, will eventually transition into and throughout the workforce. But they will now be more empathetically responsive to how the unknown can dismantle a system but can also generate the investment needed to strengthen and advance individuals for resiliency. However, this will remain a challenge for social work, inviting new professionals into an environment that aided in shaping them but not necessarily embracing them. This sounds like a familiar tune of marginalization, but it is not. The pandemic was an equal opportunity destroyer, unlike society that selects what population to marginalize. No one and no community were immune to the pandemic. All were affected, though, as is known to underrepresented individuals and communities, when the oppressed, particularly Black-Brown people, have health challenges, they are disproportionately affected. Most commonly stated and accurately framed is the statement that, when America develops a common cold, Black Americans contract the flu.

The saturation of news regarding the health rankings of neighborhoods and socialization restrictions, as well as the most recent racial injustices and unrest in years, will become as routine as mass shootings. In five years, there will be a new normalcy for recent college graduates; the repeated unjust racial macroaggressions and new and challenging public health outbreaks will no longer be novel occurrences. Current college students will then be in the probationary stage of their jobs and careers, and quite possibly dealing with the aftermath of having endured the onset of the pandemic and renewed racial confrontations. This new normalcy will challenge social work professionals to deconstruct policies so that they respond responsibly with the necessary equality and inclusiveness to public health and racial concerns.

### Construct Student Empathy

In addition to the social work profession advocating for and participating in the social-ecological approach, it would be critical to begin to engage in instructing college students with intention while they are in their relationally developmental stage.

The already-established decline of empathy levels in college-aged students generates a conduit for the needed academic arrangements for social work students. Social work students are particularly vulnerable to empathic decline because of self-identified life struggles. Students noted classroom learning to be a valuable process to build empathy levels (Williamson-Ashe, 2019). Knowing this, a specifically devised assignment strategizes to address the continuous empathy gap, a gap noted as an earlier deterioration or the new normal gap for modern-day empathy deficits in college-age students.

The documented lack of empathy and the tools of pedagogical influence (as noted in Williamson-Ashe, 2019) can provide a conceptual context that will address students with the historical spiraling empathy levels, paired with current-day movements in technology and cultural climates. In *Pedagogical Techniques That Provide Educational Value to Social Work Students through Bereavement Academics and Empathetic Advancements*, student-centered instruction (SCI), teaching through relationships, and the "sorrowful empty chair" are techniques used that produce student devotion to good work (Williamson-Ashe, 2019). This study specifically surveyed social work students; previous research documented that social work students have self-proclaimed impactful pre-college circumstances that contributed to their selection of the social work discipline (Williamson-Ashe, 2019). However, applying the pedagogical techniques to non-social work students is not a guarantee that they will be free of pre-college circumstances, but it does provide a greater probability that all students could benefit from the intentional academic plans if social work students profit.

The first technique, SCI, uses open-ended problems requiring creative critical thinking for solutions (Williamson-Ashe, 2019). As a technique, SCI requires heightened levels of student prompting, favorably demonstrated through starting the research process with current events. The empathetic social work student studies using SCI involves the research of subject matter related to the enrolled course of study. As students initiate the learning process in SCI, they will progress from a passive to an active learner (Student-Centered Learning, n.d.). Students are able to exercise control over their intended research subject through the professor's organization of activities and the student's use of critical curiosity to dissect information. This practice of student subject control may encourage confidence and reduce thoughts of uncertainty.

At this time of current-day stressors, students have been saddled with an unfamiliar loss of control over their circumstances, confining them to feelings that lead to anxiety and fear. Students will benefit from guided independent work by selecting areas of their greatest interest, critically examining them, finding logic different from their assumptions, building knowledge, and then integrating concepts for learning. Thereby, in SCI activities, students take responsibility for learning and explore their curiosities, acutely using technology productively while promoting a preparedness for their future careers as they research current events related to their discipline of study (Student-Centered Learning, n.d.) and how it has been affected by the areas previously noted, the pandemic, the racial awakenings, and the saturation of news events.

In teaching through relationships, the second technique, the professor knows where the student is intellectually and shares as a mentor, professorial exposure of experiences with the students (Williamson-Ashe, 2019). This active engagement is intimate in the connectivity of the professor and the student; the communication embraces vulnerability and trust and can be very individualized. Teaching through relationships (TTR) allows for a course mentorship from the professor to the student, where the professor has got to know the positions of students. The professor is able to support and nurture the student in the SCI process as they initiate their learning activity through current event research, and the professor guides them according to their academic position and encourages academic enhancement based on current events, current intellect, goals, and career aspirations. It is readily known that mentees often mimic the behaviors modeled and professors model critical thinking to address the student's subject of choice. In the empathic social work study, students were assigned a written research paper; it would be helpful too for students to collaborate on their research ideas in writing and integrate the concepts discovered.

And, third, an integral part of the pedagogical techniques are the reflective exercises in the sorrowful empty chair that add to the much-needed area of self-awareness, something highly practiced in the discipline of social work and necessary to the advancement of students. The "sorrowful" empty chair reflective exercise, a term coined by the author Williamson-Ashe (2019), encourages students to assume that the empty chair in the classroom was previously occupied by a recently deceased classmate. For the current-day student, this chair may be assumed to have been occupied by someone who recently succumbed to COVID-19 or the racial turmoil. In an exercise such as this one, it would be important for students to be aware of their mental health status and how they are likely to respond to certain traumas.

Self-awareness is not an exercise widely practiced by non-social work collegiate disciplines. Its usefulness and value have been attributed to the increase in student confidence and a derivative of diversity education. Targeting self-awareness, students understand what makes them unique as individuals through recognition of their strengths, habits, failings, and needs; this will aid them in adapting to life's ever-changing climate (Srivastava, 2015).

Combining SCI with TTR and the sorrowful empty chair creates the format that forces initiation, critical thinking, knowledge to application, and self-reflection. In the process of applying problem-solving techniques to current problems, students will connect the layered learnings from TTR while exercising self-reflection in self-awareness. This results in students using the independence necessary for open-ended problem-solving and creative critical thinking and applying it to the real world just as they practiced using current events. This application makes the current event a vignette and the practice role-playing for social work students. This development into self-awareness, a part of the empathetic domain of emotional intelligence, provides the lifelong learning template needed to acclimate in an ever-changing society. The methodologies of SCI, TTR, and the sorrowful empty chair are not restricted caveats for learning; they simply create one foundational template that allows learners continuous development.

### Conclusion

Considering the decline in college student empathy levels over the past few decades, an increase in the volume of tragedies that amass the airways, it is wise to believe these levels will suffer more decline. This is strengthened with the inclusion of the stages young adults are growing in and through, while a nation of advanced adults responds with as much uncertainty as the stressful occurrences impose.

The cultural shifts of health and social construct, and the immense domination of media attention, were unveiled without preparation for the amount or intensity. To address the exertions of young adults in academia, instruction may provide an avenue for constructing and framing successful methods to build empathy. SCI, TTR, and the sorrowful empty chair coincide and provide intentional reflective activities that aid students in assessing their values and positioning.

This movement toward an academic contributor is paramount because the traditional-age college student is in the primal stages of relational development and value construction. Students can assess and recognize identity caveats through the underpinnings of social identity, convened behaviors, and demeanors so the future can be framed with clarity, preventing the pitfalls orchestrated in power imbalances. These imbalances represent the misalignments explained theoretically in social identity, the ambiguities in the pandemic, and the intensities of media saturations. The development of oneself as a student while repairing empathetic levels will promote healing, relationships, creativity, and resilience; reduce stress; and foster learning and connectivity (Center for Building a Culture of Empathy, n.d.; Robbins, 2021).

To ensure that the command of the future is prepared to choreograph the next unforeseen universal storm, the health crisis will be marshaled with the public health prevention framework, the racial reckoning will have characterized understanding social identity theory, and the explosiveness of media will have a momentum equal to personal desires from a self-awareness context that exposes individual tolerance. All navigation in this territory may advance global citizenry through the platform of education. Using the empathetic strides in coursework noted above, to harness the loss of control felt from societal events, positions students to examine and halt their empathy decline for reassembly.

## Questions for Reflection

1 Consider using the exercise, the Sorrowful Empty Chair, for students. This task involves envisioning an empty chair in the classroom, but with a deceased person who could have been a classmate. The students will use this opportunity to dictate what their classmates, not themselves, may be experiencing as they reflect on the loss of a loved one/peer that should have occupied this space.
2 What is the impact of the high levels of intensity experienced by the out-groups during the global racial reckoning on social science professorial discussions, collegiate course development, and student organizations?
3 What could be the future long-term loving commitment impacts for 18–40-year-olds, having experienced disruption in the development of their intimacy versus isolation stage?

## References

Campbell, P. (2022, September 27). *Excessive News Consumption May Harm Mental and Physical Health*. Retrieved from Psychology Today. https://www.psychologytoday.com/us/blog/imperfect-spirituality/202209/excessive-news-consumption-may-harm-mental-and-physical-health

*Center for Building a Culture of Empathy*. (n.d.). Center for Building a Culture of Empathy. https://cultureofempathy.com/References/Benefits/

*COVID-19 Projections*. (2022, July 18). Institute for Health Metrics and Evaluation. https://covid19.healthdata.org/united-states-of-america?view=cumulative-deaths&t%20ab=trend

Frnka-Davis, L. (2020, April 2). *Too much media can take a toll on mental and physical health*. UT Physicians.

Janse, B. (2020). *Social Identity Theory (SIT)*. Toolshero. https://www.toolshero.com/psychology/social-identity-theory/

Kellam, W., & Degges-White, S. (2017). Introduction to student affairs and student development issues. In W. Kellam, & S. Degges-White (Eds.), *College student development: Applying theory to practice on the diverse campus* (pp. 1–13). Springer Publishing Co. https://connect.springerpub.com/content/book/978-0-8261-1816-5/part/part01/chapter/ch01

King, M. (1963/2004). Letter from the Birmingham jail. In J. Martin Luther King (Ed.), *Why we can't wait* (pp. 77–100). The Estate of Martin Luther King, Jr.

Madhav, N., Oppenheim, B., Gallivan, M., Mulembakani, P., Rubin, E., & Wolfe, N. (2017). Pandemics: Risks, impacts, and mitigation. In G. H. Jamison DT (Ed.), *Disease control priorities: Improving health and reducing poverty*. The International Bank for Reconstruction and Development/The World Bank. https://www.ncbi.nlm.nih.gov/books/NBK525302/

Magruder, K., McLaughlin, K., & Borbon, D. (2017). Trauma is a public health issue. *European Journal of Psychotraumatology, 8*(1). https://www.ncbi.nlm.nih.gov/pmc/articles/PMC5800738/

McLeod, S. (2018). *Simply psychology*. Erik Erikson's Stages of Psychosocial Development. https://www.simplypsychology.org/Erik-Erikson.html

McLeod, S. (2019). *Social identity theory*. Simply Psychology. https://www.simplypsychology.org/social-identity-theory.html

Reed, J. (2022). *Understanding racial microaggression and its effect on mental health*. Pfizer. https://www.pfizer.com/news/articles/understanding_racial_microaggression_and_its_effect_on_mental_health

Robbins, M. (2021, February 5). *Why empathy is important: How to become more empathetic*. Mike Robbins. https://mike-robbins.com/the-power-of-empathy/

Robinson, M. (n.d.). *A guide to theory: Florida state university's higher education program*. Student Development Theory Overview. https://studentdevelopmenttheory.wordpress.com/chickerings-seven-vectors/

Srivastava, G. (2015, November 25). *The importance of self-awareness*. WellBeing. https://www. whiteswanfoundation.org/mental-health-matters/wellbeing/the-importance-of-self-awareness

Statista Research Department. (2020, July 10). *Level of support among U.S. adults for the protests in response to the death of George Floyd as of June 2020, by age*. Statistica. https://www.statista.com/ statistics/1122591/support-george-floyd-protests-us-age/

*Student-Centered Learning*. (n.d.). International Society for Technology in Education (ISTE). https://www.iste.org/standards/essential-conditions/student-centered-learning

Swanbrow, D. (2010, May 27). Empathy: College students don't have as much as they used to. *Michigan News*. https://news.umich.edu/empathy-college-students-don-t-have-as-much-as-they-used-to/

Thompson, E. (2021, September 1). *How George Floyd's death changed college campuses*. The Best Schools. https://thebestschools.org/magazine/after-george-floyd-changes-college-campuses/

Unitedwaynca. (2022, April 7). *United way of the national capital area*. Surveying Americans on Empathy Burnout. https://unitedwaynca.org/blog/empathy-burnout-survey/

Williamson-Ashe, S. (2019). Pedagogical techniques that provide educational value to social work students through bereavement academics and empathetic advancements. *The Journal of Human Services, Training, Research, and Practice, 4*(1), 1–15.

# 28 The New Homeschool Movement

## What Human Services Professionals Need to Know

*Emilee Prins and Scott Shaw*

## Introduction

### Homeschool History

Homeschooling in its current form is a relatively new phenomenon with its origins traced back to the 1970s (Bartholet, 2020). The mid-19th century saw the first child labor laws, which protected children from working in harsh factory settings and consequently, helped increase the possibility of an education. Compulsory education laws and the development of free public schooling helped build the case for a child's right to an education (Bartholet, 2020). School was traditionally viewed as an advance of the greater societal good (Bartholet, 2020).

This began to shift near the end of the 20th century with the advent of homeschooling. To understand this shift, it is important to recognize the sociopolitical landscape within the United States at various historical eras, notably during the Free Love Era (1960s), the hippie movement (1970s), and the Equal Rights Act (1972). Emily Hunter McGowin writes of the key role of conservatives and Evangelical Christians during this time, "1970's and following, evangelicals were increasingly aware of the gradual displacement and marginalization of their values in the United States" (2018, p. 20). Initially in 1960, conservatives and Evangelical Christians chose to work toward ensuring the mainstay of their values, with the urge to allow school-organized prayer and Bible reading as evidenced in efforts such as "See You at the Pole" and the rise of after-school Bible clubs on school property.

Conservative Evangelicals were not the only ones concerned about sociocultural changes. These changes had come to the attention of the entire country. The White House Conference on Children and Youth highlighted concerning trends. There was a 38% increase in babies born out of wedlock in the 1970s, along with an increase in premarital sex and decreasing birth rates in general (Gaither, 2017). Divorce rates doubled between 1966 and 1976, often attributed to Reagan's no-fault divorce law (Gaither, 2017). Urie Bronfenbrenner, psychologist and creator of Ecological Systems Theory, participated in the White House Conference on Children. In an address, he shared his concerns by reading a report created by his task force, which stated,

> America's families are in trouble—trouble so deep and pervasive as to threaten the future of our nation. The source of the trouble is nothing less than a national neglect of children and those primarily engaged in their care—America's parents.
> (U.S. Department of Health, Education, and Welfare, 1971, p. 33)

DOI: 10.4324/9781003531258-33

Throughout this time, conservatives advocated for the continuation of traditional values. Their efforts were met with the 1962 and 1963 Supreme Court decisions, which outlawed school prayer and Bible reading. It is also important to note the role and response toward desegregation efforts. George Andrews, Alabama State representative, spoke on television claiming the Supreme Court "put the Negros in the schools—now they put God out of the schools" (Gaither, 2017, p. 116). Milton Gaither notes that this did not immediately result in homeschooling but in an abundance of private and church-based schools. "Many conservatives gave up, at least for the time being, on the idea of transforming the public school and sought instead to 'restore power to the local evangelical communities by creating a parallel educational culture'" (Gaither, 2017, p. 116). Eventually, due to funding and accreditation challenges, many church-based schools shuttered, which propelled families toward homeschooling.

This growing discontent with the public school system was not limited to Evangelical Christians or conservatives. The rapid growth of the public school system and awareness of its many flaws came to light, citing perceived growing bureaucracy, being less adaptive to the needs of students, and being less responsive to parents' desires (Gaither, 2017, p. 123). John Holt, author of *How Children Learn* and thought leader of the unschooling movement, is also noted by many as an unofficial, unintentional homeschool forerunner, as many parents began to link the cultural family challenges with the public school system (Bartholet, 2020; Davis, 2011).

James Dobson, founder of Focus on the Family and author of books including *Dare to Discipline* (1977), was a key player in the evangelical scene in the 1970s and 1980s. Dobson advocated for a parenting strategy that moved away from the perceived permissiveness of progressive parenting leaders. Instead, he admonished Christian parents take an intentional and structured role in parents actively disciplining their children (McGowin, 2018). As recently as 2002, he issued calls to Christians to remove their children from public schools. His work and radio shows helped promote the work of Raymond and Dorthy Moore, who were, in 1982, the most sought-after homeschool leaders in the country (McGowin, 2018). Mary Pride was also a founding leader in the homeschool movement and benefited from Dobson's platform. Pride's work was anti-feminist and a call to renounce family planning and return to family values. McGowin summarizes Pride's work with homeschooling families during this time as follows:

> While the Religious Right was mobilizing voters to win the "culture war" at the ballot box, pronatalist homeschoolers were committing themselves to a strategy of long-term, family-driven, demographic triumph. Eventually, families who eschewed family planning and practiced gender hierarchy and homeschooling would come to be called "Quiverfull" based upon their obedience to the "principles" of Psalm 127:4–5.
>
> (2018, p. 31)

Again, it is important to recall the social shifts that gave an audience to these ideologies. More mothers were home, with the average family living in a comfortable home with the resources necessary for such an undertaking.

> By the late 1970s many conservatives lived in comfortable suburban homes that could easily accommodate a homeschool. Many housewives were well-educated and committed both to their children and to staying at home. A Gallup poll in the mid-1970s showed

that 60 percent of housewives did not want to work outside of the home. Most listed "my children" as their biggest source of pride.

(Gaither, 2017, p. 119)

In considering major leaders in the early homeschool movement, Rousas Rushdoony should be mentioned. Though his name is unfamiliar, his work significantly shaped evangelical thought. His influence spread to educational circles and was popularized by homeschooling pioneer Greg Harris, father of Joshua Harris—the author of I Kissed Dating Goodbye—and E. Ray Moore of the Exodus Mandate. Rushdoony's work highlights "opposition between God's laws and man's laws," resulting in a strong belief that the government must not direct family and educational matters. These ideologies influenced the next wave of homeschool leaders, including Doug Phillips, founder of Vision Forum Ministries, Voddie Baucham, and the Botkins, proponents of the Stay at Home Daughter movement.

Bill Gothard was also an influential leader in this era. His work was not limited to the homeschooling sphere, with an estimated 300,000 people attending his conferences annually at their peak, with as many as 10,000 attendees at any given seminar. The conferences drew large crowds, and other materials and conferences were specifically launched for homeschooling families. McGowin notes that he was one of the first to link hierarchical gender norms with homeschooling and taught that God entrusted children to their parents for their education. This echoed Rushdoony's claims, with Gothard teaching that homeschooling was the only true education option for Christian parents (McGowin, 2018, p. 22).

Familiarity with the history of homeschooling and current trends will help the human services worker place their experiences in the field within the larger homeschool landscape. Two additional areas of homeschool history are especially relevant for the human services worker to guide their understanding and practice: Child abuse and neglect in homeschool settings and the work of Mary Pride in shaping homeschool attitudes toward social work and related professions.

Mary Pride is considered by many to be the "Queen of homeschooling." As a founding leader in the homeschool movement, Pride taught that society would change from the inside out as women work within their homes and raise their children, claiming this is the way to "take back control" of all spheres of society, including healthcare, social welfare, and housing (xiii). In a book titled *The Child Abuse Industry*, Pride surmises that the child welfare system is built as an anti-parental rights system that primarily exists to take children and replace traditional family, community, church, and extended family (p. 61). She warns parents that social workers can "remove your children any time they choose. All they must do is find you guilty of some trivial, undivided offense like "emotional neglect." Then your children are torn screaming from your arms and put into 'protective custody'" (1986, p. 67). Social workers are referred to as "leeches" and child abuse hotlines as "the KGB" (Pride, 1986, p. 148). Finally, she urges that reports of suspected abuse should not be made to the police except in rare circumstances. Mandated reporters should not report or at least not in a timely fashion, noting that any law that meddles with one's thoughts (i.e., suspicions of abuse) is innately wrong and should be ignored (Pride, 1986, p. 153).

It may be tempting to dismiss Pride's work as alarmist at best, with stories of CPS cases "gone awry" sprinkled throughout. However, to do so would fail to recognize the enormous influence her writing had on many homeschool families. An appendix in *The Child Abuse Industry* guides parents on how to respond to a social work visit and contains similar advice to that found in a pamphlet circulated by the Homeschool Legal Defense Association

(HSLDA) and published in Pride's *Practical Homeschooling* magazine. Chris Klicka, a senior HSLDA advisor, wrote that parents should not let social workers into their home without a warrant or court order. Parents should obtain the business card of the social worker so that an HSLDA lawyer would be able to contact them on the family's behalf. However, if the situation became hostile, families should call HSLDA's 24-hour emergency hotline and hand the phone out the door to the social worker (Klicka, 2000). Klicka also listed steps families could take to avoid investigations from CPS, which included conducting public relations with neighbors about the legality and success of homeschooling, avoiding leaving children home alone, and not spanking someone else's child (Klicka, 2000).

### Policy and Law

The history of homeschooling must also include its legal history. Harvard Law professor Elizabeth Bartholet writes that homeschooling in its current capacity exists, "not because our society through its elected representatives has decided it *should*. It exists because homeschooling advocacy groups have become an overwhelming political force and because there is no effective opposing political force" (2020).

The HSLDA was founded in 1983 and is widely viewed as the leader in homeschool law and policy. The organization, founded by Michael Farris, a law attorney and homeschooling parent, states that its mission is to "make homeschooling possible" (Homeschool Legal Defense Association, 2019a). The history section of HSLDA website notes that the organization grew out of Farris' recognition that homeschooling was one of the oldest, most effective forms of education in history (Homeschool Legal Defense Association, 2019b).

HSLDA has been largely effective in its goal of making homeschooling possible in the most literal sense. For homeschooling families, HSLDA offers what has been referred to as legal insurance. In 2022, families could become members by paying a $150 yearly membership. Membership terms include agreeing to contact HSLDA immediately about any possible legal action regarding their homeschooling practices. In turn, HSLDA will advocate for homeschooling families and provide legal representation. It was HSLDA's legal representation that turned the tide for homeschooling families. A Vanderbilt law review notes the following with reference to a 2004 Economist piece: "In the fifteen years following the founding of the HSLDA, the most powerful legal and political advocate for homeschooling, homeschooling went from being illegal 'in most states' to legal in all 50 in what has been described as a 'political miracle'" (Waddell, 2010; Economist, 2004). Farris' organization is considered the most powerful group in the realm of homeschooling and law and politics. This can be noted by its sheer dominance in political spheres, with legislators and staff testifying to the lobbying power of the organization (Brown & Jamison, 2023; Huseman, 2015). One noted that her interactions with HSLDA member families "make the anti-vaxxers seem rational" (Huseman, 2015).

Among the reasons for its success is its use of fear-mongering techniques, which have been criticized by both homeschool families and advocates and those opposed to homeschooling. Members of the HSLDA receive monthly publications from HSLDA that highlight current or recent cases, demonstrating the need for their membership. Though thanks to HSLDA, homeschooling is legal in all 50 states, they continue to post calls to action to members and supporters. Their legal action center outlines upcoming legislation, explains how this might affect homeschooling families, and encourages them to contact their local representative. Any bill aimed to protect homeschooled children and their right to an education, as outlined in the United Nations Convention on the Rights of the Child, has faced strong opposition from HSLDA. An example is its stated concerns about a Washington Senate Bill 6236, which would require homeschooling parents to file a notice of intent. HSLDA stated this bill would explicitly target homeschoolers for more regulation. It claimed the bill biased against homeschooling families as it adds "legal burdens on homeschooling families that are not shared by parents who send their children to private or public school" (Dentel, 2024). According to HSLDA, this is a prime example of bad legislation aimed at penalizing and creating red tape for homeschooling families and could serve as gateway leading to further targeting of homeschooling families. Similarly, HSLDA released a call to action with Missouri State Bill 727 regarding schools and firearms. HSLDA feared the bill contained "unclear wording in the bill would open a door for judges to rule that Missouri homeschool families are criminals simply for having firearms in the home" (Woodruff, 2024). The 2024 call to action was edited, thanking members for their support, stating that HSLDA worked to propose an amendment and told members that they are "neutral" on the bill before thanking them for their help in standing for freedom. HSLDA archives their "call to action" alerts, making them inaccessible unless printed or downloaded, as is the case for this alert (Woodruff, n.d.).

HSLDA's work centers on its claims of parental absolutism rights and the belief that state regulation of homeschooling in any form is an unconstitutional infringement of parental liberties and free exercise (Brown & Jamison, 2023; Waddell, 2010). They also have a history of representing cases that do not address homeschool rights directly, but involve parental rights and perceived government oversight (Kelly, 2021; Parker & Steffenhagen, n.d.).

As noted above, HSLDA was responsible for changing homeschool law across the United States, shifting the tide from being legal in very few states to, as of this writing, *being unregulated*. HSLDA's lobbying efforts are centered on themes of "freedom" and "parental rights." These are also central in their legal cases. One of the most significant cases in HSLDA history is De Jonge v. People. Before the 1993 Michigan Supreme Court case, all educators—including homeschooling parents—were required to have a state-issued teaching certification or equivalent (MCL 3388.553). The only exception provided by the law was ten years of teaching experience. Mark and Christine DeJonge began homeschooling in 1985, though neither parent had a teaching certificate. In their supreme court case, the DeJonges, represented by Chris Klicka and Michael Ferris, claimed that the current statutes infringed on their First Amendment rights, echoing ideas promoted by homeschool thought leaders such as Rushdoony and Gothard in the transcribed interview:

> We had been trained in the Word concerning the authority God has given to different institutions on earth, Civil, Church and the Family. Each having their own realm of authority. We thoroughly searched the Word of God and were convinced that nowhere is education given to the State but rather the State had usurped that authority. We could not agree to teacher certification because that would be denying God's authority that he has given to us as parents and allow the state control in our home in an area that God has not given them.
>
> (Michigan Christian Homeschool Network, 2021)

The case traveled through the court system, reaching the Michigan Supreme Court. Court documents quote the DeJonges as stating they believed "the major purpose of education is to show a student how to face God, not just show him how to face the world" (People v. DeJonge, 1993). The court opinion noted that the state's desire for universal education did not override First Amendment rights. HSLDA argued that the DeJonges' motivation for homeschooling was motivated by religious reasons, and the current legislation opposed their religious freedom. Additionally, the DeJonge children demonstrated no educational concerns. It is interesting to note that the court opinion cites empirical studies claiming that children's quality of education is not correlated with teacher certification, particularly in the context of homeschooling. However, Brian Ray, the author of the study and founder of the National Home Education Research Institute, has received funding from HSLDA. His research claims have been criticized for invalidity and poor methodological research methods (McCracken, 2014; Meckler, 2023). For example, in several of his major studies comparing the academic achievement of homeschooled students versus public school students, a sample of homeschooled students was selected for the specific research project, and their academic scores were self-reported. The testing completed by homeschooled students was largely parent-proctored, in-home testing. This information was then compared to national average data. The proposed findings were that homeschooled students scored in the 80th percentile or higher in all areas (Kunzman & Gaither, 2020). Furthermore, his findings are inconsistent and contradictory to findings from similar research (Martin-Chang et al., 2011; Murphy, 2014; Yu et al., 2016).

Regardless, the Supreme Court ruled in Mark and Christine DeJonge's favor. The landmark case shifted the homeschooling landscape. In Michigan, parents may homeschool their children through an umbrella school (i.e., with homeschool oversight from an existing school), operate as a private school if parents have teacher certifications, or homeschool without oversight or teacher certifications by claiming a religious exemption. There are no registration or paperwork requirements to operate as a private school with teacher certifications and no formal process required to homeschool under religious exemption. Homeschooling, for any reason and in any form, is essentially both legal and unregulated in the State of Michigan (The Revised School Code, 1976). Similar legislation can be found across the nation. Eleven states do not have enrollment requirements (Coalition for Responsible Home Education, n.d.a). In these states, parents or guardians are not required to inform local school districts or the state of their decision to homeschool. Eighteen states require written or other formal notice that the students will be homeschooled, with no other assessment or follow-up. Nineteen states require varying forms of assessments. However, in these states, multiple homeschool options exist, and assessment requirements do not apply across the board. For example, families homeschooling in Colorado can do so under the homeschooling statute. This requires an annual notice of intent to homeschool and semi-annual assessments beginning in third grade. Interventions include being required to attend school if warranted by a lack of satisfactory academic performance (at or below 13% of the national average). However, parents may also homeschool under state legislation for an independent school. If the parent or guardian has a teaching certificate, they may homeschool under the state definition of a private tutor. Neither the independent school nor private tutor options require an intent notice or any assessments or record keeping (Coalition for Responsible Home Education, n.d.a, Title 22).

New York and Hawaii are currently the only two states that enforce assessment requirements and have intervention plans in place for all homeschool options provided under the law. In Hawaii, a one-time intent to homeschool notice is required. Parents or guardians must keep a record of the curriculum taught, with records subject to review by the Department of Education in cases of suspected educational neglect (Hawaii Dept of Education, n.d.). Following the completion of grades 3, 5, 8, and 10, standardized testing and assessment should occur. If students perform below standard expectations, parents should submit a remedial intervention plan documenting intended remedial means (Coalition for

Responsible Home Education, n.d.a, 302A-1132). New York statutes differ slightly but follow a similar model of standardized tests or other assessments and remedial plans if necessary.

Ten states require that homeschooling parents hold a high school diploma, GED, or higher. Of these, five have alternate options, such as Virginia, Washington, and West Virginia, which allow superintendents to waive this requirement at their discretion. Other exemptions include homeschooling under the supervision of a certified teacher or religious exemption (Coalition for Responsible Home Education, n.d.c). Only two states currently have legislation in place that prohibits registered sex offenders from homeschooling (Coalition for Responsible Home Education, n.d.a). The range of government responses and regulations leaves much to individual homeschooling families and the States in which they reside.

## Current Trends

While we have looked at the homeschool movement of the 1970s, it is crucial to note that this movement is not representative of all homeschoolers during that time. Gaither notes that homeschooling was for some a response to increasing challenges in the public school system. Concerns regarding appropriate services and education for students with IEPs, advanced placement students, and bullying were prevalent (Gaither, 2017).

Sociologist Jane Van Galen is credited with using the terms ideologues and pedagogues to organize the types of homeschooling parents. Van Galen noted that ideologues' motivation to homeschool stemmed from a fear of government regulation and what they viewed as secular humanism. Based on Van Galen's observations, these homeschoolers tended to follow a strict curriculum and more deliberate discipline. Pedagogues, on the other hand, were more likely to homeschool for other reasons and take a wider, more effective, and innovative approach to education (Van Galen & Pitman, 1991). Regardless of the terms used, it is clear that parental reasons for homeschooling vary due to strong religious beliefs (historically conservative Christians); educational rigor or benefit; psychosocial concerns (i.e., values, bullying, school safety); and some are simply truant with little parental engagement.

Accurately understanding homeschool motivations, current trends, and educational efficacy is limited by a stark lack of research and available data. Current regulations make it nearly impossible to gather data on how many children are being homeschooled. Like in Hawaii, some have argued that greater accountability should be enforced by local school districts or state education departments. This also presents challenges for further research on homeschool motivations, needs, and outcomes. Much of the existing research comes from unreliable and personally motivated sources such as Brian Ray's work discussed above.

Historically, many viewed homeschooling as an opportunity to give their child a better education, a means to provide religious or moral instruction, or an alternative to an unsatisfactory school environment (Princiotta & Bielick, 2006, p. 13). National Center for Education Statistics (NCES) collected data as part of a National Education Household Survey in 2003 which demonstrated an estimated increase in the rate of homeschooling from 1.7% in 1999 to 2.2% in 2003 (Princiotta & Bielick, 2006, p. 13). The primary reported reasons parents chose to homeschool had not changed, though the distribution between the three reasons shifted slightly.

Consistent with the conservative, faith-based, Republican values depicted in the Michigan supreme court case, the average homeschooled student in 1999 was: more likely to be white than Black or Hispanic, have two or more siblings, and come from a two-parent household in which only one parent was in the workforce (Princiotta & Bielick, 2006).

The data from 2019 demonstrates little change in the racial makeup of homeschooled children. Survey respondents were able to select multiple applicable reasons for home-schooling, which included a concern about the school environment, a desire to provide moral instruction, an emphasis on family life, dissatisfaction with academic instruction, and a desire to provide religious instruction in order of most to least common (NCES, 2022). It is worth noting that 74.7% selected moral instruction, and 58.9% noted a desire to provide religious instruction. Because participants were allowed to choose multiple factors, it is unknown how many participants chose both. It is reasonable to wonder if combined moral and religious factors would surpass the concern of the school environment (80.3%). Another explanation is that the same families who are concerned with the school environment are also concerned with family life and moral and religious instruction. When asked to choose the most important reason for homeschooling from the same list, 25% cited concerns with the school environment, 15% cited dissatisfaction in academic instruction at other schools, and only 13% cited a desire for religious instruction (NCES, 2022).

The statistics noted here are challenging since participation in the surveys was voluntary. Lack of regulatory or registration policies makes it impossible to determine how many children are being homeschooled. However, the 2019 data provides useful insights on why some families choose to homeschool.

Lack of academic benchmarks (such as standardized testing) makes the quality of an average homeschool education indeterminable. The data does not exist to determine if and to what degree homeschooling benefits students through creating an alternative learning environment.

The risks of educational neglect, whether it may occur intentionally or unintentionally, grow as homeschooling rises in popularity. Data suggests as many as 3 million K-12 students disappeared from United States' school systems between March and October of 2020 following school closures due to the COVID-19 pandemic (Litvinov, 2021). When schools reopened, these students simply never returned. Recent data suggests that at least 230,000 of these students are still missing and are either being homeschooled or truant (Vazquez Toness & Lurye, 2023). Because many states do not require the registration of homeschooling, clearer data on how many students are truant and how many are being homeschooled is simply not available. Stanford University published research that estimates a 30% growth in homeschooled students between the school year of 2019–2020 and 2021–2022 (Dee, 2023). States with homeschool data reported high levels of homeschool growth: Florida at 41%, Pennsylvania at 53%, and New York at a 65% increase (Dee, 2023). Tracking the exact numbers of children who are home-schooled remains challenging given the paucity of data and no requirement that parents register their children as being homeschooled in most states. This significant increase in the number of homeschooled students further demonstrates the necessity of policies that protect at-risk students and ensure access to education.

Post-pandemic, homeschooling has become a growing and popular choice for primary education in the United States. Data from the Census Bureau noted that in the fall of 2020, homeschooling in households that identified as Black or African American increased by 12.8% or fivefold between May 2020 and October 2020 (Eggleston & Fields, 2021). Other racial and ethnic groups also increased between 4% and 6%.

Black families increasingly cite racism, whitewashed history, and microaggressions among their reasons for homeschooling. Parents recount their children being the only Black child in the classroom, with low levels of diversity in schools, particularly in

Christian and private schools, gaps in education, a lack of understanding of civil rights, and what has been called "pro-slavery" racist curriculum (Adams, 2023; McDonald, 2023, Parks, 2021).

While national data is not available, some state-level research has been conducted. The Washington Post reported a study on the increase in homeschooling in 2023. The study found that Washington D.C. had a 108% increase in homeschooled students from the 2017–2018 school year to the 2021–2022 school year. In the states that data was available for, the study found increases in homeschooling in all studied states, with increases ranging from 1% to the 108% increase in Washington D.C. Other states that saw a high level of increase included California (78%), South Dakota (94%), and New York (103%) (Jamison et al., 2023). Parents are increasingly citing non-religious reasons for homeschooling, including bullying (Parks, 2021; Skarpness, 2019; West, 2023) and the threat of school shootings (Chuck, 2022).

## Intervention and Recommendations

Human services professionals will undoubtedly come across homeschooling families and children in their work. The recommendations below highlight key practices when working with these individuals and family systems. It is important to note that the model listed below specifically addresses factors for consideration when working with homeschooled children and families. While not denying the need for further research and support for homeschool alumni, it is not the primary purpose of this chapter.

### Building Awareness

When working with homeschooling families, an awareness of the common homeschooling modalities and motives can provide the clinician with beginning insights into familial goals. This knowledge should serve as a framework, allowing the clinician to ask insightful questions to increase their understanding of the family's own goals, motives, and values. Finding supportive and respectful ways to engage clients who may be resistant to possible human services workers or interventions can be challenging, yet it is a vital foundation for effective interventions.

Human services workers should also be aware of existing legislation in their state, if any. While homeschooling is largely legal and unregulated throughout the United States, the competent clinician should be aware of any applicable legislation at the state level. Local school districts and state agencies may have recommended, but not required, practices surrounding record keeping and attendance of schooling or instructional benchmarks. The potential limited interaction with outside professionals should encourage the human services worker to consider where additional support or intervention may be needed to protect children if signs of suspected abuse or neglect are present.

### Respectful and Ethical Interactions

Interactions and subsequent interventions should be informed by the assessment and a familiarity with the family's goals and values. For example, families who began homeschooling due to bullying will present with different goals, strengths, and challenges than those whose motives are based on one's religious or political identity. Human services workers should take the necessary time to get to know clients and seek to understand their motivations from their own worldview. This will help to build compassion and understanding, as well as develop rapport to encourage meaningful change.

The human services worker should engage with all families with curiosity and humility, especially when working with families and groups who may have a strong distrust of human services. Many homeschool families may have negative assumptions regarding human services workers' involvement or have heard horror stories from others (real or fictitious). Questions for parents should be open-ended, aiming to better understand the family's own goals and motives, utilizing a person-centered approach (Rogers, 1961). Motivational interviewing (Miller & Rollnick, 2023) should be utilized to engage in effective communication, build hope, and promote a desire to change when ambivalence is present and a gap between actual values and current practices or behaviors. Building upon the clients' own motivations to strategize meaningful outcomes can help meet the needs of families, especially potentially vulnerable children.

Interviewing children should also be done with curiosity out of a desire to understand the child's microlevel system from their point of view. Questions should be open-ended and strengths-based, both mitigating routine questions and the possibility of receiving a dictated answer as coached by a parent or guardian. When asked in such a manner, the human services professional can more accurately ascertain strengths and challenges within the family system from the child's experiences. This also acknowledges the possibility of, and attempts to mitigate, inaccurate or incomplete reports from children out of self-preservation.

Human services professionals practice under established ethical codes for their specific credentialing, including but not limited to the ethical codes of the National Association of Social Workers (2021) and the National Organization of Human Services (2024). These codes uphold the values of non-maleficence and beneficence, simply described as doing no harm and doing the most good. Thus, the human services professional must also be committed to mitigating harm. This includes understanding that homeschooling in the United States is, at this time, largely unregulated and unsupervised and the real risks and benefits this affords families. It allows abused and neglected children to slip under the radar and remain at a significant risk, as the *Homeschool's Invisible Children* database demonstrates (Coalition for Responsible Home Education, 2024). However, lax legislation is also praised by advocates of parental absolutism and those desiring religious homeschooling without governmental oversight.

### Mitigating and Engaging

Human services workers must be aware of red flags when working with homeschooled families and children. The Coalition for Responsible Home Education has found that children are highly at risk when a parent removes a child from public or private school to homeschool immediately after receiving notification of a CPS investigation (Coalition for Responsible Home Education, n.d.b). Other concerns include stating they are homeschooling to avoid truancy charges, excessive control, and fostering social isolation, as well as instituting deliberate discipline to break a child's will. Most children who are being homeschooled do not interact with teachers and school staff on a daily basis, which may limit the contact they may otherwise have with mandated reporters.

Children may also be at risk for educational neglect, where little or inappropriate education is provided under the term "homeschooled." Parents are responsible for finding or creating their own curriculum. Some school districts may provide funding for extracurricular activities, state testing, and allow them to join sports teams. It is necessary to note that educational neglect is not a concept that is often recognized within the United States. This highlights the importance of being able to accurately understand and recognize other possible forms of abuse when present, as emotional neglect alone is often regarded as an insufficient cause for services, child removal, or other court-mandated interventions.

Human services workers should be familiar with state requirements graduation. Many states allow parents to graduate their children at will, regardless of educational achievements or lack thereof. It is often up to the parent to supply an official, unaccredited diploma, which is often purchased from an online vendor or crafted at home. Parents or alumni are also responsible for creating a transcript for college admissions if desired.

The human services worker should be familiar with local, healthy organizations and resources for families. The specific needs of each family will vary with demographics and the reason for homeschooling, often defining these needs. Clinicians should be aware of any technology-related needs, such as Chromebooks or Wi-Fi for families desiring a virtual school option. State and school districts may have funds designated for homeschooling families. The ability to participate in the local school district sports and extracurricular activities will also vary based on one's local school district. Connecting families with local libraries, community sports teams, arts, and other activities may be useful for some families. Others may benefit from support groups and sufficient homeschooling resources. The ability to connect families to local support groups, community activities, and other local resources is a valuable skill as this encourages open family systems, peer support for parents and children, and community engagement.

Finally, human services workers can minimize potential harm by advocating for safe homeschooling and legislation that protects children's rights to an adequate education and a safe environment, free from abuse and neglect (Convention on the Rights of the Child, 1989). Policies advocating for safe homeschooling and protection against missing children, such as legislation requiring homeschooling legislation and parents to maintain records of twice-yearly visits to a doctor, dentist, or other licensed professional, have received strong opposition from those who view this as in opposition to parental rights. The human services worker should be aware of the wide variety of families who are turning to homeschool to meet their child's needs (educational, preventing bullying, etc.) and advocate for policies that both protect all children and have the interest of families and children in mind, equipping them to provide the best for their homeschooled children and protecting children when they are at serious risk of education, emotional, and physical harm.

## Questions for Reflection

1 Consider your own perceptions of and experiences with homeschooling families. How might your perceptions and experiences shape the approaches you will use to connect with these families?
2 Given the growing diversity in homeschooling demographics and motivations, what cultural competencies and considerations should be utilized?
3 Become familiar with homeschool legislation in your state. What extracurriculars, testing, and other services are available for homeschooling families through the local school district that would support educational equity with your clients?

## References

Adams, C. (2023, February 8). Black families are changing the educational landscape through communal home-schooling. *NBC News.* https://www.nbcnews.com/news/nbcblk/black-families-are-challenging-educations-status-quo-home-schooling-rcna69027

Bartholet, E. (2020). Homeschooling: Parent rights absolutism vs. Child rights to education & Protection. *Arizona Law Review, 62*(1), 1–80. https://arizonalawreview.org/pdf/62-1/62arizlrev1.pdf

Brown, E., & Jamison, P. (2023, August 29). The Christian home-schooler who made "parental rights" a GOP rallying cry. *The Washington Post.* https://www.washingtonpost.com/education/2023/08/29/michael-farris-homeschoolers-parents-rights-ziklag/

Chuck, E. (2022, June 12). After Uvalde shooting, parents feel there is 'no safe place' for children. *NBC News.* https://www.nbcnews.com/news/us-news/uvalde-shooting-parents-feel-no-safe-place-children-rcna32534

Coalition for Responsible Home Education. (2024). *Homeschool's invisible children database.* https://www.hsinvisiblechildren.org/findings/

Coalition for Responsible Home Education. (n.d.a). *Inside homeschool policy.* https://responsiblehomeschooling.org/current-policy/

Coalition for Responsible Home Education. (n.d.b). *For social workers and caseworkers.* https://responsiblehomeschooling.org/advocacy/kids/a-message-for-social-workers/

Coalition for Responsible Home Education. (n.d.c). *Parent qualifications.* https://responsiblehomeschooling.org/research/current-policy/parent-qualifications/

Davis, A. (2011). Evolution of homeschooling. *Distance Learning, 8*(2), 29–35.

Dee, T. S. (2023, February). *Where kids went: Nonpublic schooling and demographic change during the pandemic exodus from public schools.* Urban Institute. https://www.urban.org/sites/default/files/2023-02/Where%20the%20Kids%20Went-%20Nonpublic%20Schooling%20and%20Demographic%20Change%20during%20the%20Pandemic%20Exodus%20from%20Public%20Schools_0.pdf

Dentel, D. (2024, February 6). Help us defend homeschool freedom this legislative season. *HSLDA.* https://hslda.org/post/help-us-defend-homeschool-freedom-this-legislative-season

Dobson, J. C. (1977). *Dare to Discipline.* Tyndale House Publishers.

The Economist. (2004, February 26). *George Bush's secret army.*

Eggleston, C., & Fields, J. (2021, March 22). *Census Bureau's household pulse survey shows significant increase in homeschooling rates in fall 2020.* United States Census Bureau. https://www.census.gov/library/stories/2021/03/homeschooling-on-the-rise-during-covid-19-pandemic.html

Gaither, M. (2017). *Homeschool: An American history* (2nd ed.). Palgrave Macmillan.

Homeschool Legal Defense Association. (2019a, September 18). *History of HSLDA.* https://hslda.org/post/history-of-hslda

Homeschool Legal Defense Association. (2019b, September 18). *Our history.* https://hslda.org/post/our-mission

Huseman, J. (2015, August 27). Small group goes to great lengths to blog homeschooling regulation. *ProPublica.* https://www.propublica.org/article/small-group-goes-great-lengths-to-block-homeschooling-regulation

Jamison, P., Meckler, L., Gordy, P., Morse, C. E., & Alcantara, C. (2023, October 31). Homeschool's rise from fringe to fastest-growing form of education. *The Washington Post.* https://www.washingtonpost.com/education/interactive/2023/homeschooling-growth-data-by-district/

Kelly, G. S. (2021). HSLDA concerned with more than just homeschool. *CUNY Academic Works.* https://academicworks.cuny.edu/gj_etds/559

Klicka, C. (2000). The social worker at your door. *Homeschool World.* https://www.home-school.com/Articles/the-social-worker-at-your-door.php

Kunzman, R., & Gaither, M. (2020). Homeschooling: An updated comprehensive survey of the research. *Other Education: The Journal of Educational Alternatives, 9*(1), 253–336. https://icher.org/files/Kunzman_and_Gaither_An%20Updated_Comprehensive_Survey.pdf

Litvinov, A. (2021). *Finding the lost students of the pandemic.* National Education Association. https://www.nea.org/advocating-for-change/new-from-nea/finding-lost-students-pandemic

Martin-Chang, S., Gould, O. N., & Meuse, R. E. (2011). The impact of schooling on academic achievement: Evidence from homeschooled and traditionally schooled students. *Canadian Journal of Behavioural Science/Revue canadienne des sciences du comportement, 43*(3), 195–202. https://doi.org/10.1037/a0022697

McCracken, C. (2014, January 15). *How to mislead with data; A critical review of Ray's "Academic achievement and Demographic Traits of homeschool students: A nationwide study" (2010).* CRHE. https://www.responsiblehomeschooling.org/wp-content/uploads/2013/12/ray-2010-for-pdf.pdf

McDonald, K. (2023, June 16). Homeschooling remains a popular option, while defying stereotypes. *Forbes.* https://www.forbes.com/sites/kerrymcdonald/2023/06/16/homeschooling-remains-a-popular-option-while-defying-stereotypes/?sh=223c73091b6f

McGowin, E. H. (2018). *Quivering families: The quiverfull movement and Evangelical theology and family.* Fortress Press.

Meckler, L. (2023, December 11). How a true believer's flawed research helped legitimize home schooling. *The Washington Post.* https://www.washingtonpost.com/education/2023/12/11/brian-ray-homeschool-student-outcomes/

Michigan Christian Homeschool Network. (2021, November29). *Interview with the De Jonge family, history of homeschooling in Michigan.* https://www.michn.org/resources/37741/history-of-homeschooling-in-michigan

Miller, W. R., & Rollnick, S. (2023). *Motivational interviewing: Helping people change and grow.* Guilford.

Murphy, J. (2014). The social and educational outcomes of homeschooling. *Sociological Spectrum, 34*(3), 244–272. https://doi.org/10.1080/02732173.2014.895640

National Association of Social Workers. (2021). *Code of ethics of the National Association of Social Workers.* https://www.socialworkers.org/About/Ethics/Code-of-Ethics/Code-of-Ethics-English

National Center for Education Statistics. (2022). *The Condition of education report: Homeschooled children and reasons for homeschooling.* https://nces.ed.gov/programs/coe/pdf/2022/tgk_508.pdf

Parker, H., & Steffenhagen, M. (n.d.). *Lobbying on many fronts: HSLDA's state-by-state fight against oversight.* When home is school, New York City News Service. https://homeschooling.nycitynewsservice.com/political-force/

Parks, C. (2021, June 14). The rise of black homeschooling. *The New Yorker.* https://www.newyorker.com/magazine/2021/06/21/the-rise-of-black-homeschooling

People v. DeJonge, 442 Mich. 266 (1993). https://law.justia.com/cases/michigan/supreme-court/1993/91479-5.html

Pride, M. (1986). *The child abuse industry: Outrageous facts about child abuse & everyday rebellions against a system that threatens every North American family.* Crossway.

Princiotta, D., & Bielick, S. (2006). *Homeschooling in the United States: 2003, (NCES 2006–042).* U.S. Department of Education, National Center for Education Statistics. https://nces.ed.gov/pubs2006/2006042.pdf

Revised School Code of 1976, Michigan Complied Laws, Section 380.1561 (2017). https://legislature.mi.gov/doc.aspx?mcl-380-1561

Rogers, C. R. (1961). *On becoming a person: A therapist's view of psychotherapy.* Houghton Mifflin.

Skarpness, L. (2019, May 3). *Sisters homeschooled after decade of bullying. It's a growing issue, MN official says.* Twin Cities Pioneer Press. https://www.twincities.com/2019/05/12/sisters-homeschooled-after-decade-of-bullying-its-a-growing-issue-mn-official-says/

U.S. Department of Health, Education, and Welfare. Office of Education. (1971). *White House conference on children - child development recommendations: Hearings before the subcommittee on children and youth of the committee on labor and public welfare United states senate.* Government Printing Office. https://files.eric.ed.gov/fulltext/ED059761.pdf

United Nations Convention on the Rights of the Child. (November 20, 1989). https://www.ohchr.org/en/instruments-mechanisms/instruments/convention-rights-child

Van Galen, J., & Pitman, M. A. (1991). *Home schooling: Political, historical, and pedagogical perspectives. Social and policy issues in education: The University of Cincinnati Series.*

Vazquez Toness, B., & Lurye, S. (2023, February 9). Thousands of kids are missing from school. Where did they go? *Associated Press News.* https://apnews.com/article/covid-school-enrollment-missing-kids-homeschool-b6c9017f603c00466b9e9908c5f2183a

Waddell, T. B. (2010). Bringing it all back home: Establishing a coherent constitutional for the re-regulation of homeschooling. *Vanderbilt Law Review, 63*(2), 541–597. https://scholarship.law.vanderbilt.edu/vlr/vol63/iss2/5/

West, T. (2023, March 9). Bullying led to bloodshed. Now Bayonne sisters are being homeschooled. *The Jersey Journal.* https://www.nj.com/hudson/2023/03/bullying-of-sisters-was-ignored-and-bayonne-girls-nose-was-broken-mom-says-now-theyre-being-homeschooled.html

Woodruff, S. A. (2024, April 9). *Correspondence with families for home education.* https://fhe-mo.org/Resources/1-295.pdf

Woodruff, S. A. (n.d.). *No more calls needed for Missouri SB 727.* Homeschool Legal Defense Association. https://www.votervoice.net/iframes/HSLDA/Campaigns/114644/Respond

Yu, M. C., Sackett, P. R., & Kuncel, N. R. (2016). Predicting college performance of homeschooled versus traditional students. *Educational Measurement: Issues and Practice, 35,* 31–39. https://doi.org/10.1111/emip.12133

# Leading Conversations about Human Services Trends

# 29 Human Service Transformations and Emergent Trends

*James C. Wadley*

## Introduction

In the United States, the human services field, which encompasses a broad range of programs and services designed to meet the social, emotional, and economic needs of individuals and families, faces a critical juncture. As the nation becomes increasingly diverse—with the U.S. Census Bureau (2020) reporting a significant increase in multiracial populations and a decline in the percentage of non-Hispanic white individuals—the need for equitable and inclusive services has become paramount. This chapter explores key trends shaping human services, including diversity, equity, and inclusion (DEI) initiatives, the ongoing struggle to provide affordable housing (with the National Low Income Housing Coalition [NLIHC, 2023] reporting a national housing wage of $28.58 per hour), the complex needs of immigrant communities, persistent disparities in healthcare access (Robertson et al., 2022), and the evolution of leadership within the field. By examining these trends and their implications for service delivery, this chapter aims to provide insights into effective strategies for meeting the diverse needs of communities.

## Diversity, Equity, and Inclusion in Human Services

The focus on DEI has become a cornerstone of modern human services, driven by ethical imperatives and the recognition that inclusive practices lead to more effective service delivery. As population needs change rapidly, leaders of organizations increasingly understand that fostering environments where diverse voices are valued and equitable outcomes are prioritized is essential.

### A More Diverse America Demands a More Inclusive Human Services System

The complexion of American demographics continues to change into a more diverse society. Demographic transformation necessitates a fundamental shift in how human services are designed and delivered. Even when agencies have strong mission statements and an array of services, some practitioners may be unprepared and less agile when it comes to service delivery.

Imagine a young Latina mother who struggles to access mental health services due to language or cultural barriers between her and her service provider. Some service providers are unable or unwilling to provide bilingual professionals to support their clients and constituents. Thus, clients find themselves disadvantaged when services are needed. Another example may be a homeless veteran who faces a complex web of challenges, unable to find

DOI: 10.4324/9781003531258-35

culturally competent support. These are just two examples of the countless individuals who fall through the cracks of a system not designed to meet their specific needs. Implementing robust DEI strategies strengthens service effectiveness and fosters trust within communities. When people feel seen, heard, and valued, they're more likely to engage with services and experience positive outcomes.

### Beyond Demographic Representation: Key Dimensions of DEI in Human Services

While demographic representation is an important starting point, true DEI in human services extends far beyond simply reflecting the community's demographics within an organization. Wiltshire et al. (2024) suggest that programs should consider focusing on topics that include culture, ethnicity, religion, ability, and/or sexual orientation. DEI program development should encompass several key dimensions that focus on creating inclusive environments and ensuring equitable outcomes.

#### *Cultural Competence*

Cultural competence, the ability to understand, appreciate, and interact effectively with people from diverse cultures, is a critical skill for human service professionals. Eden et al. (2024) suggest that cultural competence acknowledges and respects cultural backgrounds and experiences as well as the identities of constituents. Increasingly, professionals receive training to recognize and address implicit biases and enhance their cultural competence (Sue & Sue, 2016). Educators and institutions are vital in that they are responsible for engaging and preparing professionals to thrive in an array of settings (Lyu, 2024). Training may equip professionals to respond effectively to individuals from diverse cultural backgrounds' unique needs, values, and beliefs.

Tham and Solomon (2024) suggest that cultural competence also includes cultural humility. The goal is to create a culture of collaboration and partnership that acknowledges the authenticity of each individual. In addition, when members feel invested, cared for, and valued, goal acquisition becomes more attainable.

#### *Understanding Historical Trauma*

Training may explore historical trauma, the cumulative emotional and psychological wounding across generations resulting from massive group trauma. This concept is particularly relevant when working with Indigenous communities. The Indian Health Service recognizes the profound impact of historical trauma on the health and well-being of Native American and Alaska Native populations, including higher rates of substance abuse, mental health disorders, and chronic diseases compared to their white counterparts (Gone, 2013). For example, Brave Heart and DeBruyn (1998) explored the intergenerational effects of historical trauma among the Lakota people, highlighting the need for culturally sensitive interventions addressing historical grief and loss.

#### *Developing Culturally Appropriate Communication Strategies*

Effective communication is crucial in human services. Communication styles vary across cultures; for instance, avoiding direct eye contact is a sign of respect in some Asian cultures but might be interpreted as disinterest in Western cultures. Training may involve role-playing and case studies to practice navigating these cultural differences. Unfortunately, some human services agencies fail to be culturally sensitive and competent due to intended or unintended acts of discrimination, including microaggressions.

### Addressing Microaggressions

Microaggressions are subtle, often unintentional, slights or insults that are biased and communicate negative messages. Sue and Constantine (2007) found that racial microaggressions significantly negatively impact the mental health and well-being of people of color. Moreover, when microaggressions are pervasive across an agency or company, morale and production may be negatively impacted. When professionals feel targeted and marginalized, they may be less invested in positive systemic outcomes. In a qualitative study completed on therapists of color, Gonazalez Vera et al. (2024) suggested that they experienced many types of microaggressions; were significantly impacted after being microaggressed; sought and obtained support after being microaggressed; and viewed microaggressions as opportunities for growth and learning. Thus, agencies need to remain mindful and sensitive to reports of microaggressions. Staff trainings that specifically address the etiology, prevalence, and impact of microaggressions may reduce the likelihood of perpetuating these harmful interactions within human service agencies. Professionals need to know that these trainings and supports are available and accessible.

### Accessibility

Ensuring accessibility is another critical component of DEI, encompassing physical and linguistic access. Physical accessibility is crucial for individuals with disabilities. The Americans with Disabilities Act (ADA) is vital in promoting physical accessibility by establishing standards for public accommodations, including human service organizations. These standards address various aspects of physical environments, such as ramps, elevators, accessible restrooms, and signage. According to the Centers for Disease Control and Prevention (CDC, 2022), 26% of adults in the United States have some type of disability, including mobility impairments, sensory impairments (e.g., vision or hearing loss), cognitive disabilities, and other conditions that can significantly impact access to services. For instance, a study by Parish and Cloud (2006) found that physical inaccessibility of healthcare facilities was a significant barrier to healthcare utilization for people with mobility impairments. This highlights the importance of ADA compliance and proactive efforts by human service organizations to ensure their facilities are accessible to all.

Linguistic accessibility is essential for reaching individuals with limited English proficiency (LEP). The U.S. Census Bureau (2020) reported that 21.9% of people over the age of five spoke a language other than English at home, translating to over 67 million people. This substantial portion of the population requires language access services to communicate effectively with human service providers and access needed support. Providing professional interpretation and translation services is crucial for ensuring that LEP individuals can access and benefit from human services. Jacobs et al. (2004) found that providing interpreter services in healthcare settings improved LEP patients' satisfaction with their care and led to better health outcomes, including improved adherence to treatment plans and reduced hospital readmission rates. This underscores the importance of qualified interpreters, as untrained interpreters or reliance on family members can lead to miscommunication and potentially harmful consequences. For example, a case study by Flores (2005) documented a tragic instance where miscommunication due to inadequate interpretation services led to a child receiving an incorrect medication dosage. This emphasizes the need for human service organizations to prioritize professional language access services as a core component of equitable service delivery.

### Equity in Service Delivery

Achieving equitable outcomes in human services requires more than simply treating everyone equally; it necessitates recognizing and addressing systemic barriers disproportionately affecting certain groups. Equity provides tailored support and resources based on individual needs and circumstances to achieve fair and just outcomes. This section will examine disparities in mental health and child welfare as examples of systemic inequities.

### Mental Health Disparities

Although the overall prevalence rates of mental illness are similar across racial groups, significant differences exist in diagnosis and treatment. A meta-analysis by Olbert et al. (2018) found that Black individuals were diagnosed with schizophrenia at a rate 2.4 times higher than white individuals, even after controlling for socioeconomic status and other confounding factors. Similarly, data from the Substance Abuse and Mental Health Services Administration (SAMHSA, 2021) shows that, in 2021, among adults with any mental illness, 48.4% of white adults received mental health services, compared to 37.1% of Black adults and 33.1% of Hispanic adults. These statistics highlight the persistent disparities in access to mental health treatment. The disproportionate diagnosis rate of Black clients may be attributed to several factors. These factors may include implicit bias in diagnostic practices, a lack of culturally competent mental health providers, and systemic barriers to accessing appropriate care.

Implicit biases are negative attitudes and beliefs about sexual identity, age, ability, gender, socioeconomic status, and religion that fall outside of conscious awareness (Sabin, 2022). These biases influence judgment in a way that a person behaves in a discriminatory manner toward someone else. These individual practices seem to exist and organize themselves within macrolevel structures that perpetuate systemic sexism, racism, and other forms of discrimination. A professional's implicit bias may impact the assessment and diagnosis of Black clients.

Disproportionate diagnosis of Black clients may also be a product of a lack of culturally competent mental health providers. While most academic and training programs have some sort of multicultural or social justice course, professionals stay abreast of culturally competent best practices over the duration of their careers. Because the notion of diversity is constantly changing and today's consumer may have more nuanced needs, professionals have to continue to formally and informally educate themselves about cultural and community shifts. Without doing so, practitioners may make decisions based upon assumptions or ideas that are antiquated or less refined. There are too few professionals who engage in ongoing multicultural or social justice training.

Systemic barriers in human services may impact professionals' capacity to appropriately diagnose clients. Fewer qualified (licensed) professionals and inadequate staffing, bureaucratic entanglements, access to services, and inconsistent or truncated services serve as deflections to accurate assessments and diagnoses. Agencies and professionals need to continue to work toward removing systemic barriers and have more streamlined processes that may enable a more comprehensive understanding of one's presenting issue(s) as well as their mental health concerns.

### Disparities in Child Welfare

Disparities also exist within the child welfare system. Black children are disproportionately represented in foster care. According to data from The Annie E. Casey Foundation (2019), Black children represented 23% of children in foster care while comprising only 14% of the general child population. This rate may be attributed to socioeconomic disparities (compared to whites) and access to resources (e.g., information about developmentally appropriate parenting, adequate housing, access to healthcare) that impact some families to retain their children in a stable home environment. For human service and child welfare professionals, cultural competence about poverty, as well as implicit bias, may be a contributing factor to some Black families being under-resourced (Hill, 2006). For example, research has shown that families in predominantly Black neighborhoods are more likely to be investigated by child protective services compared to white families who are reported for similar types of reported concerns (Drake et al., 2011).

DEI initiatives in human services seek to eliminate these disparities by implementing culturally tailored interventions, addressing the root causes of inequity, and advocating for policy changes that promote social justice. By prioritizing these dimensions of DEI, human service organizations can create more inclusive and effective services that truly meet the needs of all community members.

### Public Housing and Affordable Living

The demand for affordable housing in the United States has reached crisis levels, with public housing programs and other initiatives struggling to provide stable living conditions for vulnerable populations. Many factors drive this crisis, including stagnant wages, rising housing costs, and a shortage of available affordable units. The National Low Income Housing Coalition's (NLIHC, 2023) "Out of Reach" report provides stark data illustrating the severity of the affordability gap on the concept of the housing wage and the affordability gap.

#### HOUSING WAGE

The national housing wage—the hourly wage a full-time worker must earn to afford a modest rental home (a two-bedroom unit)—in 2023 was $28.58. This means a worker earning the federal minimum wage ($7.25 per hour) must work nearly *four* full-time jobs to afford a modest two-bedroom rental.

#### AFFORDABILITY GAP

This national average masks significant regional variations. In high-cost metropolitan areas, the housing wage is substantially higher. For example, in San Francisco, CA, the housing wage is $61.75, and in Honolulu, HI, it is $49.81 (NLIHC, 2023). This highlights the extreme affordability challenges renters face in many parts of the country.

The consequences of this affordability crisis are far-reaching. Housing instability and homelessness are associated with a range of negative outcomes, including poor health, educational disruption, and economic instability.

POOR HEALTH

Lack of stable housing is linked to increased rates of chronic diseases, mental health issues, and substance abuse (National Health Care for the Homeless Council, n.d.). When clients struggle to find or maintain adequate housing, they may not prioritize their health in a way that allows them to access foods that are high in nutrition, get proper medical attention, or engage in consistent positive wellness practices. Adequate housing resources and information should be seen as a priority for all human service agencies.

EDUCATIONAL DISRUPTION

Children experiencing homelessness or housing instability are more likely to miss school, perform poorly academically, and drop out (National Center on Family Homelessness, 2014). Formal education sometimes isn't a priority for some adolescents and their families when there are housing challenges. Moreover, some adolescents may not be able to conceptualize or experience the long-term benefits (e.g., job acquisition and retention, exposure to different perspectives, networking opportunities) of remaining in school through high school or completing a GED.

ECONOMIC INSTABILITY

The high cost of housing can strain family budgets, leaving little room for other essential expenses like food, transportation, and healthcare. This can perpetuate cycles of poverty and make it difficult for families to achieve economic self-sufficiency.

Recent policies and programs increasingly emphasize a holistic approach by integrating social support services with housing assistance. This "housing plus services" model recognizes that addressing housing needs is often intertwined with other challenges, such as employment, healthcare, and mental health. Research consistently demonstrates that access to affordable housing reduces homelessness and improves overall health and economic stability for families (Culhane et al., 2002).

To address the affordable housing crisis, various innovative solutions are gaining traction, including:

- **Modular Housing:** This construction method offers a faster and potentially more cost-effective way to build affordable housing units.
- **Community Land Trusts:** These non-profit organizations acquire land and hold it in trust for the benefit of the community, ensuring the long-term affordability of housing built on the land.
- **Inclusionary Zoning:** These policies require developers to include a certain percentage of affordable units in new housing developments.
- **Rental Assistance Programs:** Programs like Housing Choice Vouchers (Section 8) provide rental subsidies to low-income families, helping them afford housing in the private market.

While these innovations offer promising avenues for increasing the supply of affordable housing, significant investment and policy changes are needed to address the scale of the current crisis and ensure that all individuals and families have access to safe, stable, and affordable housing.

## Immigration and Access to Services

Immigration continues to significantly shape the social, economic, and cultural landscape of the United States, presenting both opportunities and complex challenges for human services. The flow of immigrants into the United States is a dynamic process influenced by various global and domestic factors. According to recent immigration trends discussed in the Department of Homeland Security's *2021 Yearbook of Immigration Statistics* (United States Office of Immigration Statistics, 2023), in the 2021 fiscal year, approximately 740,000 individuals obtained lawful permanent resident status in the United States. This number represents a decrease compared to previous years, partly influenced by the COVID-19 pandemic and related travel restrictions. Historically, the sources of immigration have shifted, with recent decades seeing a greater influx of immigrants from Latin America and Asia.

The diverse backgrounds, languages, and experiences of immigrant populations necessitate culturally competent and linguistically accessible services. Human service providers are adapting to meet these needs by offering a range of specialized programs and services, including language support, legal assistance, and culturally sensitive programs.

### Language Support

Language barriers can significantly hinder access to essential services. Many organizations offer English as a Second Language classes, interpretation services, and translated materials to facilitate communication and ensure effective service delivery.

### Legal Assistance

Navigating the complex U.S. immigration system can be overwhelming. Legal aid organizations and attorneys specializing in immigration law support immigrants seeking legal status, understanding their rights, and accessing due process.

### Culturally Sensitive Programs

Recognizing that cultural factors influence individuals' needs and experiences, human service providers are increasingly developing culturally tailored programs. These programs consider cultural values, beliefs, and practices to ensure that services are relevant and effective. For example, a mental health program serving a specific immigrant community might incorporate culturally relevant therapeutic approaches and address culturally specific stressors.

Collaboration between the public and private sectors is crucial for effectively serving immigrant populations. Public agencies, such as the U.S. Citizenship and Immigration Services and the Office of Refugee Resettlement, are key in providing funding, setting policy, and overseeing immigration-related programs. Private non-profit organizations, community-based organizations, and faith-based groups provide direct services to immigrants, often with specialized expertise in serving particular communities. Research suggests that this public–private collaboration enhances resource availability, promotes the integration of immigrant populations, and improves service outcomes (Fix et al., 2009).

Furthermore, it's important to acknowledge the diverse experiences within immigrant communities. Refugees, asylum seekers, and undocumented immigrants face distinct challenges and require different types of support. Understanding these nuances is essential for developing effective and equitable service delivery strategies.

*Healthcare Access and Equity*

Access to quality healthcare in the United States remains inequitable. According to the U.S. Census Bureau, 27.5 million Americans lacked health insurance in 2021, disproportionately impacting Black and Hispanic populations. These disparities contribute to significant differences in health outcomes, with Black Americans experiencing infant mortality rates nearly 2.5 times higher than white Americans. Data from the Centers for Disease Control and Prevention (CDC, 2023a, 2023b) and other sources paint an even clearer picture of these inequities:

- **Health Insurance Coverage:** In 2021, uninsured rates varied significantly by race and ethnicity. According to the CDC (2023b), 10.6% of Hispanic adults were uninsured, compared to 5.4% of non-Hispanic white adults and 7.5% of non-Hispanic Black adults. This lack of insurance can create significant barriers to accessing necessary medical care.
- **Chronic Disease Prevalence:** Disparities also exist in the prevalence of chronic diseases. For example, the CDC (2023a) reports that non-Hispanic Black adults are 60% more likely than non-Hispanic white adults to be diagnosed with diabetes. Similarly, American Indian/Alaska Native adults are twice as likely as non-Hispanic white adults to be diagnosed with diabetes.
- **Maternal Mortality:** Maternal mortality rates in the U.S. also exhibit stark racial disparities. Data from the CDC (2023c) show that in 2021, the maternal mortality rate for non-Hispanic Black women was 69.9 deaths per 100,000 live births, approximately three times higher than the rate for non-Hispanic white women (26.6 deaths per 100,000 live births).

    These disparities are often rooted in a complex interplay of factors, including:
- **Socioeconomic Factors:** Poverty, lack of access to quality education, and limited employment opportunities can all contribute to poorer health outcomes.
- **Environmental Factors:** Exposure to environmental hazards, such as air and water pollution, can disproportionately impact specific communities.
- **Discrimination and Bias:** Experiences of discrimination and bias within the healthcare system can create barriers to care and contribute to mistrust.

*Medicaid Expansion*

The Affordable Care Act's Medicaid expansion has significantly increased access to health insurance for low-income individuals, particularly in states that have chosen to participate. Medicaid expansion under the ACA may have increased Medicaid coverage rates among low-income adults. Increased insurance coverage translates to improved access to healthcare services. The expansion has led to reductions in the rate of uninsurance-related medical debt and increased utilization of preventive care services such as screenings and vaccinations. Medicaid expansion may also contribute to a reduction in health disparities.

*Community Health Centers*

Community health centers (CHCs) help provide high-quality, affordable healthcare to underserved communities. CHCs are located in medically underserved areas and serve a disproportionate number of low-income individuals, racial and ethnic minorities, and individuals living in rural communities. CHCs provide various services, including primary care, preventive care, dental care, mental health, and social services. Operating on a sliding fee scale based on income, CHCs ensure patients can afford the care they need, regardless of their financial situation. By expanding access to affordable healthcare through initiatives like Medicaid expansion and supporting vital institutions like CHCs, we can work toward a more equitable and just healthcare system for all.

## Telehealth

Telehealth has emerged as a crucial tool for expanding access to medical care, particularly in rural and underserved areas. The COVID-19 pandemic significantly accelerated the adoption of telemedicine, transforming it from a niche approach to a mainstream component of healthcare delivery, as highlighted by Martin and Alarcón-Urbistondo (2024). This shift presents a significant opportunity to improve access to healthcare for vulnerable populations by overcoming geographical barriers. However, ensuring equitable access to these technology-driven services requires addressing the digital divide and promoting digital health literacy.

The digital divide refers to the unequal access to and use of information and communication technologies, including the internet and digital devices. In the context of telehealth, it encompasses disparities in internet access, digital literacy skills, and access to appropriate devices. Individuals lacking reliable internet access, who are uncomfortable with technology, or who do not possess the necessary digital skills may face significant barriers to accessing and effectively utilizing telehealth services.

Promoting digital health literacy is crucial for mitigating these disparities. Digital health literacy encompasses the skills and knowledge necessary to effectively seek, find, understand, and utilize health information from electronic sources. Individuals with strong digital health literacy are better equipped to schedule telehealth appointments, understand and adhere to online medical instructions, and access reliable health information from reputable sources. By addressing the digital divide and promoting digital health literacy, we can ensure that the benefits of telehealth are equitably distributed across all populations.

## Leadership Styles in Human Services

Leadership within human services is evolving significantly, shifting from traditional hierarchical models to more adaptive, transformational, and participatory approaches. Effective leadership is crucial for navigating uncertainty, fostering collaboration, and inspiring innovation in a field characterized by complex social problems, limited resources, and diverse stakeholder needs.

Transformational leadership emphasizes inspiring and motivating staff to achieve a shared vision. These leaders focus on creating a sense of purpose, fostering intellectual stimulation, and providing individualized support to their team members (Bass & Avolio, 1994). These leaders invite and lead their followers to be creative, imaginative, and innovative when it comes to service delivery (Bakker et al., 2023). In human services, this might involve articulating a compelling vision for addressing a specific social issue, such as homelessness or poverty, and empowering staff to develop innovative solutions.

Adaptive leadership recognizes that many challenges human service organizations face are complex and require adaptive solutions rather than simple technical fixes (Heifetz, 1994). Adaptive leaders focus on identifying the core values and beliefs that guide the organization, fostering experimentation and learning, and mobilizing stakeholders to address complex problems collaboratively.

Participatory leadership emphasizes engaging stakeholders at all levels—including staff, clients, community members, and other partners—in decision-making processes. By creating opportunities for shared governance and co-creation of solutions, participatory leadership can enhance service delivery, build stronger relationships with the community, and foster a sense of ownership and accountability (Avolio et al., 2009). Moreover, participatory leadership may also provide opportunities to solve challenges and find viable solutions (Setiadi, 2024). For example, a CHC might establish a community advisory board composed of residents to provide input on program design and service delivery. Participants may offer a variety of potential solutions and quickly determine which response may be best for the good of the whole.

There may be a positive impact on constituents if transformational, adaptive, and participatory leadership styles are considered for human service organizations. These leadership approaches can significantly enhance organizational effectiveness and contribute to positive client outcomes, including the following.

### Improved Service Delivery

When leaders truly empower their teams, encourage everyone to work together, and embrace new ideas, it makes a huge difference for the people we serve. Imagine this scenario in a community struggling with crime. Instead of just telling the police what to do, the leaders encourage them to work side-by-side with the community. They hold meetings, listen to residents' concerns, and develop solutions. This approach, called participatory leadership, leads to better outcomes. Research by Denhardt and Denhardt (2000) shows that when police leaders actively engaged community members in problem-solving and decision-making, it led to more effective crime prevention strategies and improved community satisfaction with police services. This is a powerful example of how putting people first and working together can lead to better services for everyone.

### Increased Staff Morale and Retention

Supportive and engaging leadership can enhance staff morale, reduce burnout, and improve retention rates, which is crucial in a field often characterized by high turnover. A case study by Kim (2014) explored the impact of transformational leadership in a social service agency serving individuals with developmental disabilities. The study found that when leaders focused on inspiring staff, providing individualized support, and creating a shared purpose, it significantly lowered staff turnover rates and improved job satisfaction. This underscores the importance of transformational leadership in creating a positive and supportive work environment that promotes staff retention.

### Stronger Community Relationships

Participatory leadership and community engagement can build trust and strengthen relationships between human service organizations and the communities they serve. A study by Roberts (2004) examined the role of community-based organizations in addressing homelessness. The research found that organizations that prioritized participatory leadership and actively involved homeless individuals and community members in program design and implementation were more successful in building trust and fostering community support.

This demonstrates how participatory leadership can strengthen community relationships and enhance the effectiveness of human service interventions.

*Organizational Resilience*

Organizations with strong leadership are better equipped to adapt to change, navigate challenges, and achieve their mission. A case study by Couto (1995) analyzed the leadership of a community development corporation in responding to economic downturns. The study found that community development corporations with adaptive leaders who could mobilize resources, build partnerships, and adapt their strategies to changing circumstances were more resilient and better able to continue serving their communities during times of crisis. This assertion is similar to the suggestion of Widner and Smith (2024) that adaptive leadership seeks to challenge issues of violence and chaos to build inclusive and peaceful systems. This highlights the importance of adaptive leadership in fostering organizational resilience and ensuring long-term sustainability. By embracing these evolving leadership styles, human service organizations can better address the complex social challenges of our time and create more equitable and effective services for all community members.

## Conclusion

The trends examined in this chapter—the growing emphasis on DEI, the persistent struggle for affordable housing, the complex needs of immigrant communities, disparities in healthcare access, and the evolution of leadership—are not isolated issues. They are deeply interconnected, reflecting systemic inequities requiring multifaceted, collaborative solutions.

As the U.S. population diversifies (U.S. Census Bureau, 2020), the need for culturally competent and equitable services becomes even more critical. For example, addressing the affordable housing crisis (NLIHC, 2023) is about providing shelter and improving health outcomes, educational attainment, and economic stability. Similarly, ensuring equitable access to healthcare (CDC, 2023a, 2023b) requires addressing social determinants of health and dismantling systemic barriers. Effective leadership, particularly transformational, adaptive, and participatory approaches (Avolio et al., 2009; Bass & Avolio, 1994; Heifetz, 1994), is essential for navigating these complexities and fostering collaboration to create lasting change. The human services field is pivotal, poised to perpetuate existing inequities or embrace innovation and create a more just and equitable society. Ongoing research, data-driven practice, and genuine community engagement will be crucial in shaping a future in which all individuals have the opportunity to thrive.

## Questions for Reflection

1 What are some trends that have emerged at your agency or in your community, and how have you had to adjust to meet the changing needs of your constituents?
2 Given the changing needs of the human services field and the high probability of burnout, what has self-care looked like for you, your staff, and your colleagues? How supportive has your agency been in reducing the likelihood of burnout?
3 What trends or professional innovations may emerge over the next three to five years? How might technology (e.g., the internet and access to information or AI) be a catalyst or deterrence for change in the field?

4  Given some of the ideas/trends mentioned in this chapter, if you could start your own agency, what services would you want to provide for your clients or constituents?

5  With some of the concepts of this chapter in mind, share your ideas about professional and personality traits needed by human services providers to be successful.

## References

Avolio, B. J., Walumbwa, F. O., & Weber, T. J. (2009). Leadership: Current theories, research, and future directions. *Annual Review of Psychology, 60*, 421–449. https://doi.org/10.1146/annurev.psych.60.110707.163621

Bakker, A. B., Hetland, J., Olsen, O. K., & Espevik, R. (2023). Daily transformational leadership: A source of inspiration for follower performance? *European Management Journal, 41*(5), 700–708.

Bass, B. M., & Avolio, B. J. (1994). *Improving organizational effectiveness through transformational leadership*. Sage Publications.

Brave Heart, M. Y. H., & DeBruyn, L. M. (1998). The American Indian holocaust: Healing historical unresolved grief. *American Indian and Alaska Native Mental Health Research, 8*(2), 56–78.

Centers for Disease Control and Prevention. (2022). *Disability and health promotion.*

Centers for Disease Control and Prevention. (2023a, February 23). *Maternal mortality rates in the United States, 2021.* National Center for Health Statistics. https://www.cdc.gov/nchs/data/hestat/maternal-mortality/2021/maternal-mortality-rates-2021.htm

Centers for Disease Control and Prevention. (2023b, November 17). *Health insurance coverage: Early release of estimates from the National Health Interview Survey, 2022.* National Center for Health Statistics. https://www.cdc.gov/nchs/fastats/health-insurance.htm

Couto, R. A. (1995). *An American challenge: A report to the Ford Foundation on community development corporations and social change.* Kettering Foundation.

Culhane, D. P., Metraux, S., & Hadley, T. (2002). Public service reductions associated with placing homeless persons with severe mental illness in supportive housing. *Psychiatric Services, 53*(1), 106–112.

Denhardt, J. V., & Denhardt, R. B. (2000). The new public service: Serving, not steering. *Public Administration Review, 60*(6), 549–559.

Drake, B., Jolley, J. M., Lanier, P., Fluke, J., Barth, R. P., & Jonson-Reid, M. (2011). Racial bias in child protection? A comparison of competing explanations using national data. *Pediatrics, 127*(3), 471–478.

Eden, C. A., Chisom, O. N., & Adeniyi, I. S. (2024). Cultural competence in education: Strategies for fostering inclusivity and diversity awareness. *International Journal of Applied Research in Social Sciences, 6*(3), 383–392.

Fix, M., Zimmermann, W., & Barrows, S. (2009). *All under one roof? Mixed-status families in an era of reform.* Migration Policy Institute.

Flores, G. (2005). The impact of medical interpreter services on healthcare quality: A systematic review. *Medical Care Research and Review, 62*(3), 255–299.

Gone, J. P. (2013). Redressing First Nations historical trauma: Theorizing mechanisms for indigenous culture as mental health treatment. *Transcultural Psychiatry, 50*(5), 683–706.

Heifetz, R. A. (1994). *Leadership without easy answers.* Harvard University Press.

Hill, S. A. (2006). Marriage among African American women: A gender perspective. *Journal of Comparative Family Studies, 37*(3), 421–440.

Jacobs, E. A., Shepard, D. S., & Suaya, J. A. (2004). Overcoming language barriers in health care: Costs and benefits of interpreter services. *American Journal of Public Health, 94*(5), 866–869.

Kim, S. (2014). The effects of transformational leadership on employees' work-related outcomes in a human service organization. *Administration in Social Work, 38*(2), 176–193.

Lyu, J. (2024). Cultivating Cross-Cultural Competence in Students. In *SHS Web of Conferences* (Vol. 187, p. 4006). EDP Sciences.

Martin, M. S., & Alarcón-Urbistondo, P. (2024). Digital transformation in healthcare and medical practices: Advancements, challenges, and future opportunities. In M. B. Garcia, & P. Alarcón-Urbistondo (Eds.), *Emerging technologies for health literacy and medical practice* (pp. 176–197). IGI Global.

National Center on Family Homelessness. (2014). *America's youngest outcasts: State report card on child homelessness*. National Center on Family Homelessness at American Institutes for Research.

National Health Care for the Homeless Council. (n.d.). *Health care and homelessness*. Retrieved December 27, 2023.

National Low Income Housing Coalition. (2023). *Out of reach: The high cost of housing*. https://reports.nlihc.org/oor

Olbert, C. M., Nagendra, A., & Buck, B. (2018). Meta-analysis of Black vs. White racial disparity in schizophrenia diagnosis in the United States: Do structured assessments attenuate racial disparities? *Journal of Abnormal Psychology, 127*(1), 104–115. https://doi.org/10.1037/abn0000309

Parish, S. L., & Cloud, M. (2006). Barriers to health care for people with intellectual disabilities: An ecological model. *Mental Retardation and Developmental Disabilities Research Reviews, 12*(1), 60–69.

Robertson, M. M., Shamsunder, M. G., Brazier, E., Mantravadi, M., Zimba, R., Rane, M. S., Westmoreland, D. A., Parcesepe, A. M., Marko, A. R., & Nash, D. (2022). Racial/ethnic disparities in exposure, disease susceptibility, and clinical outcomes during COVID-19 pandemic in national cohort of adults, United States. *Emerging Infectious Diseases, 28*(11), 2171–2180. https://doi.org/10.3201/eid2811.220072

Roberts, N. C. (2004). Stakeholder collaboration in government: An organizational analysis. *Public Administration Review, 64*(1), 19–28.

Sabin, J. (2022). Tackling implicit bias in health care. *The New England Journal of Medicine, 387*(2), 105–107.

Substance Abuse and Mental Health Services Administration (SAMHSA). Psychosocial Interventions for Older Adults with Serious Mental Illness. SAMHSA Publication No. PEP21-06-05-001. Rockville, MD: Substance Abuse and Mental Health Services Administration, 2021.

Setiadi, G. (2024). Analysis of principal leadership strategies in improving teacher performance. *ICCCM Journal of Social Sciences and Humanities, 3*(3), 66–72.

Sue, D. W., & Constantine, M. G. (2007). Racial microaggressions as instigators of difficult dialogues on race: Implications for student affairs educators and students. *College Student Affairs Journal, 26*(2), 136–143.

Sue, D. W., & Sue, D. (2016). *Counseling the culturally diverse: Theory and practice* (7th ed.). John Wiley & Sons, Inc.

Tham, S. S., & Solomon, P. (2024). Practicing cultural humility will achieve recovery-oriented mental health practice and service delivery. *Administration and Policy in Mental Health and Mental Health Services Research, 51*(1), 10–13.

The Annie E. Casey Foundation. (2019, June 6). What is Foster Care? Retrieved from The Annie E. Casey Foundation: https://www.aecf.org/blog/what-is-foster-care/

United States Census Bureau. (2020). *2020 Census results*. U.S. Department of Commerce. https://www.census.gov/programs-surveys/decennial-census/decade/2020/2020-census-results.html.

United States Office of Immigration Statistics. (2023). *Yearbook of Immigration Statistics*. US Department of Homeland Security, Office of Immigration Statistics.

Vera, J. G., Domenech Rodríguez, M., Navarro Flores, C., Vázquez, A., San Miguel, G., Phan, M., Wong, E., Klimczak, K., Bera, J., Papa, L., & Estrada, J. (2024). Invisible wounds: Testimony of microaggressions from the experiences of clinicians of color in training. *Training and Education in Professional Psychology, 18*(4), 331–339.

Widner, T., & Smith, R. (2024). The Mutuality of Adaptive Leadership and Integral Peace Leadership. *Journal of Leadership Studies, 18*(3), 76–82.

Wiltshire, J., Epps, A. S., Gutta, J., Yeager, V. A., & Menachemi, N. (2024). Implementing simple interventions to advance DEI in a dealth administration program. *Journal of Health Administration Education, 40*(2), 315–328.

# Index

Note: **Bold** page numbers refer to tables, *italic* page numbers refer to figures.

21st-century issues: and culturally competent interventions 251–266
2020 CLAS Physician Survey 154

Abrahams, H. 237
abuse: economic 40–41; emotional 16, 21, 45, 256; pediatric 53–56; physical 16; sexual 16; *see also* child abuse; partner abuse
Academy to Innovate Human Resources (AIHR) 28, 30
access: to community support services 260; to funding 283; healthcare 227–229, 231, 348; to health services 258; to services 347
accessibility 135–136, 152–156, 343–344
adaptive coping 206, **207**
adaptive leadership 349–351
adolescents: AI art for 279; discovery of AI art to assist 279–282; grief process 205 *see also* grief and bereavement; loss/death/bereavement; in marginalized communities 279
adult grief 206–208; *see also* grief and bereavement; loss/death/bereavement
adverse childhood experiences (ACEs) 19, 53–55, 199, 201
adversity: child maltreatment 16–17; cumulative 164; overview 15–17; and trauma 15–17, 199
advocacy 233, 305; animal 112; community 72; defined 99; models of 94; and safety 61–62; theory 99–100; training 98
affordability gap 345
Affordable Care Act (ACA) 152, 228, 348
affordable living 345–346
African Americans 288, 303; artistic expression 305; community 279, 303–313; perceptions 304
algorithms 107; and Incel communities 70–71; for other people and populations 71; social media 69
alienation 95, 215–216, 219

Allen, H. K. 140
Allen, K. A. 25
altered books 9–10
America: diverse 341–342; inclusive human services system 341–342
American College Health Association (ACHA) 141
American Psychological Association (APA) 127, 144, 208, 304
Americans with Disabilities Act (ADA) 131, 132, 343
Amyotrophic Lateral Sclerosis (ALS) 203
Andrews, George 326
Angelou, Maya 289
anti-racist language 290
antiretroviral therapy (ART) 171
Arbery, Ahmaud 160
artificial intelligence (AI) art 275–283; for adolescents in marginalized communities 279; awareness and outreach 283; COVID-19 278–279; discovery of AI art to assist adolescents 279–282; Hurricane Katrina 277–278; innovative community building 282; integrating with Maslow's hierarchy of needs 276; reflection and history 276–277; and trauma-informed care 275–276
Atewologun, D. 236
attachment dilemma 7
attachment injury 80
Autism Hiring Program 33
Autistic Self-Advocacy Network 131
Axline, Virginia 57

Baker, L. 6–7
Bane Frizzell, L. 94
Bartholet, E. 328
Behavior Assessment System for Children (BASC-3) 163
Beloved Community: creating 286–292; and human service organizations 286
Benoit, Yasmin 192

Bergman, M. E. 289
betrayal trauma 44, 79–80; disclosure 86; early recovery 83–87; and escape cycles 83–85, *84–85*; format for therapy 81–83; late recovery 88–89; middle recovery 87–88; treating 80–89; *see also* trauma
bisexuals 146, 189, 192
Black developers 282
Black, Indigenous, People of Color (BIPOC) 129, 140, 166, 213, **225**, 225–233
Black Lives Matter (BLM) movement 33, 288, 317
*The Blackpill* 68
Bloomquist, K. 192–193
Bloom's taxonomy 254, *254*, 306
Bordere, T. 238
Bowlby, J. 200
Bradford, J. H. 192
brain: and trauma 42–44; and violence 42–44
Braun, V. 240
Bressi, S. K. 6
bridging capital 142
Bronfenbrenner, U. 107–108, 239, 252, 325
Buehler, S. 188–189, 192, 194
building awareness 194, 333
bullying 215, 261–264, 331
Burger, W. R. 99

capital/capitalism 106, 130; bonding 142; bridging 142; influence on human rights 130; social 33, 67, 142–143, 146
Carter, G. 99
Carver, N. 98
cascading collective trauma 158–166; and adolescent development 159–160; adolescents at risk of 163; and COVID-19 pandemic 160–161; cultural and socioeconomic factors 166; described 158; direct and media-based exposure 161–162; evidence-based direct interventions for 165–166; historical context and theoretical foundations 158–159; role of school-based human services professionals 162–163; school shootings 161; supporting students 163–165
celebration 215, 216, 236
Centers for Disease Control and Prevention (CDC) 94–95, 127, 258, 262, 343, 348
chameleon effect 216
Champions of Science organization 305
Chan, S. 78, 80
Chaudhari, P. 219
Chaudoir, S. R. 176
Chaudry, R. 98
Chickering, Arthur 316, 317
child abuse: pediatric abuse and trauma 53–56; play therapy in 52–63; *see also* abuse
*The Child Abuse Industry* (Pride) 327

Child Abuse Prevention and Treatment Act 61
child and family welfare: "real-world" social work analysis of 251–266
childhood grief 200; *see also* grief and bereavement; loss/death/bereavement
child maltreatment 16–17, 256–257
child protection services (CPS) 21, 61, 118
Child PTSD Symptom Scale 163
children: assessment and treatment planning 57–59; chronic stress 45; developing trust and safety with 59; and domestic violence 44–45
children's comprehension of death 200–201; concrete operations 201; preoperational stage 200–201
Children's Defense Fund 261, 279
Children's Defense Fund Report 255
Child Trauma Screen 163
Child Welfare League of America (CWLA): National Blueprint 265; National Blueprint for Excellence in Child Welfare 260
child welfare system 118–125; CBT techniques 122–123; DBT techniques 123; dignity-centered approaches 123–124; disparities 345; family resilience 119; overview 118–119; parental challenges in 119–120; resilience theory 120–121; systems theory 121–122; theoretical frameworks for family resilience 120–121
chronic disease prevalence 348
Civil Rights Act 152
Clarke, V. 240
Coalition for Responsible Home Education 334
Coates, T. 289
code-switch 143, 290
Coenen, C. 6
coercive control 38–39
Cognitive Behavioral Interventions for Schools (CBITS) 165
cognitive-behavioral therapy (CBT) 122–123, 125, 182–183
college-age students: challenge and growth 317–320; current landscape 315–317; empathy deficits in 315–323; student empathy 320–322; utilizing social work pedagogy amid social shifts 315–323
colonization 105–106
common humanity 134
common sexual stereotypes 189–190
communication strategies 22, 342–343
community building: Black developers 282; community partnerships 282; innovative 282; mental health professionals 282
community health centers (CHCs) 348–349
community land trusts 346
community partnerships 232, 282
community relationships 350–351

complexity 63, 107, 215, 219, 265, 318
Compulsive Sexual Behavior Disorder (CSBD) 79
Conceptual Team Belonging Framework 31
Connected Recovery™ model 80–81
consensual non-monogamy (CNM) 193
"Consent Is Sexy!" Campaign 191
Conservative Evangelicals 325
Constantine, M. G. 343
Constantinides, D. M. 189
Corrado, M. 136
cotherapy 81
course goals 305–306
course student learner outcomes (CSLOs) 306–313
COVID-19 pandemic 6, 33, 53, 98–99, 140, 258–259, 272, 274, 278–279, 287, 295, 319–320, 332, 347, 349; and cascading collective trauma 160–161; lockdown 315
creative agency 216
Crenshaw, K. 144–145
Critical Race Theory (CRT) 236, 238–241
cultural competence models 296–297, 342
cultural/ethnic-heritage identity processes 217
culturally appropriate communication strategies 342–343
culturally competent interventions: to address 21st-century issues 251–266; importance of theories in addressing 252–255; importance of theories in comprehending 252–255
culturally focused 21st-century response 264–266
culturally relevant pedagogy (CRP) 146
culturally sensitive programs 347
culture 5, 28, 30–32, 45, 80, 134, 275–283
Curtis, Lois 131
Curtis, M. A. 86

*Dare to Discipline* (Dobson) 326
data analysis 307–308
data plan 307–310
dating violence 46–47
Davis, A. S. 28–29, 32
Davis, L. J. 129
deep listening 110–112
DeJonge, Christine 329–330
DeJonge, Mark 329–330
demographic representation 342–351
Department of Homeland Security's *2021 Yearbook of Immigration Statistics* 347
*Diagnostic and Statistical Manual (DSM-5)* 43, 190–191
dialectical behavioral therapy (DBT) 22, 123, 125
dignity-centered approaches 123–124
direct education of the race discourses 221
disability: medical model 131–132; present conceptualizations of 131; social model 132–133; universal design 133

disability rights activists 131
disabled persons 127–137
discourses: of color blindness 221; of denial 221; direct education of the race 221; of normative whiteness 221; racial binary 220–221
discovery of AI art to assist adolescents 279–282
discrimination 26, 43, 46, 55, 140, 143–145, 147–148, 152, 175, 192–193, 226, 230–232, 259, 277, 286, 289, 296, 303, 305, 307, 308, 318, 343–344
disenfranchised grief 198–199
disparities 127–137; in access to healthcare 227–229; in child welfare 345; health 102, 171, 226, **226**, 227, 230, 232, 344; HIV demographic 171; mental health 344–345
Displaced Behavior Theory 262
diversity, equity, and inclusion (DEI): accessibility 343–344; community health centers (CHCs) 348–349; community relationships 350–351; cultural competence 342; culturally appropriate communication strategies 342–343; culturally sensitive programs 347; disparities in child welfare 345; equity in service delivery 344; healthcare access and equity 348; historical trauma 342; in human services 341–351; immigration and access to services 347; key dimensions of 342–351; language support 347; leadership styles in human services 349–350; legal assistance 347; Medicaid expansion 348; mental health disparities 344–345; microaggressions 343; organizational resilience 351; public housing and affordable living 345–346; service delivery 350; staff morale and retention 350; telehealth 349
diversity, equity, inclusion, and, most recently, belonging (DEIB) principles 28–30, *29,* 32–34
Dobson, J. 326
Doka, K. J. 199
Dolezal, C. 174
domestic violence 39; and children 44–45; LGBTQ+ population 46; male victims 45; people with disabilities 46; *see also* violence
Drucker, Peter 30

Early, T. J. 100
Earnshaw, V. A. 176
echo chambers: defined 71; and Incel communities 71–72; for other people and populations 72
ecological systems theories 107, 109, 112, 236, 238–241, 246, 325
economic abuse 40–41
economic instability 346

edge dancers 213–222; academic departments 219–221; experience in higher education 216–217; and human services departments 221–222; identity negotiations on campus 217–218; mixed-race/ethnic persons 214–216; mixed-race/ethnic students 219–221; multiracial/ethnic identity development 218–219; overview 213–214
"Edge Dancers: Mixed Heritage Identity, Transculturalization, and Public Policy and Practice in Health and Human Services" (Houston and Hogan) 214
"Edge Dancing: Campus Climate Experiences and Identity Negotiation of Multiracial College Students of Multiple Minoritized Ancestry" (Misa-Escalante) 216
educational disruption 345, 346
Eisenberger, N. I. 207–208
Elder, M. Q. 97
Emond, M. 191
emotional abuse 16, 21, 45, 256
emotional contagion 71
emotional expression 56–62
emotionally focused therapy (EFT) 87–88
empathy: deficits 315–323; student 320–322
Enzlin, P. 193
Equal Employment Opportunity Commission 135
Equal Rights Act (1972) 325
equity: and healthcare access 348; in service delivery 344; *see also* diversity, equity, and inclusion (DEI); health equity
Erickson, Erik 316
essentialist anti-Black racism 220
ethical non-monogamy (ENM) 193
Evangelical Christians 325, 326
Exodus Mandate 327

Facebook 276, 277
family resilience 118–125; CBT techniques 122–123; DBT techniques 123; systems theory 121–122; theoretical frameworks for 120–121
Farris, Michael 328
fawn response 42
Felberbaum, S. 6
Felitti, V. J. 199
Ferris, Michael 329
Finkelhor, D. 199
Finnerty, P. S. 101
fishbowl effect 257
Floyd, George 160, 288, 317
Focus on the Family 326
Foster, T. 101
Free Love Era 325
Freyd, J. 44
friendship 82, 159, 199, 253, 272–274

Gabbay, N. 87
Gaither, M. 326
Galton, Sir Francis 253
Ganesh, K. 33
gender: and human immunodeficiency virus (HIV) 172, 177–179; as a social construct 189
Gibson, I. J. 253
Goodwyn, E. 237
Gothard, Bill 327, 329
graphs 309–313
Great Recession 272
grief and bereavement: cross-cultural issues of 236–248; CRT 239–241; cultural contexts 238; ecological systems theory 239–241; human services practice 247–248; literature review 237; religious and cultural practices 241–242; stages of 86–87; theology 243–244; theoretical framework 238–239; therapists' 5–10
grief therapy: for adolescents 205–206; for adults 208–209; for children 201–204
group therapy 183–184
Gunaratne, D. 144
gun violence 259–261

Habitat for Humanity 286
Hajighasemi, A. 295–298
Hamako, E. 213
Harris, Greg 327
Harris, Joshua 327
Harvard Trauma Questionnaire (HTQ) 163
healthcare access and equity 348
health disparities 102, 171, 226, **226**, 227, 230, 232, 344
health equity **225**, 225–233; disparities in access to healthcare 227–229; health inequalities 227; intersectionality of social justice concerns in healthcare inequality 230; overview 226–227; population health model 230–231; social determinants of health 227
health inequalities 55, 227, 230
health insurance coverage 348
Hegazi, A. 176
Herring, B. 80
Hierarchy of Needs 87
Highly Active Antiretroviral Therapy (HAART) 173–176
hippie movement 325
Historically Black College (HBCU) 106–107
historical trauma 43, 159, 342
Hodson, R. 262
Hogan, M. 214–216, 219; "Edge Dancers: Mixed Heritage Identity, Transculturalization, and Public Policy and Practice in Health and Human Services" 214
Holt, John 326
homelessness and poverty 257–258

homeschool history 325–328
homeschooling: building awareness 333;
    current trends 331–333; intervention and
    recommendations 333–335; mitigating and
    engaging 334–335; policy and law 328–331;
    respectful and ethical interactions 333–334
Homeschool Legal Defense Association
    (HSLDA) 327–330
*Homeschool's Invisible Children* database 334
housing wage 345
Houston, H. R. 214–216, 219; "Edge
    Dancers: Mixed Heritage Identity,
    Transculturalization, and Public Policy and
    Practice in Health and Human Services" 214
Hovick, S. R. 191
*How Children Learn* (Holt) 326
human immunodeficiency virus (HIV)
    171–185; age and racial differences
    179–180; cognitive-behavioral therapy
    (CBT) 182–183; demographic disparities
    171; diagnoses 172; effective prevention of
    vertical HIV transmission 173; and gender
    172; gender differences 177–179; global and
    national landscape of 171; group therapy
    183–184; historical data and trends 172–173;
    hypnotherapy 184–185; interventions to
    decline transmission rates 173; locus of
    control in 175, 177–179; mediating role
    181; medication and treatment adherence
    in perinatal transmission 173–174;
    mental and behavioral health challenges
    in 174–175; mindfulness-based cognitive
    therapy (MBCT) 183; perinatal HIV
    transmission 172; PHIV+ youth and adults
    176; psychoanalytic and psychodynamic
    therapies 181–182; psychoeducation 184;
    psychotropic medications 184; quality of life
    and challenges for people living with 174,
    177–179; socioeconomic status 179; stigma
    175–181; in United States 171
human rights 55; fundamental 128; influence of
    capitalism on 130
human services: curriculum 109–110;
    diversity, equity, and inclusion (DEI) in
    341; internalized White supremacy in
    272–274; leadership styles in 349–350;
    multiculturalism in 294–298; professionals
    325–335; and public health 93, 96–99
human service conversations: cultural
    considerations 275–283; social
    justice 275–283
human service transformations: demographic
    representation 342–351; diversity, equity,
    and inclusion (DEI) 341; and emergent trends
    341–352; inclusive human services system
    341–342; key dimensions of DEI in human
    services 342–351

Huntington, R. 237
Hurricane Katrina 276–278, 280–281
hypnotherapy 184–185

I Kissed Dating Goodbye (Harris) 327
immigration and access to services 347
imperfect human 136–137
Incel beliefs: classification 68; overview 67–68
Incel communities: algorithms 70–71; and
    echo chambers 71–72; identifying with
    69–73; mental health 66–67; misapplied
    science scholarship 72–73; overview 65–69;
    pornography use 67; and therapy 68–69;
    vulnerability 69–70
inclusionary zoning 346
individual barriers 31
individual-level facilitators 32
infinite losses 208
innovative community building 282
installation work 10
Institute of Medicine 226
Integrative Treatment of Complex Trauma for
    Children (ITCT-C) 165
intentionality 216, 290
intergenerational trauma 43
Internal Family Systems (IFS) 89
internalized White supremacy in human services
    272–274
International Disability Alliance 127, 137
interpersonal sexual communication (ISC) 191
interpersonal violence 38
interprofessional collaboration: barriers to 31;
    conceptualization of 27; defined 25; ethical
    considerations 33–34; facilitation of 32–33;
    sense of belonging in 25–35
Interprofessional Education Collaborative
    (IPEC) 25–28, *28*
intersectional approach 144–145
intersectionality 58, 144, 147, 230, 232, 236,
    238, 241, 246–248, 289
intimate terrorism 39
*Is There No Place on Earth for Me?* (Sheehan) 9

Jencius, M. 101
Job Accommodation Network 136
Johnson, J. 25
Johnston, M. P. 39, 213, 219
Johnston-Guerrero, M. P. 219

Kamau, C. 174
Keegan, J. 100
Keeping Children and Families Safe Act 61
King, Martin Luther, Jr. 286, 292, 317
Klein, M. 54
Klicka, Chris 328, 329
Kondrat, D. C. 100
Kowalewska, E. 78–79

Krupa, T. 99
Kupershmidt, S. 34

Lafontaine, M.-F. 87
land-based care work 105–106, 110–113
land-based theory 107–109
language: assistance 152–154; support 347
law of error 129
leadership styles in human services 349–350
Lee, C.D. 222
legal assistance 347
legislation 135–136
Levine, A. 144
Levine, E. 8
Lew-Starowicz, M. 78–79
LGBTQ+ adolescents 160
LGBTQ+ affirmative therapy model 193
LGBTQ+ population 140; dating violence 46;
    mental health of 192; partner abuse 46
Lieberman, M. D. 207–208
Limited English Proficiency (LEP) 151–156;
    problematic conceptualization of 153–154;
    theoretical and political recommendations
    154–155
linguistic accessibility 343
Lonergan, M. 80
*Lookism* 68
loss/death/bereavement 197–209; adaptive
    coping 206, 207; adolescent grief 205;
    adult grief 206–208; childhood grief
    200; children's comprehension of death
    200–201; cohorts and history 197–198;
    disenfranchised grief 198–199; grief and loss
    across lifespan 199–209; grief therapy for
    adolescents 205–206; grief therapy for adults
    208–209; grief therapy for children 201–204;
    life course perspective 197–199; life events
    and turning points 198; overview 197;
    transitions and trajectories 198; trauma 199;
    *see also* grief and bereavement
*Loving vs. the Commonwealth of Virginia* 214
Lumb, P. 144

Machette, A. T. 191
Macionis, J. J. 251
Mahalingam, R. 236
Malaney-Brown, V.K. 219–220
Malee, K. M. 174
male victims 45
marginalization 58, 130, 140, 143–144, 147,
    236, 320, 325
marginalized communities 279
Maslow, A. H. 26, 253
Maslow's hierarchy of needs 254; integrating AI
    art with 276
maternal mortality 348
McGowin, Emily Hunter 325–326

Medicaid expansion 131, 228, 348, 349
medical model 131–132
meet/exceed ethical standards 136
mental health 303; advocate 304–305; in
    African American community 303–313;
    course goals 305–306; course student learner
    outcomes 313; creative means to address
    303–313; data plan 307–310; disparities
    344–345; history of 95; professionals 282;
    qualitative inquiry 306; research questions
    306–307; stigma of 95
mental illness 303–304; signs of 141
metaphorical play 59
Metcalf, P. 237
microaggressions 143–145, 147, 176, 215, 343;
    creativity of 319; multiracial 219
mindfulness-based cognitive therapy (MBCT) 183
Miners, A. 174
Misa-Escalante, Kim 216–217; "Edge Dancing:
    Campus Climate Experiences and Identity
    Negotiation of Multiracial College Students
    of Multiple Minoritized Ancestry" 216
Missouri State Bill 727 329
*Mixed Blood: Intermarriage and Ethnic Identity
    in Twentieth-Century America* (Spickard) 214
mixed-race/ethnic people: academic departments
    219–221; in academic programs 213;
    bridging 218; contextualizing 218; described
    215; homesteading 218; institutional support
    for 218; racial and ethnic differences 215;
    research literature on 214–216; sitting 218;
    in U.S. population 216
model minority myth and mental health 229
modular housing 346
Mohajeri, Orkideh 219, 220
monoracial imperative 213–214
monoracism 213–214, 217, 220
Montgomery-Vestecka, G. 191
Moon, B. L. 7
Moore, Dorthy 326
Moore, E. Ray 327
Moore, Raymond 326
Morrill Act 108
Morrison, J. 98
Moskalenko, S. 68–69
Multicultural Counseling Competencies (MCC)
    model 294
multiculturalism: cultural competence models
    296–297; in human services 294–298;
    literature review 295–297; solutions or
    strategies 297–298
multiracial/ethnic consciousness development
    220
multiracial microaggressions 219
Murray, S. 263
mutual violent control 39
Myspace 277

Nachega, J. B. 176
Nadel, K. L. 213, 219
NAMI 305
National Association of Social Workers (NASW) 264, 295, 334
National Association of Social Workers (NASW) Code of Ethics 101, 295
National Center for Education Statistics (NCES) 331
National Center for Injury Prevention and Control 259
National Child Traumatic Stress Network 163
National Home Education Research Institute 330
National Low Income Housing Coalition (NLIHC) 345
National Organization for Human Services (NOHS) 136, 334
neglect 16, 21, 32, 54, 118, 256, 260, 325, 332, 335
new homeschool movement 325–335
Non-English Language Preference (NELP) 154
normalcy 129–130

Office for Civil Rights 135
Office of Refugee Resettlement 347
Ohene-Ntow, Spencer 232
Oliver, Mike 132
one-drop rule 213–214, 221
One Health Initiative 109
organizational barriers 31
organizational facilitators 32–33
organizational resilience 351
Ortega, P. 156
Ouellette, L. 263

pansexual 134, 189
Pantelic, M. 176
participatory action research (PAR) 110
participatory leadership 350, 351
partner abuse: betrayal trauma 44; in dating relationship 38–47; dating violence 46–47; in domestic relationship 38–47; forms of 39–42; LGBTQ+ population 46; in married/cohabitating relationships 44; power and control 38–39; trauma 42–44
*Pedagogical Techniques That Provide Educational Value to Social Work Students through Bereavement Academics and Empathetic Advancements* 320
pedagogy: culturally relevant pedagogy (CRP) 146; social work 315–323
pediatric abuse 53–56; *see also* child abuse
Pediatric Emotional Distress Scale 163
pentad assessment process for childhood bereavement 202
people living with HIV (PLWH) 175–176
people with disabilities 46

Percy, P. E. 7
Perel, Esther 78
perinatal HIV transmission 172; interventions to decline 173; medication and treatment adherence in 173–174; mental and behavioral health challenges in 174–175
perinatally acquired HIV (PHIV) 174–176
Phillips, Doug 327
photography 9
physical abuse 16, 39
Piaget, J. 201, 282
play therapy: in child abuse cases 52–63; emotional expression and trauma processing 56–62; pediatric abuse and trauma 53–56; safety and advocacy 61–62; self-expression 59; social determinants of health 55–56; therapeutic art and storytelling 59–61
Pliske, M. 199
policy and law 328–331
poor health 346
population health model 225–227, 230–233; fundamentals of 230–231; importance of 231; strategies for implementation 231
posttraumatic play 54
poverty and homelessness 257–258
power and control 38–39
*Practical Homeschooling* magazine 328
predominately white institutions (PWIs) 143
pre-level consciousness 220
Pride, Mary 327–328
Primary Care PTSD Screen for DSM-5 (PC-PTSD-5) 163
problematic sexual behaviors (PSBs): background 78–79, 79; early recovery 83–87; format for therapy 81–83; late recovery 88–89; middle recovery 87–88; treating 80–89; understanding 79–80
professionalism 272–274
protective factors for bereaved children **204**
psychoeducation 181
psychological first aid (PFA) 165
psychotropic medications 181
public health: history of 94–95; and human services 93, 96–99; overview 93–94
public housing 345–346

qualitative inquiry 306

racial binary discourse 220–221
*Racially Mixed People in America* (Root) 214
racial trauma 43
racism 286–292
radical approach to unlearning racism 286–292
Ray, Brian 330
reality television 261–264
real-world social work analysis of child and family welfare 251–266

Reckford, Jonathan 286
Rehabilitation Act of 1973 131
relational counseling 78, 81, 87
relational-cultural play therapy 57–58
religious and cultural practices at death
    241–242
Rennie, R. 80
rental assistance programs 346
research questions 306–307
resilience 20–21, 145–146, 216
respectful and ethical interactions 333–334
reunification 118
Riessman, C. K. 240
right to self-determination 135
Rodriguez, Favianna 111
Rogers, Natalie 279
Rokach, A. 78, 80
Root, Maria 214; *Racially Mixed People in
    America* 214
Rosenblatt, P. C. 238
Rubinsky, V. 192
Rushdoony, Rousas 327, 329

safe-harboring behaviors 84
Santamaria, E. K. 174
school shootings 161
Schreiber, S. 238
Schut, H. 237
Schwartz, M. 144
Scull, A. 129
self-expression 59
Semansky, R. 97
sense of belonging: barriers to 31; within
    college/university 219; ethical considerations
    33–34; evaluation of current models 29–30;
    facilitation of 32–33; in interprofessional
    collaboration 25–35; and social identity
    theory 26–27
service delivery 344, 350
sexual abuse 16
sexual assault 40
sexuality and clients 188–195; chronic illness
    193–194; common sexual stereotypes
    189–190; "Consent Is Sexy!" Campaign 191;
    disabilities 193–194; discussing sex in clinical
    spaces 194; issues 190; issues with DSM
    190–191; mental health clinicians 194–195;
    overview 188–189; perceived sexlessness
    193–194; sex positivity 190; sexual minority
    stressors 192–193
sexually transmitted infections (STIs) 190
sexual minority stressors 192–193
sexual orientation 81, 88, 143–145, 189, 192,
    295, 342
sexual trauma 88–89, 188, 190
sexual violence 40, 46, 191
sex worker 192–193

Shah, S. S. 175
Shally-Jensen, M. 96
Shapiro, F. 282
Sheehan, Susan: *Is There No Place on Earth for
    Me?* 9
Silver, N. 191
Silverman, G. S. 237
Silvers, S. A. 97
Simultaneous Language Acquisition 153
Sins Invalid 129
situational couple violence 39
social capital 33, 67, 142–143, 146
social determinants of health (SDOH) 55–56,
    **225**, 227
social identity theory 26–27, 318
socialization 251–252
social justice 97, 99, 220–221, **225**, 227, 230,
    264, 275–283, 286, 317, 344–345
social media 261–264
social model 132–133
social services organizations 298
social shifts 315–323
social work pedagogy 315–323
socioeconomic status 20, 55, 144, 165, 175,
    179, **225**, 226, 344
Solomon, P. 342
Some, S. 246
Spickard, Paul 214; *Mixed Blood: Intermarriage
    and Ethnic Identity in Twentieth-Century
    America* 214
Sprankle, E. 192–193
*The Squeaky Wheel* 134
staff morale and retention 350
Stark, Evan 38
Stay at Home Daughter movement 327
Steffens, B. 80
stereotypes about pain tolerance 229
stereotypes of non-compliance 229
stigma 304
storytelling 59–61, 110
Strayhorn, T. L. 25
stress response 17–19, *17–19*
Stroebe, M. 237
"strong Black woman" stereotype 229
structural facilitators 32–33
student-centered instruction (SCI) 320–322
student empathy 320–322
Successive Language Acquisition 153
Sue, D. W. 343
systemic racism 71, 106, 166, **225**, 226, 233
system-level barriers 31
system-level facilitators 32–33
Sztompka, P. 158

Tajfel, H. 26
Taylor, Breonna 160
teaching through relationships (TTR) 321–322

technology 261–264, 273
telehealth 33, 349
Terr, L. 54
Tham, S. S. 342
therapeutic art 59–61
therapists' grief: creative processes 9–10;
    creativity as natural grief response 6–7;
    ethical underpinnings 5–6; overview 5;
    visual art making 7–8; *see also* grief and
    bereavement; loss/death/bereavement
"Therapy for Black Girls" (podcast) 192
Thorpe, S. 190
Tovar-Blank, Z. G. 101
toxic stress 16, 18
transformational leadership 349–350
trauma 199; and adversity 15–17; betrayal
    44, 79–89; and brain 42–44; child
    maltreatment 16–17; chronic/complex 16;
    exposure and populations 17; historical
    43; intergenerational 43; lasting impacts of
    19–20; overview 15–17; and pediatric abuse
    53–56; and play therapy 56–62; racial 43;
    and violence 42–44
Trauma and Life Events Checklist (TALE) 163
Trauma Assessment for Adults and Children
    (TAA/TAAC) 163
trauma-focused cognitive-behavioral therapy
    (TF-CBT) 165
trauma-informed approach 15
trauma-informed care: and AI art 275–276
trauma-informed human service practices:
    communication strategies 22; lasting impacts
    of trauma 19–20; reporting considerations
    21–22; resilience 20–21; stress response
    17–19, *17–19*; trauma-informed approach 15
Trauma Screening Questionnaire (TSQ) 163
Trauma Symptom Screening for Children and
    Adolescents 163
Traumatic Events Screening Inventory-Parent
    Report Revised (TESI-PRR) 163
Turner, J. C. 26

Underrepresented Graduate Students (UGS)
    140–148; case study 146–147; challenges for
    142–144; exclusionary practices in graduate
    education 144–146; faculty as gatekeepers

of mental health 141–142; mental health
    landscape for 140–141; signs of mental
    illness 141
Union of Physically Impaired Against
    Segregation (UPIAS) 132
United Nations Convention on the Rights of the
    Child 328
universal design (UD) 131, 133
U.S. Access Board 136
U.S. Census Bureau 341, 348
U.S. Citizenship and Immigration Services 347
U.S. Department of Justice 135, 151

Vaden, E. R. 6
Van Galen, Jane 331
vertical HIV transmission 173
violence: and brain 42–44; dating 46–47;
    domestic 39, 44–46; gun 259–261; sexual 40,
    46, 191; situational couple 39; and trauma
    42–44; youth 259–261
violent resistance 39
visual art making 7–8
vulnerability and Incel communities 69–70

Wallace, B. R. 238
Warach, B. 78
Warne, D. 94
Washington Senate Bill 6236 329
Watson, N. 130
Wei, H. 29, 34
Wellness Model 100–101
Westernized mental healthcare 304
White House Conference on Children and
    Youth 325
White supremacy: internalized 272–274
Wijeyesinghe, C. 219
Wilson, Elaine 131
Wood, S. M. 175
World Health Organization (WHO) 27, 95, 105

Yager, G. G. 101
youth violence 259–261
Yung, A. 98

Zeifman, D. M. 87
Zoom 33, 277